T0293253

A Clinician's Guide to Non-Alcoholic Fatty Liver Disease

A Clinician's Guide to Non-Alcoholic Fatty Liver Disease

Editor: Heidi Hamlin

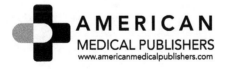

AMERICAN
MEDICAL PUBLISHERS
www.americanmedicalpublishers.com

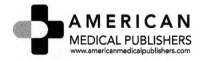

Cataloging-in-Publication Data

A clinician's guide to non-alcoholic fatty liver disease / edited by Heidi Hamlin.
      p. cm.
Includes bibliographical references and index.
ISBN 978-1-63927-577-9
1. Fatty liver. 2. Fatty liver--Treatment--Diagnosis. 3. Fatty liver--Treatment.
4. Liver--Diseases. 5. Fatty degeneration. 6. Hepatitis. I. Hamlin, Heidi.
RC848.F3 C55 2023
616.362--dc23

American Medical Publishers,
41 Flatbush Avenue,
1st Floor, New York,
NY 11217, USA

ISBN 978-1-63927-577-9 (Hardback)

Contents

Preface

I am honored to present to you this unique book which encompasses the most up-to-date data in the field. I was extremely pleased to get this opportunity of editing the work of experts from across the globe. I have also written papers in this field and researched the various aspects revolving around the progress of the discipline. I have tried to unify my knowledge along with that of stalwarts from every corner of the world, to produce a text which not only benefits the readers but also facilitates the growth of the field.

Non-alcoholic fatty liver disease (NAFLD) refers to a group of diseases including inflammatory non-alcoholic steatohepatitis (NASH), hepatic cirrhosis, simple hepatic steatosis and developing stages of fibrosis. It is also connected to other medical conditions such as obesity, diabetes, metabolic syndrome and cardiovascular disease. It can be diagnosed through various methods such as by studying the medical history, conducting a physical examination and through different tests. A few of the tests which can help in the diagnosis of non-alcoholic fatty liver disease are blood tests, imaging tests and liver biopsy. Disease progression differs from individual to individual and is related to a variety of risk factors. A few of the major risk factors linked with NAFLD are hepatic oxidative stress, reduced very low-density lipoprotein secretion, imbalanced diet and lifestyle, and influx of free fatty acids to the liver from adipose tissue due to insulin resistance. The management of NAFLD can be done through reducing weight and improving physical activity. This book provides significant information to help develop a good understanding of non-alcoholic fatty liver disease. It aims to shed light on some of the unexplored aspects of this disease. The extensive content of this book provides the readers with a thorough understanding of this medical condition.

Finally, I would like to thank all the contributing authors for their valuable time and contributions. This book would not have been possible without their efforts. I would also like to thank my friends and family for their constant support.

Editor

Periostin Circulating Levels and Genetic Variants in Patients with Non-Alcoholic Fatty Liver Disease

Carlo Smirne [1],*[iD], Violante Mulas [1], Matteo Nazzareno Barbaglia [1][iD],
Venkata Ramana Mallela [1][iD], Rosalba Minisini [1][iD], Nadia Barizzone [2], Michela Emma Burlone [1],
Mario Pirisi [1][iD] and Elena Grossini [1][iD]

[1] Department of Translational Medicine, Università del Piemonte Orientale, via Solaroli, 17,
28100 Novara, Italy; viola.mulas@gmail.com (V.M.); matteo.barbaglia89@gmail.com (M.N.B.);
vramana6565@gmail.com (V.R.M.); rosalba.minisini@med.uniupo.it (R.M.);
michela.burlone@med.uniupo.it (M.E.B.); mario.pirisi@med.uniupo.it (M.P.);
elena.grossini@med.uniupo.it (E.G.)

[2] Department of Health Sciences, Università' del Piemonte Orientale, via Solaroli, 17, 28100 Novara, Italy;
nadia.barizzone@med.uniupo.it

* Correspondence: carlo.smirne@med.uniupo.it

Abstract: Circulating periostin has been suggested as a possible biomarker in non-alcoholic fatty liver disease (NAFLD) in Asian studies. In the present study, we aimed to test its still controversial relevance in a Caucasian population. In patients with histologically-proven NAFLD (N. = 74; 10 with hepatocellular carcinoma, HCC) plasma periostin concentrations were analyzed. POSTN haplotype analysis was based on rs9603226, rs3829365, and rs1029728. Hepatitis C patients (N. = 81, 7 HCC) and healthy subjects (N. = 27) were used as controls. The median plasma periostin concentration was 11.6 ng/mL without differences amongst groups; it was not influenced by age, liver fibrosis or steatosis. However, possession of haplotype two (rs9603226 = G, rs3829365 = C, rs1028728 = A) was associated with lower circulating periostin compared to other haplotypes. Moreover, periostin was higher in HCC patients. At multivariate analysis, HCC remained the only predictor of high periostin. In conclusion, plasma periostin concentrations in Caucasians NAFLD patients are not influenced by the degree of liver disease, but are significantly higher in HCC. Genetically-determined differences may account for some of the variability. These data suggest extreme caution in predicting a possible future role of periostin antagonists as a rational therapeutic alternative for NAFLD, but show a potential periostin role in the management of NAFLD-associated HCC.

Keywords: periostin; biomarker; non-alcoholic fatty liver disease; non-alcoholic steatohepatitis; hepatocellular carcinoma; liver steatosis; liver fibrosis; single nucleotide polymorphism; metabolic syndrome; extracellular matrix

1. Introduction

Non-alcoholic fatty liver disease (NAFLD), the major cause of chronic liver disease worldwide, includes a spectrum of chronic diseases ranging from simple steatosis (SS) to non-alcoholic steatohepatitis (NASH). Some patients with NASH are likely to develop into cirrhosis and even hepatocellular carcinoma (HCC) [1]. The mechanisms that lead to NAFLD development are complex and multifactorial, and have not yet been fully clarified. They range from environmental factors to genetic variants resulting in a disturbed lipid homeostasis and an excessive accumulation of triglycerides (TG) and other lipid species in hepatocytes [2–5].

During the last years, a major focus in the deeper understanding of pathogenesis of this condition allowed the discovery of several novel mediators and promising targets. Amongst the factors that have a potential role in driving aberrant accumulation of TGs in the liver, emerging evidence indicates that the dysfunction of periostin (PN) expression plays a prominent action. PN, also known as osteoblast-specific factor 2 (OSF-2), is a 90 kDa multifunctional extracellular matrix (ECM) protein, coded by periostin (POSTN) gene and mainly secreted by osteoblasts [6]. It has pleiotropic activities far beyond simple bone remodeling; as a matter of fact, it is also involved—amongst others—in the pathophysiology of arthritis, atherosclerosis, and inflammatory diseases [7]. Actually, one of the target organs in which PN has been shown to play a crucial role is the liver, where it can modulate the cell fate determination and proliferation, inflammatory responses, ECM remodeling, even tumorigenesis [8–12]. In this respect, the strongest evidence so far concerns its pivotal role in the onset of metabolic disease (such as obesity and glucose or lipid disorders) by suppression of fatty acid oxidation in the liver [13]. As a matter of fact, in obese mice the overexpression of PN in the liver was shown to induce hepatic steatosis and hypertriglyceridemia through the downregulation of peroxisome proliferator-activated receptor (PPAR)-α, which activates the fatty acid oxidation in mitochondria and peroxisomes [14]. Conversely, the genetic knockout of PN significantly improved those conditions [13] and was able to protect mice against dietary-induced NAFLD [15]. In detail, PN could exert its protective effects against hypertriglyceridemia and liver steatosis through the interaction with the subtype $\alpha6\beta4$ of the integrins family and the subsequent activation of an intracellular pathway involving Ras-related C3 botulinum toxin substrate (Rac) 1 and c-JUN. Those events would lead to the inhibition of the PPAR-α promoter, RAR-related orphan receptor (ROR) α, and to the downregulation of PPAR-α itself [13].

Considering human studies, the relationship between PN and hepatic steatosis, which is the basis of the present study, was first proposed by Lu et al. [13], showing an upregulation of hepatic PN expression in NAFLD patients, with a good correlation with hepatic TG content. Moreover, serum PN levels were found to be increased in the same subjects, although without a significant correlation with hepatic TGs. Additionally, in the studies from Zhu et al. and Yang et al. higher plasma PN concentrations were observed in NAFLD patients in comparison to healthy controls, although without significant differences between the ultrasound degrees of NAFLD [16,17]. In addition, circulating PN was strongly associated with lipid metabolism, chronic inflammation and insulin resistance [17,18], and the serum and liver tissue levels of PN were closely related to the decline in liver function and to the pathological stage in NAFLD patients [8,17]. It is important to note, that plasma PN analysis—performed through the same enzyme linked immunosorbent assay (ELISA) kit of the research from Zhu et al. on Chinese subjects—failed to find any association between circulating PN and hepatic steatosis on a small but histologically-confirmed casuistry of NAFLD European patients, while there was a statistically significant trend for PN level decrease in more severe fibrosis stages [19].

Besides steatosis, PN has been demonstrated to mediate also hepatic inflammation and fibrosis, probably through both direct and indirect mechanisms related to the concomitant release of pro-inflammatory and pro-fibrotic factors and inhibition of adiponectin, an insulin-sensitizing and anti-inflammatory adipokine. Despite this experimental evidence, there are currently limited data for PN in human NAFLD evolved to NASH or hepatic fibrosis/cirrhosis (which could be expected to present higher PN levels than SS patients) [8,20].

The same lack of data applies to another possible NAFLD complication, i.e., HCC. To the best of our knowledge, in fact, no specific evidence already exists for a PN role. However, it is reasonable to assume that, at least in principle, many of the considerations that have been made for HCCs in general are valid. Regarding this issue, an important PN expression has been shown in the tumor stroma, associated with a greater co-expression of vascular endothelial growth factor (VEGF), and a reduced overall, and disease-free, survival [10,21]. Additionally, circulating levels of PN were demonstrated to be higher in HCC patients compared to healthy controls [22].

Coming back to NAFLD, taking into account the aforementioned discordant results found by researchers in circulating PN levels, and assuming that they were at least in part related to ethnic differences, it is interesting to note that the *POSTN* gene, like many others, has some known genetic variants. In particular, four major and two minor haplotypes could be identified (initially, in the Japanese population). The former ones were mainly determined by three tag single nucleotide polymorphisms (SNPs), which were located at intron 66 bp upstream of exon 21 (rs9603226, alleles G>A), 5′ untranslated region (rs3829365, alleles G>C), and at promoter region (rs1028728, alleles A>T) [23]. The four major *POSTN* haplotypes obtained, respectively, from these three SNPs were: AGA (haplotype one), GCA (haplotype two), GGT (haplotype three), and GGA (haplotype four). These SNPs were then studied in different human disorders, mainly in the cardiology and pulmonology fields, and the results seem to suggest a possible role of PN and of its allelic variants in identifying patients at increased risk of disease progression [24,25]. However, to the best of our knowledge, no specific evidence has been yet provided for liver diseases, including NAFLD.

Based on these premises, in the present study we aimed to provide implications and mechanisms of PN in the pathogenesis of NAFLD, confirming (or denying) the possible association between circulating PN and this specific disease (in all its stages including HCC), and evaluating—for the first time in hepatology—the role of genetic factors as possible contributors to the observed variability in the plasma concentration of this protein.

2. Materials and Methods

2.1. Patients

For this retrospective cross-sectional study over a period of nine years (2008–2016), patients with NAFLD confirmed diagnosis were recruited, including some subjects complicated with HCC. CHC subjects, again including some with HCC, and healthy volunteers were used as control groups. The research was conducted at the Liver Clinic of Novara University Hospital, which is a large tertiary center (serving a population of about 1,000,000). The study protocol was carried out in accordance with the declaration of Helsinki. Written informed consent for the storage of biological material (blood) and clinical, histological and laboratory data processing was obtained from all the participants.

2.1.1. NAFLD Patients

Inclusion criteria were: (1) adult age; (2) clinical diagnosis of NAFLD, confirmed by liver biopsy in the case of disease not complicated by cancer, and by instrumental and/or histological means when an HCC was present; (3) availability of a blood sample with authorization to carry out the genetic investigation (*POSTN* genotyping); (4) availability of a fasting blood sample collected no more than seven days after the liver biopsy with authorization to perform PN ELISA quantification. Exclusion criteria were as follows: (1) hepatitis C virus (HCV) positive serology; (2) Australia antigen (HBsAg) positivity; (3) excessive alcohol use at the biopsy time and/or in the previous 6 months (more than one drink per day for women and two drinks per day for men, and more than one drink per day for individuals over the age of 65) [26,27]; (4) other concomitant causes of liver disease.

Based on these criteria, of the 107 subjects with NAFLD that were initially identified at different stages (i.e., fatty liver alone, non-alcoholic steatohepatitis (NASH), cirrhosis, and liver cancer) 33 were then excluded: 3 for HBsAg positivity, 5 for habitual excess alcohol consumption, and 25 for non-availability of whole blood and/or plasma samples. The tested population was therefore of 74 Caucasian subjects, 10 of whom with HCC at the time of diagnosis. All subjects underwent a liver biopsy, except for 5 HCC subjects who were diagnosed on the basis of radiological imaging, as required by the 2011 EASL-EORTC (European Association for the Study of the Liver, EASL; the European Organization for Research and Treatment of Cancer, EORTC) guidelines [28]. HCC staging was according to Barcelona clinic liver cancer (BCLC) guidelines [28,29]. Non-tumor patients had their grading and staging histological assessment according to Kleiner NAFLD Activity Score [30]. Moreover, a non-invasive assessment of liver fibrosis was performed in the same patients both through transient elastography (TE) (FibroScan®, Echosens, Paris, France), which measures liver stiffness (LS), and NAFLD fibrosis score (NFS) [31]. Only TE measurements taken no more than six months after liver biopsy were taken into account; furthermore, examinations were considered valid as long as they were technically feasible and satisfied the known quality criteria as previously described [32]. Whenever the correct probe was available, TE device was used to assess, at the same time, LS, which as previously reported is related to liver fibrosis, and the CAP, indicative of the degree of liver steatosis [33].

A systematic data collection was carried out by review of all medical records at baseline (time of liver biopsy or HCC radiological diagnosis). Age, gender, race, height, and weight were documented, and BMI was calculated as weight (in kilograms) divided by the square of the height (in meters). History of diabetes mellitus, hyperglycemia, or hyperlipidemia was ascertained. Laboratory data included, amongst others, the following: blood count, serum AST, ALT, GGT, alkaline phosphatase, total bilirubin, albumin, total protein, creatinine, prothrombin time, international normalized ratio, fasting glucose, fasting insulin, and lipid panel. Liver biopsy, TE and blood tests were performed within 3 months in more than 80% of subjects, and between 3 and 6 months in the remaining cases.

2.1.2. HCV Control Patients

A control population comprising age- and sex-matched Caucasian CHC patients was studied. Inclusion and exclusion criteria were the same as for NAFLD patients (except for inclusion criterion # 2 and exclusion criterion # 1). Of the 97 subjects initially identified, 7 were excluded for habitual excess alcohol consumption, and 9 for non-availability of whole blood and/or plasma samples, resulting in 81 patients included in the study. This population included 7 subjects with HCC at the time of diagnosis: two underwent a liver biopsy, and five were diagnosed on the basis of radiological imaging and staged similarly to NAFLD patients. CHC histological evaluation of non-tumor patients included grading and staging assessment using the Ishak classification [34], and fat percentage quantification. Subjects underwent TE for non-invasive assessment of liver fibrosis, when technically feasible, with the same considerations for validity and CAP measurement as for NAFLD patients.

The above considerations for the data collection described for NAFLD subjects also apply in this context, but with the addition of HCV genotype and viremia at the time of biopsy. HCV RNA was detected by COBAS AMPLICOR HCV Test, v2.0 (Roche Molecular Systems, Pleasanton, CA, USA).

2.1.3. Healthy Controls

Twenty-seven Caucasian subjects in apparent good health and between 24 and 54 years old were studied. They were not age- and sex-matched with the patients, but selected according to the following criteria: normal weight ($18.5 \leq$ BMI < 25 kg/m^2), no medical history of liver disease, asthma, diabetes, allergic syndromes, and/or high risk alcohol consumption as reported above. All underwent TE liver stiffness measurement, which was less than 7.0 kPa in all subjects, allowing to exclude the presence of advanced liver fibrosis. CAP was also measured in all, and was indicative of the absence of significant steatosis [33].

2.2. POSTN Genetic Studies

Genomic DNA was extracted from whole blood or buffy coat, using a commercial kit (Invitrogen, Carlsbad, CA, USA), according to the manufacturer's instructions. DNA was then amplified by polymerase chain reaction (PCR). We analyzed three different polymorphism of *POSTN* gene (rs9603226, rs3829365 and rs1028728) using restriction fragment length polymorphism-PCR. The PCR primer sequences used for *POSTN* amplification were as follows: rs9603226 forward: 5′-ATGAATTGGTGACCTTGGTG-3′, reverse: 5′-CAATCTATTGTTCATTTCCATACC-3′; rs3829365 forward: 5′-TTCAGGTTGATGCAGTGTTCC-3′, reverse: 5′-CCGACCCCTGATACGACT-3′; rs1028728 forward: 5′-GCAGCCAATATTGGAAGCAAG-3′, reverse: 5′-GGATGGTGTGCAGCTTGTTTATTC-3′. The PCR products of rs9603226, rs3829365 and rs1028728 were digested using the enzymes AhdI, Eam1104I (Life Technologies, Thermo Fisher Scientific, Carlsbad, CA, USA) and AgsI (SibEnzyme Ltd., Novosibirsk, Russia), respectively. All samples were amplified twice; when discordant, they were run a third time. The lab technicians performing the genetic studies were blinded about the case/control state of the subjects enrolled. As an additional check, some samples were sequenced by GATC Biotech AG (European Custom Sequencing Service, Cologne, Germany). The haplotypes were obtained using the program Beagle 4.1 [34,35]. For each patient, two haplotypes were assigned, based on the SNP association, as shown in Table 1. The haplotype analysis was performed using the software Haploview (Broad Institute of MIT and Harvard, Cambridge, MA, USA). Appendix A Table A1 reports the diplotypes obtained from haplotype combinations and found in the studied population.

Table 1. *POSTN* gene haplotypes based on the allelic variants of the three polymorphisms analyzed.

	rs9603226	**rs3829365**	**rs1028728**
Haplotype 1	A	G	A
Haplotype 2	G	C	A
Haplotype 3	G	G	T
Haplotype 4	G	G	A
Haplotype 5	A	C	A
Haplotype 6	G	C	T

POSTN: periostin.

2.3. Plasma Periostin Concentration Dosage

Plasma samples were obtained from the recruited patients and healthy controls, and stored at −80 °C. The determination of plasma PN concentration (diluted 1:25) was performed by ELISA immunoassay on a 96-well plate (Human Periostin/OSF-2 DuoSet ELISA, R&D Systems Inc., Minneapolis, MN, USA) according to manufacturer's instructions. Each sample was analyzed in duplicate and compared with a standard curve obtained by using different PN concentrations. The reading was performed through a spectrometer at 450 nm (Victor X4 Perkin Elmer, Milan, Italy).

2.4. Statistical Analysis

The statistical analysis was conducted with the help of Stata statistical software, version 13.1 (StataCorp LP, College Station, TX, USA). The test used to verify the normality of the data was that of Shapiro–Wilk, which confirmed that, for almost all of the continuous variables and as expected for the vast majority of biological parameters (in both health and disease conditions), the data distribution deviated significantly from the normal one. The centrality and data dispersion measures for the continuous variables were therefore median and IQR. The categorical variables were presented as frequencies (percentage of the total). For the continuous variables, the differences between the groups were analyzed with the Mann–Whitney (in the case of two independent groups) and Kruskal–Wallis (in the case of more than two independent groups) tests. The association between the categorical variables was explored using Fisher's exact test or Pearson's chi-square test, as appropriate. An extension of the Wilcoxon rank-sum test as proposed by Cuzick et al. was used to handle the situations in which a variable was measured for individuals in three or more (ordered) groups and a non-parametric test for trend across these groups was desired [36]. The strength and direction of the monotonic relationship between two ordinal variables was measured by Spearman's Rho correlation coefficient. The concordance between invasive (histopathological examination) and non-invasive (NFS, TE) measures of liver fibrosis was assessed by calculating Cohen's kappa index. The differences in a dependent variable (e.g., plasma PN values) among groups, taking into account its variability explained by one or more covariates, were tested through the analysis of covariance (ANCOVA). Finally, a set of variables (*POSTN* diplotype, age, sex, HCC, and platelet count) was analyzed in a maximum-likelihood logit regression model as a predictor of high plasma PN values (defined by belonging to the last quintile of the study population). For all the tests used, the value chosen to indicate the statistical significance threshold was 0.05 (two tailed).

3. Results

3.1. Patients and Healthy Controls

As extensively described in the Materials and Methods section, the study was centered on 74 patients with confirmed diagnosis of NAFLD. Hepatitis C virus (HCV) infected patients (N. = 81) and healthy individuals (N. = 27) were used as controls. Thus, the total sample consisted of 182 subjects (155 patients with chronic liver diseases and 27 healthy controls). NAFLD and HCV groups included a proportion of subjects affected by HCC, 10 (two stage zero, two stage A, five stage B, one stage C) and seven (two stage zero, two stage A, two stage B, one stage D), respectively. The main characteristics of the patients and the healthy controls included in the study are shown in Table 2; Table 3, respectively. The distribution of NAFLD patients according to the Kleiner classification system is detailed in Appendix A Table A2.

Table 2. Comparison of the main demographic and clinical features of the studied population according to the etiology of liver disease. Data are presented as medians (range) for continuous variables, and as frequencies (%) for categorical variables. The p value refers to the comparison between NAFLD and HCV groups.

Parameter	NAFLD (N. = 74)	HCV (N. = 81)	p	All Patients (N. = 155)
Age, years	56 (47–66)	55 (45–64)	0.532	56 (45–66)
Male/female sex, N.	37 (50)/37 (50)	40 (49)/41 (50)	1.000	77 (50)/78 (50)
Body Mass Index, kg/m^2	28.2 (26.8–33.2)	23.1 (21.3–27.4)	**<0.001**	27.1 (24.4–30.9)
Obese subjects, N.	31 (42)	11 (14)	**<0.001**	42 (27)
Diabetic/prediabetic subjects, N.	20 (27)/38 (51)	14 (17) 28 (35)	**0.003**	34 (22)
Liver stiffness, kPa [1]	9.1 (7.2–13.3)	8.4 (6.5–11.6)	0.536	8.8 (6.2–12.0)
CAP [2], db/m	300 (265–328)	251 (214–289)	**0.032**	280 (227–311)
Advanced histological fibrosis, N. [3]	24 (38)	24 (32)	0.593	48 (31)
Severe histological steatosis, N. [4]	13 (20)	3 (4) [5]	**0.006**	16 (10)
NFS, value	−0.625 (−1.534–0.468)	N.A.		N.A.
NFS > 0.676 [6], N.	17 (23)	N.A.		N.A.
HCC, N.	10 (14)	7 (9)	0.442	17 (11)
Platelets, ×10^9/L	182 (153–236)	185 (144–233)	0.617	183 (146–234)
AST, U/L	36 (24–52)	56 (35–84)	**<0.001**	41 (29–67)
ALT, U/L	49 (30–75)	77 (50–113)	**<0.001**	62 (36–98)
AST/ALT ratio	0.75 (0.58–0.97)	0.70 (0.58–0.93)	0.878	0.73 (0.58–0.95)
Bilirubin, mg/dL	0.7 (0.5–1.0)	0.8 (0.6–1.1)	0.113	0.8 (0.6–1.0)
Albumin, g/L	43 (40–45)	43 (41–46)	0.904	43 (40–46)
Total cholesterol, mg/dL	170 (145–199)	158 (134–185)	**0.023**	165 (137–189)
Triglycerides, mg/dL	129 (87–170)	98 (82–121)	**0.002**	108 (83–139)
Glucose, mg/dL	114 (100–140)	100 (93–110)	**<0.001**	105 (94–117)
Creatinine, mg/dL	0.8 (0.7–0.9)	0.7 (0.7–0.9)	**0.050**	0.77 (0.67–0.90)

NAFLD: non-alcoholic fatty liver disease; HCV: hepatitis C virus; CAP: controlled attenuation parameter; NFS: NAFLD fibrosis score; HCC: hepatocellular carcinoma; AST: aspartate aminotransferase; ALT: alanine aminotransferase; N.A.: not applicable. [1] Available and with technically valid results in 102/155 patients (N. = 50 NAFLD and N. = 52 HCV). [2] Available for 25 NAFLD and 24 HCV patients. [3] Defined as Kleiner stage ≥ 3 or Ishak stage ≥ 4 for NAFLD and HCV subjects, respectively. HCC patients are not included. [4] Defined as a percentage of steatotic hepatocytes greater than 66%. HCC patients are not included. [5] Two HCV genotypes 1b and one genotype 3. [6] Predictive of severe fibrosis (Kleiner stage ≥ 3). Bold values denote statistical significance at the $p < 0.05$ level.

Table 3. Main demographic and clinical features of the healthy controls (N. = 27). Data are presented as medians (range) for continuous variables, and as frequencies (%) for categorical variables.

Parameter	Parameter
Age, years	25 (25–29)
Male/female sex, N.	11 (41)/16 (59)
Body Mass Index, kg/m^2	21.7 (19.4–23.4)
Obese subjects, N.	0 (0)
Liver stiffness, kPa	4.4 (3.9–5.4)
CAP, db/m	196 (177–230)

CAP: controlled attenuation parameter.

Patients' biochemical parameters were obtained after at least 8 h of fasting. As can be seen, these were subjects that can be considered reasonably representative of the type of patients who typically accesses a hepatology unit for the diagnosis and treatment of the respective pathologies. As far demographic characteristics are concerned, the two groups were similar, both for median age and the sex ratio. Metabolic parameters such as glycaemia, total cholesterol and triglycerides were significantly more elevated in the NAFLD group. The same applies for the frequencies of obesity, diabetes or prediabetes. Specularly, it appears consistent with belonging to the HCV group, that the levels of aspartate aminotransferase (AST) and alanine aminotransferase (ALT) were higher in this subpopulation, which is more commonly characterized by increased cytonecrotic damage.

Considering only non-cancer patients (N. = 138), the cases of advanced fibrosis (defined as a stage ≥3 or ≥4 according to Kleiner or Ishak classifications, respectively) (N. = 48) showed similar proportions between the two groups, although with some excess prevalence in the NAFLD group. The same considerations applied for the liver stiffness. Concerning the frequency of HCV patients with advanced fibrosis, it is consistent with the estimates of disease stage distribution in Italy (and, more generally, in Europe) before the spread of direct antiviral agents (DAA). Focusing only on patients with established cirrhosis (defined as a stage four or six according to Kleiner or Ishak classifications, respectively) (N. = 16), they were more prevalent in NAFLD than in HCV group (19% vs. 5%, respectively, $p = 0.01$); all subjects had Child-Pugh score A, and the median score (interquartile range, IQR) of the Model for End-Stage Liver Disease (MELD) was eight (seven to eight). With regard to hepatic steatosis, the NAFLD group (N. = 64), as expected, had significantly higher controlled attenuation parameter (CAP) values than the chronic hepatitis C (CHC) subset (N. = 74) ($p = 0.003$). Additionally, histological steatosis, quantified as the percentage of steatotic hepatocytes (up to 33%, between 33 and 66%, and more than 66%), was significantly more severe in NAFLD patients compared to HCV subjects: 21 (33%), 30 (47%), and 13 (20%) vs. 67 (91%), 4 (5%), and 3 (4%) patients, respectively ($p < 0.001$). In particular, the NAFLD group had a higher prevalence of severe (i.e., more than 66%) steatosis ($p = 0.006$).

3.2. Plasma Periostin Concentrations

3.2.1. Periostin Concentrations and Disease Etiology

The median plasma PN value (IQR) in the study population (N. = 182) was 11.6 ng/mL (8.7–13.3). In particular, it was 10.9 ng/mL (7.7–14.6) in the NAFLD group (N. = 74), 12.0 ng/mL (9.8–16.5) in the HCV group (N. = 81), and 12.0 ng/mL (9.1–16.3) in the healthy subject group (N. = 27), respectively, with a trend toward statistical significant differences amongst groups ($p = 0.06$). Figure 1 shows the scatterplot of the distribution of plasma PN values among the different disease etiologies. The red symbols identify cases of HCC; it can be observed that these subjects had PN concentrations that were always equal to or higher than the median of the respective groups -with the exception of one single NAFLD case ($p = 0.006$ and 0.004 for NAFLD and HCV patients, respectively) (also see Table 4).

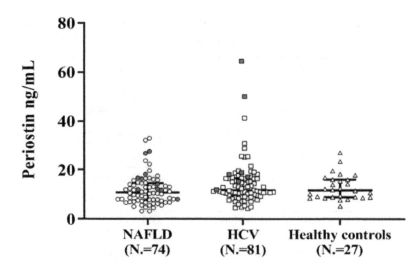

Figure 1. Scatterplot of the distribution of plasma periostin values according to the different disease etiologies. The red symbols identify cases of HCC. NAFLD: non-alcoholic fatty liver disease; HCV: hepatitis C virus.

Table 4. (a): plasma periostin concentrations according to the severity of liver disease. Data are presented as medians (range). The p value refers to the differences between the four considered disease stages. (b): differences of PN circulating levels within the various fibrosis stages in non-HCC individuals. p values are reported. (c): differences of PN circulating levels between HCC and non-HCC patients divided according to the various fibrosis stages. p values are reported.

(a)	Plasma Periostin (ng/mL)				
	No/mild fibrosis (N. = 79) [1]	Moderate fibrosis (N. = 38) [2]	Severe fibrosis (N. = 48) [3]	HCC (N. = 17)	p
Total population (N. = 182)	10.5 (8.1–15.0)	12.0 (10.8–15.5)	11.1 (8.4–15.7)	16.8 (12.2–22.9)	**0.001**
NAFLD (N. = 74)	9.9 (6.8–13.1)	10.9 (7.1–11.3)	10.2 (7.7–14.7)	15.4 (12.1–18.3)	**0.045**
HCV (N. = 81)	10.4 (7.8–14.4)	13.1 (10.9–16.5)	11.4 (8.9–18.2)	18.2 (15.5–50.1)	**0.013**
Healthy controls (N. = 27)	12.0 (9.1–16.3)	-	-	-	N.A.

(b)	Differences in plasma periostin concentrations, p value			
	Moderate vs. no/mild fibrosis [1,2]	Severe vs. no/mild fibrosis [1,3]	Severe vs. moderate fibrosis [2,3]	Cirrhosis [4] vs. pre-cirrhosis [5]
Total non-HCC subjects (N. = 165)	0.101	0.424	0.548	0.937
Non-HCC NAFLD (N. = 64)	0.952	0.535	0.696	0.238
Non-HCC HCV (N. = 74)	0.073	0.254	0.889	0.535

(c)	Differences in plasma periostin concentrations, p value		
	HCC vs. no/mild fibrosis [1]	HCC vs. moderate fibrosis [2]	HCC vs. severe fibrosis [3]
Total patients (N. = 155)	**<0.001**	**0.002**	**0.004**
NAFLD (N. = 74)	**0.008**	**0.01**	**0.04**
HCV (N. = 81)	**0.007**	**0.004**	**0.03**

NAFLD: non-alcoholic fatty liver disease; HCV: hepatitis C virus; HCC: hepatocellular carcinoma; N.A.: not applicable. [1] Defined as Kleiner stage ≤ 1 or Ishak stage ≤ 1 for NAFLD and HCV subjects, respectively. Number of patients: 34 NAFLD, 18 HCV. [2] Defined as Kleiner stage = 2 or Ishak stages 2–3 for NAFLD and HCV subjects, respectively. Number of patients: 6 NAFLD, 32 HCV. [3] Defined as Kleiner stage ≥ 3 or Ishak stage ≥ 4 for NAFLD and HCV subjects, respectively. Number of patients: 24 NAFLD, 24 HCV. [4] Defined as Kleiner stage 4 or Ishak stage 6 for NAFLD and HCV subjects, respectively. Number of patients: 12 NAFLD, 4 HCV. [5] Defined as Kleiner stage 3 or Ishak stages 4–5 for NAFLD and HCV subjects, respectively. Number of patients: 12 NAFLD, 20 HCV. Bold values denote statistical significance at the $p < 0.05$ level.

Considering all patients (N. = 155), differences among sexes with regard to PN levels did not reach statistical significance, either considering them as a whole (median in males: 11.9 ng/mL, IQR 8.2–16.8; median in females 11.1 ng/mL, IQR 8.5–14.8, p = 0.196), or separately analyzing the two subgroups, i.e., HCV (median in males: 12.9 ng/mL, IQR 10.7–17.4; median in females 11.3 ng/mL, IQR 9.2–16.0, p = 0.275) and NAFLD (median in males: 11.8 ng/mL, IQR 7.8–16.1; median in females 10.5 ng/mL, IQR 7.1–13.3, p = 0.418).

3.2.2. Periostin Concentrations and Hepatic Steatosis Degree

Additionally, no differences could be found between circulating PN levels and the degree of hepatic steatosis in cancer-free patients (N. = 138), quantified as the following percentages of steatotic hepatocytes: up to 33%, between 33 and 66%, and more than 66% (for the number of individual groups, see Section 2.1). For what concerns NAFLD group (N. = 64), median values were 10.4 (8.0–13.0), 11.0 (7.5–14.6), and 8.1 (7.0–13.8) ng/mL, respectively (p = 0.553). Hepatitis C patients (N. = 74) had the following concentrations: 11.2 (8.6–15.3), 13.1 (9.2–16.7), and 11.5 (10.5–15.5) ng/mL, respectively (p = 0.763). Similarly, no correlation was observed between plasma PN levels and the three degrees of steatosis both in NAFLD (Spearman Rho = −0.089, p = 0.488) and HCV (Spearman Rho = 0.139, p = 0.236) subjects. Finally, no correlation was found between PN and CAP values in the NAFLD, HCV and healthy control subjects (Spearman Rho = 0.084, −0.303, and −0.252, respectively; p = 0.688, 0.151, and 0.215, respectively).

3.2.3. Periostin Concentrations and Hepatic Fibrosis

Table 3 panel a shows the values of PN soluble concentrations according to the severity of the disease in the various study groups, including healthy controls: significant differences were found within total and patient populations. Table 3 panel b describes the comparisons of PN plasmatic levels within the various fibrosis stages in non-HCC individuals (again, including healthy controls): no significant differences could be found. Table 3 panel c shows the comparison of PN plasmatic levels in HCC vs. non-HCC patients (NAFLD and HCV) divided according to the various fibrosis stages: HCC subjects showed always significantly higher PN values compared to any stages of fibrosis in their respective groups.

For what concerns non-HCC patients, no correlation was observed between plasma PN levels and the three stages of fibrosis both in NAFLD (N. = 64) (Spearman Rho = 0.079, p = 0.534) and HCV (N. = 74) (Spearman Rho = 0.139, p = 0.237) subjects.

As regards HCC patients, no significant differences were found between NAFLD (N. = 10) and HCV (N. = 7) subjects (p = 0.187) (Figure 2 panel a). Additionally, no differences were found amongst various BCLC HCC stages (p = 0.27) (Figure 2 panel b), although there was a trend for increased PN levels in more advanced stages: 14.9 (11.9–17.6) vs. 18.3 (14.4–38.8) ng/mL in stages 0–A vs. B–C–D, respectively (Figure 2 panel c) (p = 0.09).

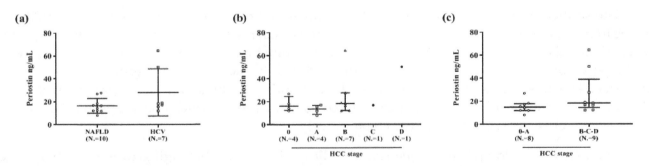

Figure 2. Scatterplot of the distribution of plasma periostin values in HCC patients. NAFLD: non-alcoholic fatty liver disease; HCV: hepatitis C virus. (**a**): periostin concentrations according to HCC etiology. (**b**): periostin concentrations according to HCC stages. (**c**): periostin concentrations according to combined (0–A and B–C–D) HCC stages.

Always with regard to HCC patients, a further analysis was conducted on serum alpha-fetoprotein, which was dosed, as clinical practice, in all HCC patients at the same time of PN sampling. The concentrations were as follows in the different BCLC stages: 31.9 (8.9–79.8), 18.7 (2.6–672.0), 19.9 (4.0–601.0), 276.3 (276.3–276.3), and 9.2 (9.2–9.2) ng/mL, for stages 0, A, B, C and D, respectively. No significant differences were found in alpha-fetoprotein concentrations within the total HCC population ($p = 0.834$) or when HCC stages were grouped as 0–A (23.1 (4.5–79.8) ng/mL) and B–C–D (19.9 (4.7–438.6) ng/mL) ($p = 0.704$), as performed for the analysis of PN. Finally, a correlation was observed between circulating PN and alpha-fetoprotein levels (Spearman Rho = −0.487, $p = 0.047$).

3.2.4. Periostin Concentrations and Main Demographic and Clinical Variables

When PN concentrations were analysed according to the main clinical variables of the entire study population (N. = 182), no statistically significant associations were observed among the various age groups (<40, 40–60, >60 years; $p = 0.356$), sex ($p = 0.203$), and body mass index (BMI) ($p = 0.521$) categorized, according to the cutoffs indicated by the World Health Organization [37]. PN levels had a trend to be inversely related to BMI (Spearman Rho = −0.134, $p = 0.086$), and did not vary in relation to age (Spearman Rho = 0.064, $p = 0.392$).

A similar analysis was conducted within the patient population (NAFLD and HCV groups, N. = 155). considering glucose metabolism status (normal glucose tolerance, prediabetes, diabetes) and some main laboratory variables: ALT (cutoffs: <40, 40–99, ≥100 IU/L), creatinine (cutoffs: <1.0, 1.0–1.4, ≥1.5 mg/dL), total cholesterol (cutoffs: <200, 200–240, ≥240 mg/dL), triglycerides (cutoffs: <80, 80–149, ≥150 mg/dL) and platelets (cutoffs: ≥150, 100–149, <100 × 109/L). No statistically significant associations could be identified for the first five studied parameters ($p = 0.749, 0.810, 0.715, 0.543$, and 0.861, respectively). Instead with regard to the aforementioned platelet cutoffs—commonly used in clinical practice to indicate a mild or a moderate thrombocytopenia—a progressive significant decrease in the plasma levels of PN was observed ($p = 0.007$): 15.2 (11.9–18.3) ng/mL (N. = 115), 13.1 (10.5–17.7) ng/mL (N. = 27), and 11.0 (7.99–16.3) ng/mL (N. = 13) for platelets ≥150, 100–149, <100 × 109/L, respectively. However, no correlation was found between the individual PN and platelet levels (Spearman's Rho = 0.102, $p = 0.205$). Finally, when adjusted for the concentrations of serum glucose and serum TGs, plasma PN levels (after logarithmic transformation) were significantly higher in the HCV group (N. = 74) than in the NAFLD group (N. = 64) (geometric mean ± standard deviation (SD): 12.9 ± 1.6 vs. 10.2 ± 2.5 ng/mL, respectively; $p < 0.001$).

3.3. POSTN Genotyping

3.3.1. Genotypic Frequencies

The studied population was in Hardy–Weinberg equilibrium for all three (rs9603226, rs3829365 and rs1028728) POSTN gene SNPs ($p = 0.135, 0.224$, and 0.580, respectively). Table 5 reports the specific locus of each SNP (obtained from the website www.ncbi.nlm.nih.gov/snp) and shows the distributions of the polymorphisms in the entire study population and in each individual group (NAFLD, HCV, controls). The most frequent genotypes for each SNP, both globally and in single groups, were G/G, C/C and A/A, respectively (thus being considered as homozygous wild types). Specularly, the less common variants were A/A, G/G and T/T, respectively.

The POSTN haplotype full sequences are shown in Table 1 belonging to the Materials and Methods section.

Table 5. Distribution of *POSTN* gene polymorphisms in the total studied population and in the three distinct groups. Data are presented as frequencies (%). The *p* value refers to the comparison between genotypes in the different study groups.

SNPs	Genotype			*p*
rs9603226—chr13:37569449 (GRCh38.p12)	G/G	G/A	A/A	
Total (N. = 182)	132 (72)	49 (27)	1 (1)	
NAFLD (N. = 74)	53 (72)	21 (28)	0 (0)	
HCV (N. = 81)	58 (72	23 (28)	0 (0)	0.153
Healthy controls (N. = 27)	)21 (78)	5 (18)	1 (4)	
rs3829365—chr13:37598759 (GRCh38.p12)	C/C	C/G	G/G	
Total (N. = 182)	168 (92)	13 (7)	1 (1)	
NAFLD (N. = 74)	70 (95)	4 (5)	0 (0)	
HCV (N. = 81)	71 (88)	9 (11)	1 (1)	0.224
Healthy controls (N. = 27)	27 (100)	0 (0)	0 (0)	
rs1028728—chr13:37599679 (GRCh38.p12)	A/A	A/T	T/T	
Total (N. = 182)	106 (58)	64 (35)	12 (7)	
NAFLD (N. = 74)	44 (59)	25 (34)	5 (7)	
HCV (N. = 81)	46 (57)	29 (36)	6 (7)	0.968
Healthy controls (N. = 27)	16 (59)	10 (37)	1 (4)	

POSTN: periostin; SNP: single nucleotide polymorphism; NAFLD: non-alcoholic fatty liver disease; HCV: hepatitis C virus.

3.3.2. Periostin and *POSTN* Gene Polymorphisms

Plasma PN concentrations were evaluated as a function of the three *POSTN* gene polymorphisms. Table 6 shows the median concentrations (IQR) of PN, both in the total studied population and in the three groups. No statistically significant correlations were observed between the genotype of the single polymorphisms and PN circulating levels.

Table 6. Periostin plasmatic concentrations according to *POSTN* gene polymorphisms. Median and interquartile range are reported. The *p* value refers to the correlation between the genotype of the single polymorphisms and periostin circulating levels.

SNPs	Genotype and Plasmatic Periostin (ng/mL)			
rs9603226	G/G	G/A	A/A	*p*
Total (N. = 182)	11.9 (9.0–16.3)	11.1 (8.2–15.6)	9.1 (9.1–9.1)	0.491
NAFLD (N. = 74)	11.4 (7.7–15.8)	9.7 (8.0–12.3)	–	0.232
HCV (N. = 81)	12.2 (9.8–16.5)	11.2 (9.2–16.8)	–	0.742
Healthy controls (N. = 27)	12.0 (9.3–16.2)	15.6 (8.7–19.8)	9.1 (9.1–9.1)	0.710
rs3829365	C/C	C/G	G/G	*p*
Total (N. = 182)	11.8 (8.6–16.4)	10.5 (8.7–13.0)	64.6 (64.6–64.6)	0.121
NAFLD (N. = 74)	11.2 (7.7–14.8)	9.6 (7.2–11.7)	–	0.430
HCV (N. = 81)	12.5 (10.1–16.8)	10.5 (9.2–13.2)	64.6 (64.6–64.6)	0.119
Healthy controls (N. = 27)	12.0 (9.1–16.3)	–	–	NA
rs1028728	A/A	A/T	T/T	*p*
Total (N. = 182)	11.4 (8.0–15.6)	11.1 (9.11–15.9)	15.1 (10.3–19.1)	0.153
NAFLD (N. = 74)	9.8 (6.9–13.3)	11.9 (9.4–15.8)	11.8 (8.1–17.7)	0.206
HCV (N. = 81)	12.3 (9.2–16.5)	11.2 (10.3–16.5)	16.0 (13.1–19.4)	0.394
Healthy controls (N. = 27)	13.3 (10.2–16.2)	9.2 (8.7–12.6)	17.1 (17.1–17.1)	0.232

POSTN: periostin; SNP: single nucleotide polymorphism; NAFLD: non-alcoholic fatty liver disease; HCV: hepatitis C virus.

Dominant and recessive genetic models were then calculated by referring to the allele frequency, considering the most frequent allele as the major one (M), and the least frequent allele as the minor one

(m) [38]. Table 7 panel a shows plasma PN concentrations as a function of a dominant model (thus comparing MM versus Mm + mm): no statistically significant differences in PN levels with regard to the aforementioned variant alleles in the whole patient population were reported (N. = 155). The same also happened when applying a recessive model, and comparing MM + Mm versus mm (Table 7 panel b).

Table 7. Periostin levels as a function of *POSTN* gene SNPs in NAFLD and HCV patients (N. = 155), see text for details. Median and interquartile range are reported. The *p* value refers to the differences of periostin plasma levels between the various *POSTN* genotypes. (a): dominant model (MM versus Mm + mm). (b): recessive model (MM + Mm versus mm). * = any of the two possible nucleotides for each of the conditions of interest.

	POSTN SNPs	*POSTN* Genotypes [1] and Periostin Levels ng/mL		*p*
(a)	rs9603226	G/G 11.9 (9.0–16.3)	A/* 11.1 (8.2–16.6)	0.301
	rs3829365	C/C 11.8 (8.6–16.4)	G/* 10.5 (8.7–13.1)	0.521
	rs1028728	A/A 11.5 (8.0–15.6)	T/* 11.9 (9.1–16.7)	0.153
(b)	rs9603226	G/* 11.7 (9.7–16.3)	A/A 9.1 (9.1–9.1)	0.714
	rs3829365	C/* 11.5 (8.7–16.2)	G/G 64.6 (64.6–64.6)	0.085
	rs1028728	A/* 11.3 (8.6–15.8)	T/T 15.1 (10.3–19.1)	0.091

POSTN: periostin; SNP: single nucleotide polymorphism. [1] Dominant and recessive models were calculated by referring to the allele frequency, considering the most frequent allele as the major one and the least frequent allele as the minor one.

3.3.3. Periostin and *POSTN* Gene Diplotypes

We analyzed the frequencies of the *POSTN* gene haplotypes in the entire study population and in the individual groups. In all cases (in the total studied population, NAFLD patients, HCV subjects, and healthy controls, respectively) haplotype two (allelic frequencies of 0.596, 0.602, 0.574, 0.648) was significantly more prevalent than haplotype one (not detected), haplotype three (frequencies of 0.003, 0, 0.006, 0), haplotype four (frequencies of 0.025, 0.020, 0.037, 0), haplotype five (frequencies of 0.137, 0.142, 0.136, 0.130), and haplotype six (frequencies of 0.239, 0.236, 0.247, 0.222).

An analysis was then conducted of circulating PN values as a function of the diplotypes (i.e., matched pairs of haplotypes on homologous chromosomes), considering the most frequent haplotype (number two, as previously mentioned) as the major one. Diplotype 2/* (i.e the combination of haplotype two and a haplotype other than 2), was the most frequent, both in the total study population and in the NAFLD, HCV and healthy controls groups (Table 8). In no case it was possible to detect any statistically significant difference amongst the groups in plasma PN levels. However, when analyzing patients carrying haplotype two (i.e., diplotypes 2/2 and 2/*) against other diplotypes, the former ones had more frequently plasma PN levels that were lower than the last quintile of the total studied population (130/156 vs. 16/26, respectively; *p* = 0.01).

Significant differences in steatosis grading and fibrosis staging were found between different diplotypes (either applying dominant and recessive models): *p* was <0.001 in all cases, both in the total studied population and in the NAFLD group.

Table 8. Plasma periostin values as a function of the *POSTN* gene diplotypes. * = any other haplotype different from haplotype 2. Median and interquartile range are reported. The *p* value refers to the differences of periostin plasma levels between the various *POSTN* diplotypes.

Group	POSTN Gene Diplotypes and Periostin Levels ng/mL			*p*
	Diplotype 2/2	Diplotype 2/*	Diplotype */*	
Total (N. = 182)	11.7 (7.9–16.2) (N. = 61)	11.1 (8.7–15.6) (N. = 95)	11.9 (8.9–18.8) (N. = 26)	0.253
NAFLD (N. = 74)	10.4 (6.8–15.0) (N. = 25)	11.1 (8.1–14.2) (N. = 39)	11.2 (8.1–17.7) (N. = 10)	0.447
HCV (N. = 81)	11.7 (9.3–16.5) (N. = 25)	11.2 (9.2–16.5) (N. = 43)	13.2 (11.0–19.4) (N. = 13)	0.233
Healthy controls (N. = 27)	12.4 (10.8–16.2) (N. = 11)	10.4 (9.0–18.1) (N. = 13)	9.1 (8.7–17.1) (N. = 3)	0.460

POSTN: periostin; NAFLD: non-alcoholic fatty liver disease; HCV: hepatitis C virus.

3.4. Multivariate Analysis of Factors Associated with High Periostin

Multivariate analysis among those variables with $p < 0.10$ at univariate analysis was performed to identify possible predictors of high plasma levels of PN (i.e., those included in the last quintile) in the whole patient population (N. = 155). The set of covariates included *POSTN* diplotype (categorized as 2/2 plus 2/* versus */*), age, sex, HCC, and platelet count. The significant predictor variables found were *POSTN* diplotype and HCC (Table 9 panel a). The same results were confirmed when the analysis was restricted to the two single patient groups (i.e., NAFLD and HCV, Table 9 panels b and c, respectively), with the exception of *POSTN* diplotype in NAFLD subjects.

Table 9. Predictive parameters of high plasma periostin (i.e., last quintile) values. Both odds ratios (OR) with the corresponding 95% confidence intervals (CI) and statistical significance (*p* values) are reported of a maximum-likelihood logit regression model with high (i.e., belonging to the last quintile) plasma periostin as dependent variable, and *POSTN* diplotype (categorized as 2/2 plus 2/* versus */*), age, sex, HCC, and platelet count as predictor variables. (a): all patients. (b): NAFLD patients. (c): HCV patients.

Variable	(a) All Patients (N. = 155)		(b) NAFLD (N. = 74)		(c) HCV (N. = 81)	
	OR (95% CI)	*p*	OR (95% CI)	*p*	OR (95% CI)	*p*
Diplotype 2/2 + 2/*	0.25 (0.09–0.70)	**0.008**	0.37 (0.07–2.00)	0.219	0.25 (0.07–0.97)	**0.041**
Age, years	0.98 (0.95–1.02)	0.338	0.97 (0.92–1.03)	0.342	0.99 (0.95–1.04)	0.808
Male/female sex	1.98 (0.79–4.96)	0.144	1.67 (0.39–7.11)	0.519	2.74 (0.80–9.35)	0.113
HCC, N.	6.76 (1.73–26.38)	**0.006**	7.46 (1.19–56.02)	**0.022**	15.64 (2.15–113.87)	**0.001**
Platelets, ×10⁹/L	0.99 (0.98–1.00)	0.230	1.00 (0.99–1.01)	0.399	1.00 (0.99–1.01)	0.883

NAFLD: non-alcoholic fatty liver disease; HCV: hepatitis C virus; OR: odds ratio; CI: confidence interval; HCC: hepatocellular carcinoma. Bold values denote statistical significance at the $p < 0.05$ level.

4. Discussion

This is the first study aiming to examine PN plasma levels and polymorphisms in NAFLD and other different pathologic conditions (namely CHC and HCC), and their possible relations with the progression of liver disease. The results shown evidence a poor association between circulating PN levels and the etiology of liver disorders. In addition, no correlation was shown with the severity of NAFLD or its fibrotic evolution. Interestingly, however, the results obtained showed that plasma PN was influenced by genotype and HCC.

PN is a known important factor in metabolic disease pathogenesis, and is directly and indirectly involved in hepatic steatosis and hypertriglyceridemia, which are key determinants of NAFLD. The evidence coming from the first studies which demonstrated the important role played by the protein in cellular and animal models [13–15] was then confirmed in human research, at least in Asian subjects [8,17,18]. Obviously, NAFLD pathogenesis cannot be reduced to fat accumulation alone. For instance, chronic inflammation should never be omitted, being a known contributor to the progression to NASH [39]. In this respect, many studies have suggested a close relationship between PN and liver fibrosis. In particular, hepatic inflammation and fibrosis were significantly inhibited in PN-knockout mice, mainly through a transforming growth factor (TGF)-β1 and TGF-β2 dependent mechanism, revealing a potential role of PN in NASH [9,15]. More recently, researchers have further conducted discussions on the intrinsic mechanisms of PN-induced hepatic fibrosis: collectively, PN has been shown to play an important role in activated hepatic stellate cells, aggravating the accumulation of fiber and matrix, ultimately inducing liver fibrosis [40–42]. As regards these issues, it should be emphasized that PN belongs to the so called "liver matrisome", which identifies the whole of ECM and non-fibrillar proteins that interact or are structurally affiliated with the ECM, and are involved in the regulation of tissue homeostasis and organ function. In the liver, maladaptive changes of matrisome in response to any stress or injury—including liver inflammation and damage caused by a buildup of fat in the liver, the so-called NASH—can eventually lead to hepatic fibrosis [43]. The role of PN as a profibrotic agent through the liver matrisome modulation could be related to its direct actions on key molecules or proteins of ECM or on enzymes involved in the collagen stabilization and matrix integrity and elasticity, such as lysyl oxidases (LOX) and LOX like enzymes (LOXL). Hence, PN was shown to cause collagen expression in HSCs via integrin αvβ3 and the activation of the phosphoinositide 3-kinase (PI3K)-related phosphorylation of small mother against decapentaplegic (SMAD) 2/3. In turn, this would lead to LOXL1–3 activation and collagen production and cross-linking [44].

In our study, NAFLD patients had all the classic features of the metabolic syndrome, which shares an insulin resistance state, as shown by high BMI, glycemia, cholesterol, triglycerides and increased incidence of obesity and prediabetic/diabetic conditions [45]. On the contrary, AST/ALT values were slightly but significantly higher in HCV patients, which is consistent with the predominantly cytonecrotic mechanisms at the basis of HCV-related liver damages. As regards these clinical and demographic variables, our study could not demonstrate a correlation with circulating PN; in particular, no associations were found with BMI, diabetes, hypercholesterolemia and hypertriglyceridemia. Consequently, from these data, it could be stated that—at least in our casuistry—there was no pathophysiological relation between the typical NAFLD metabolic profile and soluble PN, and vice versa. These data are in contrast with those reported in the clinical Asian study conducted by Zhu et al. who showed significant positive associations between serum PN and many important metabolic parameters such as weight, fasting plasma glucose, waist circumference (WC) and hip circumference [16]. In another Chinese study (but, in this case, on overweight and obese patients), PN levels were again positively and significantly associated with WC, fasting insulin, homeostasis model assessment-insulin resistance (HOMA-IR), AST, ALT, and γ-glutamyltranspeptidase (GGT). However, similarly to our case, it was not possible to identify significant correlations with age, impaired fasting glucose, impaired glucose tolerance or BMI [17]. The authors hypothesized that it is above all the accumulation of visceral fat (which correlates well with the measurement of WC), rather than BMI, that could influence the levels of soluble PN. So, the fact that the former anthropometric parameter was not measured in our study could represent a possible limitation. It should be noted that Asian populations are notoriously subject to a greater risk of cardiovascular complications and development of type 2 diabetes mellitus—also at lower BMI values—than Caucasian populations, emphasizing the role played by racial/ethnic differences in this context, as below discussed [46–48]. In any case, to the best of our knowledge, there are currently no other studies besides ours which have focused on these correlations in the specific context of Caucasian populations, and that could help to better clarify the cited discrepancies.

The present study did not also identify a significant association between PN levels and the presence of NAFLD. As matter of fact, PN plasma median concentrations did not show statistically significant differences amongst the three studied groups (NAFLD, HCV, and healthy controls). Again, Chinese studies reached different conclusions, identifying a close association with NAFLD. For instance, Lu et al. found increased serum PN levels in NAFLD patients vs. normal subjects [12]. Similarly, Zhu et al. correlated increased levels of PN with the presence of NAFLD, after adjustment for age, gender, BMI and waist-to-hip ratio, even proposing a possible role of the protein as a biomarker in NAFLD management [16]. Yang et al., on the other hand, showed that, in overweight and obese patients, serum PN was associated with a higher risk for NAFLD, regardless of other risk factors such as insulin resistance [17]. Although a clear explanation for these discrepancies with our study cannot be given, it is reasonable to postulate again, that differences in populations and ethnicity, as well as in sample size, may be crucial. In this regard, it is interesting to note that—when confronted with a previous study conducted on a Caucasian population (therefore similar to ours)—comparable results were obtained with our research [19]. The authors indeed evidenced that that concentrations of circulating PN in NAFLD were not higher than in healthy controls; likewise, PN levels were not statistically different between simple steatosis subjects, NASH patients, and controls. This study is also important because it evidences how also methodological differences (e.g., the performance or not of a liver biopsy) could influence the discrepancies between our study and Asian research. The latter investigations were, in fact, conducted only on ultrasound-diagnosed NAFLDs, unlike ours and that of Polyzos et al. where the diagnosis was rigorously made with the current gold standard, i.e., liver biopsy. In this context, it therefore appears that a strength of our study includes having almost all histological diagnoses, even if the sample size was not particularly high. Moreover, it may constitute an element of innovation the fact that, to our knowledge, no comparisons existed—until now—between patients with NAFLD and other liver diseases.

Another message that emerged from our study is that in NAFLD subjects, no correlation was observed between plasma PN levels and the histological disease stage (including cirrhosis). The same applied for the HCV control group, although a trend of increased PN levels was observed in moderate fibrosis vs. no/mild fibrosis. Additionally, PN levels did not change in relation to a greater or lesser degree of steatosis (again, ascertained and quantified at liver biopsy). These particular aspects are currently not yet sufficiently clarified in the available literature. The Asian papers mentioned above simply did not explore this topic [13,16,17], while that from Polyzos et al. reported a somewhat apparently paradoxical fact: reduced PN levels, in correlation with BMI or WC, were able to predict F2 and F3 fibrosis stages with a sensitivity and specificity of 100%. With PN also being related to hepatic fibrogenesis, the authors hypothesized that down-regulation of protein expression may occur as fibrosis progresses, as a defense mechanism against further damage progression [19]. Instead, the report that PN levels were similar within other histological lesions (steatosis grade, ballooning, lobular, and portal inflammation) was in accordance with ours.

What clearly emerged from our study is, instead, that plasma levels of PN were significantly higher in patients with HCC than in all the other stages of the disease, including cirrhosis, both considering the entire study population, and NAFLD or HCV patients separately. Moreover, at multivariate analysis, HCC was an independent predictive variable for high plasma levels of PN. Our finding is in accordance with data showing that PN is not only involved in bone metabolism, but also in modulating cell proliferation and tumorigenesis in many other tissues and organs, including liver [49]. For example, Zinn et al. found that PN levels are positively correlated with tumor phenotype in glioblastoma patients and orthotopic xenografts [50]. Furthermore, higher PN expression in pancreatic neuroendocrine tumors can facilitate their revascularization by up-regulating fibroblast growth factor [51]. PN is also upregulated in non-small cell lung cancer, and its overexpression could enhance signal transducer and activator of transcription (Stat) 3 and Ak strain transforming (Akt) phosphorylation and survivin expression [52]. As regarding liver, PN, that could be released by cancer-associated fibroblasts and/or hepatic stellate cells, has been found to be associated with a high metastatic capability of HCC, being able to promote adhesion, migration and invasion of liver cancer cells, as well as angiogenesis [10]. Increased PN expression would also contribute to tumor cell survival during hypoxia through the overexpression of hypoxia-inducible factor (HIF)-1α [53]. As a likely consequence of these changes in the biological characteristics of HCCs, it was reported that tumors with PN positive expression showed more frequent multicentricity, microvascular invasion, Edmondson grade III–IV, and TNM stages III–IV than HCCs with PN negative expression. Additionally, further assessment demonstrated that overall survival and disease-free survival were better in patients without PN expression: both Kaplan–Meier and multivariate analysis showed that the expression of PN was an independent predictor of poor prognosis. For all these reasons, PN is now considered as an important prognostic biomarker of tumor recurrence and as a tool to distinguishing HCC patients from non-malignant liver diseases [10,22,54]. Overall, while taking into account the important size limits of this study with regard to the HCC arm (only 17 patients studied in total, of which 10 NAFLD), our findings seem to support the above-mentioned evidence, and would highlight the role of PN as a soluble biomarker potentially useful for the management of HCC patients, similarly to what already happens in current clinical practice for alpha-fetoprotein, as would be suggested by the good correlation between the two proteins that we found in our casuistry. It should also be noted that—although this study was not specifically designed to study HCC—it is the first to have analyzed HCCs specifically due to NAFLD. Although the data are preliminary and need further validation, it would seem that the modulation of PN circulating levels is not strictly dependent on the HCC etiology, being similar also in the HCV control group.

In consideration of the above-mentioned possible changes of PN expression in relation to ethnicity, in the present study we performed a genetic analysis by examining the main polymorphisms of *POSTN* gene in our population. In this regard it has to be said that the association between these genetic variables and chronic disease liver diseases has not been studied previously, unlike what (partially) happened for other disorders. The SNPs which have more literature solid data and, therefore, that were selected by us are rs9603226, rs3829365, and rs1028728. The most convincing research so far was conducted on Japanese patients, and investigated if these SNPs had any relationship with plasma PN concentrations and the clinical severity of bronchial asthma [23]. The study demonstrated that high PN levels were associated with worse pulmonary function tests, and that certain genotypes of rs3829365 and rs9603226 (but not of rs1028728) resulted in higher plasma PN concentrations and a more rapid decline in respiratory function, respectively. The authors hypothesized that the rs3829365 G/G genotype may be implicated in the mRNA stability of PN, consequently leading to changes in the circulating levels of the protein. The minor A allele of rs9603226 could instead up-regulate the binding capacity of the PN to other ECM proteins, thereby facilitating greater airway remodeling. Additionally, a study conducted on Chinese patients affected by heart failure showed an independent correlation between the C/G and G/G genotypes of rs3829365 and the disease, both in terms of risk and severity; rs1028728 was also not relevant in this context [55] [54]. When focusing on Caucasian subjects, however, other studies failed to confirm a predictive role of these SNPs in disease progression: for instance, rs3829365 and rs1028728, as well as their haplotype combinations, were not associated with atherosclerosis or coronary collateral circulation in subjects with coronary artery disease [24,25].

For what concerns our study, we did not find any correlation between *POSTN* polymorphisms and PN levels in NAFLD subjects; the same happened for HCV control patients. No correlations were found for the haplotypes, when analyzed separately. This is, therefore, not in agreement with what Japanese researchers found, albeit in a different disease model. However, it has to be said that our Caucasian subjects had a substantial different genetic pattern from that study population. As a matter of fact, the frequencies of the minor alleles reported by Kanemitsu et al. were 0.136, 0.278, and 0.330, for rs1028728, rs3829365, and rs9603226, respectively [23]. These frequencies were reported to be similar in Chinese subjects, taking into account the evidence provided by the aforementioned studies even if not directly focused on population genetics [13,16,17]: 0.052, 0.320, and 0.278, respectively [56–58]. In our population, the same frequencies were instead 0.242, 0.041, and 0.140, respectively, and comparable to what was reported in the general European population (0.263, 0.070, and 0.106, respectively) [56–58]. The same considerations can be made for the haplotype frequencies identified, respectively, by the Japanese researchers and us: haplotype one, 0.322 vs. 0; haplotype two, 0.278 vs. 0.596; haplotype three, 0.133 vs. 0.003; haplotype four, 0.267 vs. 0.025; haplotype five, 0 vs. 0.137; haplotype six, 0 vs. 0.239 [23].

So, ethnicity is also confirmed in our study to play an obvious major role in genetic patterns, and this could partially account for the reported by us absence of correlation with PN expression. A greater weight of genetics among Asian populations in determining protein expression and thus PN-mediated development of liver steatosis may also be hypothesized. On the contrary, in the Caucasian population, which certainly presents a greater prevalence of the major recognized risk factors for NAFLD (obesity, insulin resistance, high-fat diets, sedentary lifestyle), the role of environmental factors would be predominant in the development of the disease, and this would explain the similar results of this study and that conducted on Greek patients [19]. In addition to the previous analyses, the homo- or heterozygous diplotype was taken into consideration for the most common haplotype in the studied population (number two). New information that emerged from our study was that the subjects with this haplotype, either as homozygote or heterozygote, had lower PN levels in comparison with all other diplotypes. However, at multivariate analysis, diplotype */* (i.e., with both alleles different from haplotype two) failed to be an independent predictive variable for high plasma levels of PN in NAFLD patients. Moreover, our study evidenced, for the first time, significant differences in steatosis grading and fibrosis staging among different diplotypes, which would confirm a role of the genetic pattern of PN expression in the onset of liver disease and its severity. Hence, since up to now no information is available in the literature about this issue, our data—although needing to be validated in larger casuistries—would be of particular relevance.

This study obviously has some important limitations. First of all, only patients referring to a single center were recruited, even if it was a large tertiary referral hospital. Another issue, as said before, is related to the number of patients. Although the size of population was properly calculated by means of specific statistical power analysis, increasing the number could have improved the strength of results obtained. Moreover, only subjects with histological evidence of disease were selected for this research, which could represent both a strength and a selection bias: in any case, it should not be forgotten that in the vast majority of the previous studies NAFLD was diagnosed only by ultrasound. In addition, the cross-sectional design of the study could not prove if increased levels of protein expression at baseline were associated with an increased risk of HCC development, taking into account that it was not possible to observe a trend for PN increase in the more severe stages of NAFLD disease and that patients already with HCC were recruited at a single time point (i.e., at diagnosis). Finally, the study lacks an assessment of PN mRNA expression at the tissue level, in order to verify whether a specific expression pattern correlates with different SNP genotypes.

In conclusion, this study does not support the hypothesis that circulating PN is a useful biomarker of NAFLD in the Caucasian population (as regards both fibrosis and steatosis). However, increased plasma PN levels could be predictive for specific *POSTN* genotypes and NAFLD/NASH-derived HCC. So, PN confirms itself as a potential diagnostic and prognostic marker for HCC, also for what concerns NAFLD. To better address this issue, further studies could be organized in populations of HCC Caucasian and Asian patients stratified as concerning *POSTN* polymorphisms (haplotype), liver disease etiology and severity of the tumor disease. PN could also be quantified in the liver (from bioptic samples or resections) as protein expression and/or mRNA in order to better clarify its relations with the variables just mentioned. The comparison between tissue expression and plasma levels could also add information about the "dynamics" of PN release and its real role as a reliable circulating marker for HCC. Moreover, on the ground of the results of this study showing a correlation between plasma PN and alpha fetoprotein, it could be worth examining the correlations with other circulating HCC markers (including those being validated in liquid biopsies such as glypican-3 and glutamine synthetase) in order to strengthen the power of PN as a biomarker for this disease.

The clinical implications of the results obtained about plasma PN in HCC could be related to outcome parameters normally used by clinicians in common clinical practice (e.g., survival rate, event-free survival or reintervention rate) or to the results of different therapeutic approaches, which could involve PN itself. In this context, the role of PN could become of higher importance considering the existence of PN antagonists, aptamers, which are modified nucleic acids that specifically bind PN and inhibit its function. To date, PN antagonists have been investigated in breast and gastric cancer; however, a wider understanding of the role and mechanisms of PN in hepatic inflammation and fibrosis may make PN antagonists an innovative therapeutic approach for HCC and, maybe, also for NASH, when the stigmata of the metabolic syndrome are prevalent due to PN's known pathophysiological role [59].

Author Contributions: Conceptualization, M.P., V.M. and C.S.; methodology, M.P.; software, M.N.B. and N.B.; validation, R.M., V.M., M.N.B. and N.B.; formal analysis, M.P. and C.S.; investigation, V.M., M.N.B. and V.R.M.; resources, R.M.; data curation, V.M., M.E.B. and C.S.; writing—original draft preparation, C.S., V.M. and E.G.; writing—review and editing, C.S. and E.G.; visualization, C.S.; supervision, M.P. and E.G.; project administration, R.M.; funding acquisition, C.S. All authors have read and agreed to the published version of the manuscript.

Abbreviations

NAFLD	Non-alcoholic fatty liver disease
SS	Simple steatosis
NASH	Non-alcoholic steatohepatitis
HCC	Hepatocellular carcinoma
TG	Triglyceride
PN	Periostin
OSF-2	Osteoblast-specific factor 2
ECM	Extracellular matrix
POSTN	Periostin
PPAR	Peroxisome proliferator-activated receptor
Rac	Ras-related C3 botulinum toxin substrate
ROR	RAR-related orphan receptor
ELISA	Enzyme Linked Immunosorbent Assay
VEGF	Vascular Endothelial Growth Factor
SNP	Single nucleotide polymorphism
HCV	Hepatitis C virus
EASL-EORTC	European Association For The Study Of The Liver and the European Organization for Research and Treatment of Cancer
CAP	Controlled attenuation parameter
NFS	NAFLD fibrosis score
AST	Aspartate aminotransferase
ALT	Alanine aminotransferase
N.A.	Not applicable
DAA	Direct antiviral agents
SD	Standard deviation
IQR	Interquartile range
MELD	Model for End-Stage Liver Disease
CHC	Chronic hepatitis C
BCLC	Barcelona Clinic Liver Cancer
BMI	Body mass index
M	Major allele
m	Minor allele
OR	Odds ratio
CI	Confidence interval
TGF	Transforming growth factor
LOX	Lysyl oxidases

LOXL	LOX like enzymes
PI3K	Phosphoinositide 3-kinase
SMAD	Small mother against decapentaplegic
WC	Waist circumference
HOMA-IR	Homeostasis model assessment-insulin resistance
GGT	γ-glutamyltranspeptidase
Stat	Signal transducer and activator of transcription
Akt	Ak strain transforming
HIF	Hypoxia-inducible factor
HBsAg	Australia antigen
TE	Transient elastography
NFS	NAFLD fibrosis score
PCR	Polymerase chain reaction

Appendix A

Table A1. *POSTN* gene diplotypes based on the 6 haplotype combinations found in the studied population. One out of the two haplotypes present on the chromosome pair is written in italics.

		rs9603226	rs3829365	rs1028728
Diplotype 2/2	Haplotype 2	G	C	A
	Haplotype 2	G	C	A
Diplotype 2/4	Haplotype 2	G	C	A
	Haplotype 4	G	G	A
Diplotype 2/5	Haplotype 2	G	C	A
	Haplotype 5	A	C	A
Diplotype 2/6	Haplotype 2	G	C	A
	Haplotype 6	G	C	T
Diplotype 4/2	Haplotype 4	G	G	A
	Haplotype 2	G	C	A
Diplotype 4/4	Haplotype 4	G	G	A
	Haplotype 4	G	G	A
Diplotype 4/5	Haplotype 4	G	G	A
	Haplotype 5	A	C	A
Diplotype 4/6	Haplotype 4	G	G	A
	Haplotype 6	G	C	T
Diplotype 5/2	Haplotype 5	A	C	A
	Haplotype 2	G	C	A
Diplotype 5/4	Haplotype 5	A	C	A
	Haplotype 4	G	G	A
Diplotype 5/5	Haplotype 5	A	C	A
	Haplotype 5	A	C	A
Diplotype 5/6	Haplotype 5	A	C	A
	Haplotype 6	G	C	T
Diplotype 6/2	Haplotype 6	G	C	T
	Haplotype 2	G	C	A
Diplotype 6/3	Haplotype 6	G	C	T
	Haplotype 3	G	G	T
Diplotype 6/5	Haplotype 6	G	C	T
	Haplotype 5	A	C	A
Diplotype 6/6	Haplotype 6	G	C	T
	Haplotype 6	G	C	T

Table A2. Distribution of NAFLD patients (N. = 64) according to Kleiner classification system. HCC subjects are not included.

	N.	%	Cumulative Frequency
NAFLD Activity Score (NAS)			
0	1	1.56	1.56
1	8	12.50	14.06
2	8	12.50	26.56
3	11	17.19	43.75
4	16	25.00	68.75
5	16	25.00	93.75
6	1	1.56	95.31
7	3	4.69	100.00
Fibrosis stage			
0	18	28.13	28.13
1	15	23.44	51.56
2	6	9.38	60.94
3	13	20.31	81.25
4	12	18.75	100.00

NAFLD: non-alcoholic fatty liver disease; HCC: hepatocellular carcinoma.

References

1. Michelotti, G.A.; Machado, M.V.; Diehl, A.M. NAFLD, NASH and liver cancer. *Nat. Rev. Gastroenterol. Hepatol.* **2013**, *10*, 656–665. [CrossRef]

2. Brunt, E.M.; Wong, V.W.S.; Nobili, V.; Day, C.P.; Sookoian, S.; Maher, J.J.; Bugianesi, E.; Sirlin, C.B.; Neuschwander-Tetri, B.A.; Rinella, M.E. Nonalcoholic fatty liver disease. *Nat. Rev. Dis. Prim.* **2015**, *1*, 15080. [CrossRef]

3. Arab, J.P.; Arrese, M.; Trauner, M. Recent Insights into the Pathogenesis of Nonalcoholic Fatty Liver Disease. *Annu. Rev. Pathol. Mech. Dis.* **2018**, *13*, 321–350. [CrossRef]

4. Musso, G.; Gambino, R.; Cassader, M. Recent insights into hepatic lipid metabolism in non-alcoholic fatty liver disease (NAFLD). *Prog. Lipid Res.* **2009**, *48*, 1–26. [CrossRef] [PubMed]

5. Dowman, J.K.; Tomlinson, J.W.; Newsome, P.N. Pathogenesis of non-alcoholic fatty liver disease. *QJM* **2009**, *103*, 71–83. [CrossRef] [PubMed]

6. Takeshita, S.; Kikuno, R.; Tezuka, K.; Amann, E. Osteoblast-specific factor 2: Cloning of a putative bone adhesion protein with homology with the insect protein fasciclin I. *Biochem. J.* **1993**, *294*, 271–278. [CrossRef] [PubMed]

7. Conway, S.J.; Izuhara, K.; Kudo, Y.; Litvin, J.; Markwald, R.; Ouyang, G.; Arron, J.R.; Holweg, C.T.J.; Kudo, A. The role of periostin in tissue remodeling across health and disease. *Cell. Mol. Life Sci.* **2014**, *71*, 1279–1288. [CrossRef]

8. Jia, Y.; Zhong, F.; Jiang, S.; Guo, Q.; Jin, H.; Wang, F.; Li, M.; Wang, L.; Chen, A.; Zhang, F.; et al. Periostin in chronic liver diseases: Current research and future perspectives. *Life Sci.* **2019**, *226*, 91–97. [CrossRef]

9. Huang, Y.; Liu, W.; Xiao, H.; Maitikabili, A.; Lin, Q.; Wu, T.; Huang, Z.; Liu, F.; Luo, Q.; Ouyang, G. Matricellular protein periostin contributes to hepatic inflammation and fibrosis. *Am. J. Pathol.* **2015**, *185*, 786–797. [CrossRef]

10. Lv, Y.; Wang, W.; Jia, W.D.; Sun, Q.K.; Li, J.S.; Ma, J.L.; Liu, W. Bin; Zhou, H.C.; Ge, Y.S.; Yu, J.H.; et al. High-level expression of periostin is closely related to metastatic potential and poor prognosis of hepatocellular carcinoma. *Med. Oncol.* **2013**, *30*, 385. [CrossRef]

11. Wu, T.; Huang, J.; Wu, S.; Huang, Z.; Chen, X.; Liu, Y.; Cui, D.; Song, G.; Luo, Q.; Liu, F.; et al. Deficiency of periostin impairs liver regeneration in mice after partial hepatectomy. *Matrix Biol.* **2018**, *66*, 81–92. [CrossRef] [PubMed]

12. Graja, A.; Garcia-Carrizo, F.; Jank, A.M.; Gohlke, S.; Ambrosi, T.H.; Jonas, W.; Ussar, S.; Kern, M.; Schürmann, A.; Aleksandrova, K.; et al. Loss of periostin occurs in aging adipose tissue of mice and its genetic ablation impairs adipose tissue lipid metabolism. *Aging Cell* **2018**, *17*, e12810. [CrossRef] [PubMed]

13. Lu, Y.; Liu, X.; Jiao, Y.; Xiong, X.; Wang, E.; Wang, X.; Zhang, Z.; Zhang, H.; Pan, L.; Guan, Y.; et al. Periostin promotes liver steatosis and hypertriglyceridemia through downregulation of PPARα. *J. Clin. Investig.* **2014**, *124*, 3501–3513. [CrossRef] [PubMed]

14. Reddy, J.K.; Rao, M.S. Lipid metabolism and liver inflammation. II. Fatty liver disease and fatty acid oxidation. *Am. J. Physiol. Gastrointest. Liver Physiol.* **2006**, *290*, G852–G858. [CrossRef] [PubMed]

15. Li, Y.; Wu, S.; Xiong, S.; Ouyang, G. Deficiency of periostin protects mice against methionine-choline-deficient diet-induced non-alcoholic steatohepatitis. *J. Hepatol.* **2015**, *62*, 495–497. [CrossRef]

16. Zhu, J.Z.; Zhu, H.T.; Dai, Y.N.; Li, C.X.; Fang, Z.Y.; Zhao, D.J.; Wan, X.Y.; Wang, Y.M.; Wang, F.; Yu, C.H.; et al. Serum periostin is a potential biomarker for non-alcoholic fatty liver disease: A case–control study. *Endocrine* **2016**, *51*, 91–100. [CrossRef]

17. Yang, Z.; Zhang, H.; Niu, Y.; Zhang, W.; Zhu, L.; Li, X.; Lu, S.; Fan, J.; Li, X.; Ning, G.; et al. Circulating periostin in relation to insulin resistance and nonalcoholic fatty liver disease among overweight and obese subjects. *Sci. Rep.* **2016**, *6*, 37886. [CrossRef]

18. Luo, Y.; Qu, H.; Wang, H.; Wei, H.; Wu, J.; Duan, Y.; Liu, D.; Deng, H. Plasma Periostin Levels Are Increased in Chinese Subjects with Obesity and Type 2 Diabetes and Are Positively Correlated with Glucose and Lipid Parameters. *Mediat. Inflamm.* **2016**, *16*, 6423637. [CrossRef]

19. Polyzos, S.A.; Kountouras, J.; Anastasilakis, A.D.; Papatheodorou, A.; Kokkoris, P.; Terpos, E. Circulating periostin in patients with nonalcoholic fatty liver disease. *Endocrine* **2017**, *56*, 438–441. [CrossRef]

20. Polyzos, S.A.; Anastasilakis, A.D. Periostin on the road to nonalcoholic fatty liver disease. *Endocrine* **2016**, *51*, 4–6. [CrossRef]

21. Lee, J. Il Role of periostin in hepatocellular carcinoma: The importance of tumor microenvironment. *Gut Liver* **2016**, *10*, 871–872. [CrossRef] [PubMed]

22. Lv, Y.; Wang, W.; Jia, W.D.; Sun, Q.K.; Huang, M.; Zhou, H.C.; Xia, H.H.; Liu, W.B.; Chen, H.; Sun, S.N.; et al. High preoparative levels of serum periostin are associated with poor prognosis in patients with hepatocellular carcinoma after hepatectomy. *Eur. J. Surg. Oncol.* **2013**, *39*, 1129–1135. [CrossRef] [PubMed]

23. Kanemitsu, Y.; Matsumoto, H.; Izuhara, K.; Tohda, Y.; Kita, H.; Horiguchi, T.; Kuwabara, K.; Tomii, K.; Otsuka, K.; Fujimura, M.; et al. Increased periostin associates with greater airflow limitation in patients receiving inhaled corticosteroids. *J. Allergy Clin. Immunol.* **2013**, *132*, 305–312. [CrossRef] [PubMed]

24. Duran, J.; Olavarría, P.S.; Mola, M.; Götzens, V.; Carballo, J.; Pelegrina, E.M.; Petit, M.; Abdul-Jawad, O.; Otaegui, I.; del Blanco, B.G.; et al. Genetic association study of coronary collateral circulation in patients with coronary artery disease using 22 single nucleotide polymorphisms corresponding to 10 genes involved in postischemic neovascularization. *BMC Cardiovasc. Disord.* **2015**, *15*, 37. [CrossRef] [PubMed]

25. Hixson, J.E.; Shimmin, L.C.; Montasser, M.E.; Kim, D.K.; Zhong, Y.; Ibarguen, H.; Follis, J.; Malcom, G.; Strong, J.; Howard, T.; et al. Common variants in the periostin gene influence development of atherosclerosis in young persons. *Arterioscler. Thromb. Vasc. Biol.* **2011**, *31*, 1661–1667. [CrossRef] [PubMed]

26. U.S. Department of Health and Human Services and U.S. Department of Agriculture. 2015–2020 Dietary Guidelines for Americans. 8th Edition; December 2015. Available online: http://health.gov/dietaryguidelines/2015/guidelines/ (accessed on 28 September 2020).

27. Center for Substance Abuse Treatment (CSAT) and Substance Abuse and Mental Health Services Administration (SAMHSA). *Substance Abuse Among Older Adults*; Treatment Improvement Protocol (TIP) Series, No. 26; Report No.: (SMA) 98-3179; 1998. Available online: https://www.ncbi.nlm.nih.gov/books/NBK64419/ (accessed on 28 September 2020).

28. Dufour, J.F.; Greten, T.F.; Raymond, E.; Roskams, T.; De, T.; Ducreux, M.; Mazzaferro, V.; Governing, E. Clinical Practice Guidelines EASL—EORTC Clinical Practice Guidelines: Management of hepatocellular carcinoma European Organisation for Research and Treatment of Cancer. *J. Hepatol.* **2012**, *56*, 908–943.

29. Llovet, J.M.; Brú, C.; Bruix, J. Prognosis of hepatocellular carcinoma: The BCLC staging classification. *Semin. Liver Dis.* **1999**, *19*, 329–338. [CrossRef]

30. Kleiner, D.E.; Brunt, E.M.; Van Natta, M.; Behling, C.; Contos, M.J.; Cummings, O.W.; Ferrell, L.D.; Liu, Y.C.; Torbenson, M.S.; Unalp-Arida, A.; et al. Design and validation of a histological scoring system for nonalcoholic fatty liver disease. *Hepatology* **2005**, *41*, 1313–1321. [CrossRef]

31. Angulo, P.; Hui, J.M.; Marchesini, G.; Bugianesi, E.; George, J.; Farrell, G.C.; Enders, F.; Saksena, S.; Burt, A.D.; Bida, J.P.; et al. The NAFLD fibrosis score: A noninvasive system that identifies liver fibrosis in patients with NAFLD. *Hepatology* **2007**, *45*, 846–854. [CrossRef]

32. Friedrich-Rust, M.; Poynard, T.; Castera, L. Critical comparison of elastography methods to assess chronic liver disease. *Nat. Rev. Gastroenterol. Hepatol.* **2016**, *13*, 402–411. [CrossRef]

33. Mikolasevic, I.; Orlic, L.; Franjic, N.; Hauser, G.; Stimac, D.; Milic, S. Transient elastography (FibroScan®) with controlled attenuation parameter in the assessment of liver steatosis and fibrosis in patients with nonalcoholic fatty liver disease—Where do we stand? *World J. Gastroenterol.* **2016**, *22*, 7236–7251. [CrossRef] [PubMed]

34. Ishak, K.; Baptista, A.; Bianchi, L.; Callea, F.; De Groote, J.; Gudat, F.; Denk, H.; Desmet, V.; Korb, G.; MacSween, R.N.M.; et al. Histological grading and staging of chronic hepatitis. *J. Hepatol.* **1995**, *22*, 696–699. [CrossRef]

35. Browning, S.R.; Browning, B.L. Rapid and accurate haplotype phasing and missing-data inference for whole-genome association studies by use of localized haplotype clustering. *Am. J. Hum. Genet.* **2007**, *81*, 1084–1097. [CrossRef] [PubMed]

36. Cuzick, J. A wilcoxon-type test for trend. *Stat. Med.* **1985**, *4*, 87–90. [CrossRef] [PubMed]

37. World Health Organization, Regional Office for Europe. Body Mass Index—BMI. Available online: https://www.euro.who.int/en/health-topics/disease-prevention/nutrition/a-healthy-lifestyle/body-mass-index-bmi (accessed on 28 September 2020).

38. Horita, N.; Kaneko, T. Genetic model selection for a case-control study and a meta-analysis. *Meta Gene* **2015**, *5*, 1–8. [CrossRef]

39. Liang, W.; Lindeman, J.H.; Menke, A.L.; Koonen, D.P.; Morrison, M.; Havekes, L.M.; Van Den Hoek, A.M.; Kleemann, R. Metabolically induced liver inflammation leads to NASH and differs from LPS-or IL-1β-induced chronic inflammation. *Lab. Investig.* **2014**, *94*, 491–502. [CrossRef]

40. Sugiyama, A.; Kanno, K.; Nishimichi, N.; Ohta, S.; Ono, J.; Conway, S.J.; Izuhara, K.; Yokosaki, Y.; Tazuma, S. Periostin promotes hepatic fibrosis in mice by modulating hepatic stellate cell activation via αv integrin interaction. *J. Gastroenterol.* **2016**, *51*, 1161–1174. [CrossRef]

41. Chackelevicius, C.M.; Gambaro, S.E.; Tiribelli, C.; Rosso, N. Th17 involvement in nonalcoholic fatty liver disease progression to non-Alcoholic steatohepatitis. *World J. Gastroenterol.* **2016**, *22*, 9096–9103. [CrossRef]

42. Amara, S.; Lopez, K.; Banan, B.; Brown, S.K.; Whalen, M.; Myles, E.; Ivy, M.T.; Johnson, T.; Schey, K.L.; Tiriveedhi, V. Synergistic effect of pro-inflammatory TNFα and IL-17 in periostin mediated collagen deposition: Potential role in liver fibrosis. *Mol. Immunol.* **2015**, *64*, 26–35. [CrossRef]

43. Arteel, G.E.; Naba, A. The liver matrisome—Looking beyond collagens. *JHEP Rep.* **2020**, *2*, 100115. [CrossRef]

44. Kumar, P.; Smith, T.; Raeman, R.; Chopyk, D.M.; Brink, H.; Liu, Y.; Sulchek, T.; Anania, F.A. Periostin promotes liver fibrogenesis by activating lysyl oxidase in hepatic stellate cells. *J. Biol. Chem.* **2018**, *293*, 12781–12792. [CrossRef] [PubMed]

45. Dietrich, P.; Hellerbrand, C. Non-alcoholic fatty liver disease, obesity and the metabolic syndrome. *Best Pract. Res. Clin. Gastroenterol.* **2014**, *28*, 637–653. [CrossRef] [PubMed]

46. Sun, H.J.; Jae, W.S.; Park, J.; Lee, S.Y.; Ohrr, H.; Guallar, E.; Samet, J.M. Body-mass index and mortality in Korean men and women. *N. Engl. J. Med.* **2006**, *355*, 779–787.

47. Haffner, S.M.; Bowsher, R.R.; Mykkänen, L.; Hazuda, H.P.; Mitchell, B.D.; Valdez, R.A.; Gingerich, R.; Monterossa, A.; Stern, M.P. Proinsulin and specific insulin concentration in high-and low-risk populations for NIDDM. *Diabetes* **1994**, *43*, 1490–1493. [CrossRef]

48. Lee, W.Y.; Park, J.S.; Noh, S.Y.; Rhee, E.J.; Kim, S.W.; Zimmet, P.Z. Prevalence of the metabolic syndrome among 40,698 Korean metropolitan subjects. *Diabetes Res. Clin. Pract.* **2004**, *65*, 143–149. [CrossRef]

49. González-González, L.; Alonso, J. Periostin: A matricellular protein with multiple functions in cancer development and progression. *Front. Oncol.* **2018**, *8*, 225. [CrossRef]

50. Zinn, P.O.; Singh, S.K.; Kotrotsou, A.; Hassan, I.; Thomas, G.; Luedi, M.M.; Elakkad, A.; Elshafeey, N.; Idris, T.; Mosley, J.; et al. A coclinical radiogenomic validation study: Conserved magnetic resonance radiomic appearance of periostin-expressing glioblastoma in patients and xenograft models. *Clin. Cancer Res.* **2018**, *24*, 6288–6299. [CrossRef]

51. Keklikoglou, I.; Kadioglu, E.; Bissinger, S.; Langlois, B.; Bellotti, A.; Orend, G.; Ries, C.H.; De Palma, M. Periostin Limits Tumor Response to VEGFA Inhibition. *Cell Rep.* **2018**, *22*, 2530–2540. [CrossRef]

52. Hu, W.; Jin, P.; Liu, W. Periostin contributes to cisplatin resistance in human non-small cell lung cancer A549 cells via activation of Stat3 and Akt and upregulation of survivin. *Cell. Physiol. Biochem.* **2016**, *38*, 1199–1208. [CrossRef]

53. Liu, Y.; Gao, F.; Song, W. Periostin contributes to arsenic trioxide resistance in hepatocellular carcinoma cells under hypoxia. *Biomed. Pharmacother.* **2017**, *88*, 342–348. [CrossRef]

54. Jang, S.Y.; Park, S.Y.; Lee, H.W.; Choi, Y.K.; Park, K.G.; Yoon, G.S.; Tak, W.Y.; Kweon, Y.O.; Hur, K.; Lee, W.K. The combination of periostin overexpression and microvascular invasion is related to a poor prognosis for hepatocellular carcinoma. *Gut Liver* **2016**, *10*, 948–954. [CrossRef] [PubMed]

55. Wang, F.; Song, Y.; Jiang, Y.; Yang, C.; Ding, Z. Associations among periostin gene polymorphisms, clinical parameters and heart failure: A case-control study in 1104 Chinese individuals. *J. Cardiovasc. Med.* **2011**, *12*, 469–474. [CrossRef] [PubMed]

56. NIH/NCBI. dbSNP Short Genetic Variations. rs1028728. ALFA Allele Frequency (New). Available online: https://www.ncbi.nlm.nih.gov/snp/rs1028728#frequency_tab (accessed on 17 November 2020).

57. NIH/NCBI. dbSNP Short Genetic Variations. rs3829365. ALFA Allele Frequency (New). Available online: https://www.ncbi.nlm.nih.gov/snp/rs3829365#frequency_tab (accessed on 17 November 2020).

58. NIH/NCBI. dbSNP Short Genetic Variations. rs9603226. ALFA Allele Frequency (New). Available online: https://www.ncbi.nlm.nih.gov/snp/rs9603226#frequency_tab (accessed on 17 November 2020).

59. Kudo, A. Clinical Applications Targeting Periostin. *Adv. Exp. Med. Biol.* **2019**, *1132*, 207–210. [PubMed]

Usefulness of Different Imaging Modalities in Evaluation of Patients with Non-Alcoholic Fatty Liver Disease

Karolina Grąt [1,*]**, Michał Grąt** [2] **and Olgierd Rowiński** [1]

[1]   Second Department of Clinical Radiology, Medical University of Warsaw, 02-097 Warsaw, Poland;
     olgierd.rowinski@wum.edu.pl
[2]   Department of General, Transplant and Liver Surgery, Medical University of Warsaw, 02-097 Warsaw,
     Poland; michal.grat@gmail.com
*   Correspondence: karolina.grat@gmail.com

Abstract: Non-alcoholic fatty liver disease (NAFLD) and non-alcoholic steatohepatitis (NASH) are becoming some of the major health problems in well-developed countries, together with the increasing prevalence of obesity, metabolic syndrome, and all of their systemic complications. As the future prognoses are even more disturbing and point toward further increase in population affected with NAFLD/NASH, there is an urgent need for widely available and reliable diagnostic methods. Consensus on a non-invasive, accurate diagnostic modality for the use in ongoing clinical trials is also required, particularly considering a current lack of any registered drug for the treatment of NAFLD/NASH. The aim of this narrative review was to present current information on methods used to assess liver steatosis and fibrosis. There are several imaging modalities for the assessment of hepatic steatosis ranging from simple density analysis by computed tomography or conventional B-mode ultrasound to magnetic resonance spectroscopy (MRS), magnetic resonance imaging proton density fat fraction (MRI-PDFF) or controlled attenuation parameter (CAP). Fibrosis stage can be assessed by magnetic resonance elastography (MRE) or different ultrasound-based techniques: transient elastography (TE), shear-wave elastography (SWE) and acoustic radiation force impulse (ARFI). Although all of these methods have been validated against liver biopsy as the reference standard and provided good accuracy, the MRS and MRI-PDFF currently outperform other methods in terms of diagnosis of steatosis, and MRE in terms of evaluation of fibrosis.

Keywords: NASH; NAFLD; liver stiffness; liver steatosis; controlled attenuation parameter; transient elastography; MRI PDFF; MR spectroscopy

1. Introduction

Non-alcoholic fatty liver disease (NAFLD) is a chronic liver condition with globally increasing incidence rates. It is associated with the worldwide increasing prevalence of overweight, obesity, and metabolic syndrome, and is becoming one of the most important health system issues in the developed countries [1,2]. NAFLD, which is defined as an excessive accumulation of fat in hepatocytes, may progress to non-alcoholic steatohepatitis (NASH), and further into fibrosis, with all of its complications—the development of liver cirrhosis, portal hypertension, and hepatocellular carcinoma [3]. It has also been proven that patients with NAFLD have a higher risk for the occurrence of cardiovascular incidents [4–6] and increased risk for developing chronic kidney disease [7]. Remarkably, it is estimated that up to 35% of citizens of the United States of America (USA) are affected by NAFLD, which makes it the most prevalent liver disease in the USA [8]. Accordingly, end-stage liver disease in the course of NASH has already become one of the most common indications for liver transplantation in the USA. Importantly, recent analyses predict a further increase in the prevalence of NASH, with more than 60% of Americans estimated to be affected by the year 2030 [9,10]. Therefore, major effects on the access to liver transplantation, pre-transplant-mortality, wait-list dynamics, and the general outcomes of liver transplant recipients are expected. As grafts with excessive fat accumulation are not suitable for transplantation, increasing prevalence of NASH influences the donor pool. Recently various techniques, such as hypothermic oxygenated machine perfusion, have been proposed to improve the quality of grafts (Figure 1).

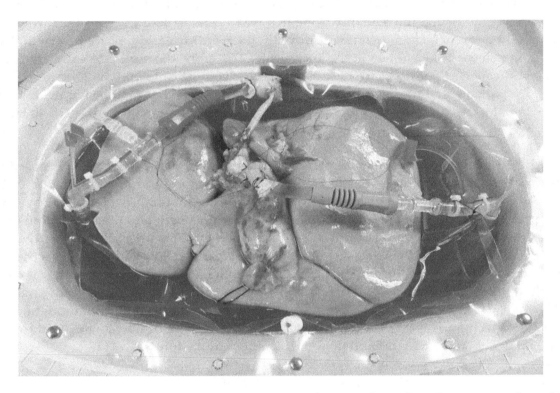

Figure 1. Liver allograft with extensive steatosis undergoing hypothermic oxygenated machine perfusion. Image from the authors' department.

Histopathological evaluation of liver biopsy still remains the gold standard for the diagnosis of NAFLD and NASH. Liver biopsy is also used as the reference standard for the assessment of other methods, despite several disadvantages. Due to the invasive character, it is associated with the risk of potentially severe complications. Further, the costs of frequent liver biopsies are relatively high [11–13]. What is more, some authors suggest that the results might be misleading, as the specimen may not be representative of the whole organ, especially in relatively benign changes. Therefore, alternative non-invasive methods of more representative assessment of liver steatosis have been proposed and validated in the recent years. Ideally, those should be non-invasive, widely available and cost-effective. As there are many ongoing clinical trials on new therapies for patients with NAFLD and NASH, new methods should be particularly characterized by the clinical utility to perform regular follow-up in order to verify treatment results. Moreover, it should also enable precise quantitative evaluation of the current status of liver parenchyma.

This is a narrative review aimed at presenting the current information on various methods used for the assessment of liver steatosis and fibrosis. Further, available data on their prognostic role in patients with NAFLD are discussed. The choice of the articles for this narrative review was made after evaluation by the authors following screening of abstracts in the PUBMED database, using the following search terms: "NASH diagnosis", "NAFLD diagnosis", "liver steatosis", "liver spectroscopy", "PDFF", "proton density fat fraction", "computed tomography liver steatosis", "liver elastography", "controlled attenuation parameter".

2. Techniques Using Computed Tomography

Computed tomography (CT) scans provide valuable information on the extent of liver steatosis, basing on the analyses of the organ density. The most basic techniques, which are simply based either on the measurement of the liver density on non-contrast enhanced scans or comparisons between the density of the liver to the density of the spleen [14], can accurately detect liver steatosis exceeding 20%, but fail to provide sufficient accuracy in patients with hepatic steatosis of lesser extent [15]. In a metanalysis performed by Bohte et al., the overall specificity of CT in the diagnosis of any liver steatosis (with biopsy used as the reference standard) was as low as 46–72%, with the lowest accuracy observed for mild forms of fat accumulation. Currently, there are no algorithms for precise and accurate quantitative assessment of fat content in the liver tissue. Therefore, the use of CT seems rather limited to general stratification of patients and it is not a suitable diagnostic modality in long term follow-up; for example, in patients undergoing treatment for NAFLD/NASH. Even extensive steatosis of more than 50% of hepatocytes can present with a density higher than the standard cut-off of 40 Hounsfield units, as shown on Figure 2.

Nevertheless, several variations of the standard scanning technique have been proposed in order to enhance the diagnostic accuracy of the CT scans. One is the use of a standardized calibration phantom, placed beneath the patients back during the CT examination. In a recent study from 2020, Guo et al. provided evidence that the utilization of this protocol enables the calculation of hepatic steatosis far more accurately, with sensitivity and specificity of 76% and 85%, respectively, for the detection of mild steatosis (involving at least 5% of hepatocytes), and 85% and 98%, respectively, for the detection of moderate steatosis (involving at least 14% of hepatocytes) [16]. The clinical usefulness of this method is especially supported by relatively high positive and negative predictive values of 78% and 83%, respectively, for mild steatosis, and 82% and 97%, respectively, for moderate steatosis. Importantly, this technique needs to be adjusted for particular type of CT scanner, as the basic liver density in Hounsfield units may differ between different manufacturers.

Computed tomography fails to detect early stages of liver fibrosis, and can only show signs of advanced stages, for example nodular shape of the liver, evidence of portal hypertension etc. Nevertheless, some authors have proposed advanced algorithms for the assessment of liver fibrosis on CT scans—for example, analysis of liver texture [17], analysis of the nodularity of the liver surface [18,19] or incorporating data from the CT into an multiparametric tool (data from the CT scans combined with laboratory tests) [20]. All of these have succeeded in providing good accuracy, especially in higher stages of fibrosis. In a study of 556 patients, Lubner et al. created a model based on a combination of four factors indicating liver texture, which provided and area under the receiver operating curve of 0.82, 0.82 and 0.86 for the diagnosis of any ($\geq$F1), significant ($\geq$F2), and severe ($\geq$F3) fibrosis, respectively [17]. While liver surface nodularity analysis provided excellent areas under the curve for the detection of both mild and severe fibrosis, the findings seem limited by almost identical cut-off values of 2.8, 2.77 and 2.9 for significant ($\geq$F2) fibrosis, severe ($\geq$F3) fibrosis and cirrhosis (F4), respectively [19]. Although the corresponding cut-offs were more separated in another study on liver surface nodularity, the overlapping values in patients with different stages of fibrosis remained as a major limitation of its clinical utility [18]. Regarding inclusion of computed tomography features into a multiparametric model, a combination of nine factors assessed on CT with Fibrosis-4 score [21] and aspartate transaminase-to-platelets ratio index [22] was proposed. It resulted in moderate improvement in the diagnostic accuracy with respect to mild (F1), moderate (F2), and severe (F3) fibrosis in a study performed on 469 patients, yet with hepatitis C virus infection [20].

a.

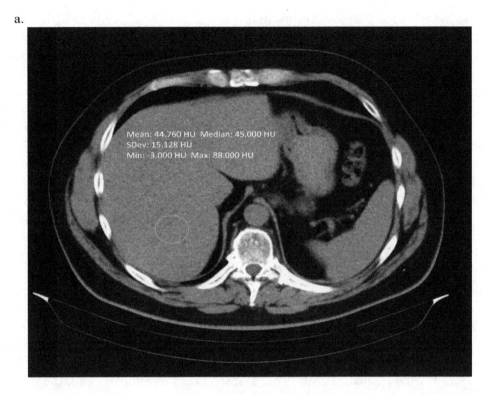

b.

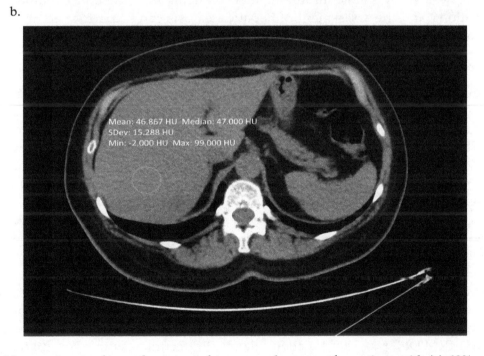

Figure 2. Non-contrast enhanced computed tomography scan of a patient with (**a**) 60% of hepatic steatosis (**b**) 80% of hepatic steatosis. In both cases simple measurement of the liver density was not suggestive on such severe changes. Images from the authors' department.

In addition to evaluation of the status of liver parenchyma, many studies have shown that computed tomography is a good diagnostic modality for the purpose of analyzing patients' body composition, in particular the amount of visceral and subcutaneous fat, and this may be especially important in patients dealing with obesity (which is the case in the vast majority of NASH/NAFLD patients), as the simple Body Mass Index (BMI) has been shown to provide insufficient accuracy [23]. For instance, in a study performed on 76 patients with liver cirrhosis, more than 20% of patients with normal body mass index had an increased amount of adipose tissue, whereas 40% of overweight patients were found to have normal amount of adipose tissue [24]. The amount of fat tissue may be measured on a single CT scan (usually on the level of the body of the third lumbar vertebra), based on the threshold of Hounsfield units, which is a fast and easy technique. There is no consensus on the optimal cut-off points. What is more, some authors define their proposed cut-off values as simple area (not adjusted for the height), which can significantly impair wide use in different populations. Notably, even in homogeneous populations, the cut-off values differ significantly; for example, in different studies on the Korean population, authors proposed values for the visceral fat area ranging from 92.6 cm^2 to 140 cm^2 for men and from 75 to 100 cm^2 for women [25–29]. The measurement can be also propagated on the whole abdominal scans (manually or by using advanced algorithms) [30,31] to calculate the whole visceral fat tissue volume. It is, however, unclear, whether evaluation of the latter provides any benefits over single-scan assessments and this should be elucidated further, yet the arguments for the use of volume over surface analyses include: independence from bowel movement and patients' breathing, individual constitutional characteristics or bowel capacity. Previous studies have shown that excess amounts of fat tissue (both visceral and subcutaneous) play an important role in carcinogenesis, and also in hepatocellular carcinoma (HCC) [24,32]. Therefore, it seems reasonable to routinely evaluate the amount of fat tissue in patients undergoing CT scans, especially in a group of NASH patients, who can progress to liver cirrhosis and develop HCC.

Obviously, one of the biggest disadvantages of CT scans is patient exposure to radiation, which precludes its regular, repeated, and life-long use, for example during regular follow-up for the assessment of NAFLD progression. However, CT scans are much more available than the MR scans and their cost is lower. What is more important, many patients are undergoing computed tomography for other indications, and the assessment of hepatic steatosis can be performed at the same time to provide additional, valuable clinical information.

3. Magnetic Resonance Imaging Techniques

New techniques in magnetic resonance imaging (MRI) have been proven to provide good specificity and sensitivity in detecting liver steatosis and are now the reference standard to which other diagnostic imaging modalities should be compared. The most promising method with excellent results and—very importantly—standard examination technique, not requiring any additional equipment, is the chemical shift-encoded MRI proton density fat fraction (MRI-PDFF). The examination can be performed on both 1.5 T and 3.0 T scanners [33,34], which are widely available at most hospitals. The technique is usually based on acquisition of 6-echo chemical-shift-encoded gradient-echo sequences, but it has been shown that acquisition of less—for example 2 or 4 echo sequences—provides nearly identical results. However, in some cases—for instance in patients with iron deposition in the liver parenchyma—the results may be influenced in case of dual-echo or triple-echo methods, which is not the case with multi-echo [35]. MRI-PDFF method has been validated in comparison to magnetic resonance spectroscopy [34,36–38] and also provides excellent intra-examination repeatability [34] and inter-examination repeatability [39]. Importantly, the results are highly comparable among different fields and scanner manufacturers [40].

A recent meta-analysis by Gu et al., including studies with biopsy as the reference standard, has shown that MRI-PDFF provides excellent diagnostic accuracy, with a sensitivity of 93% for the detection of any grade of steatosis (defines as affecting at least 5% of hepatocytes) and a corresponding specificity of 94% [41]. Further, utilization of MRI-PDFF enables classification into different grades of hepatic steatosis with sensitivity and specificity of 74% and 87–90%, respectively, regarding the diagnosis of higher-grade steatosis. Another study performed by Middleton et al. has shown that MRI-PDFF performs well also in terms of monitoring patients during treatment, in particular in the assessment of discrete changes in liver steatosis in patients with decrease or increase in steatosis grade [42]. Importantly, the MRI-PDFF assessment was highly concordant with liver biopsy assessment regarding changes in liver histology, as 71% of patients with increasing steatosis were diagnosed as such with MRI-PDFF. Further, MRI-PDFF assessment showed an improvement in 91% of patients with decreasing steatosis. Only minor changes in MRI-PDFF assessment were noted in patients with stable histopathological findings. Figure 3 presents an example of two MRI-PDFF examinations in one patient, showing improvement in the degree of hepatic steatosis.

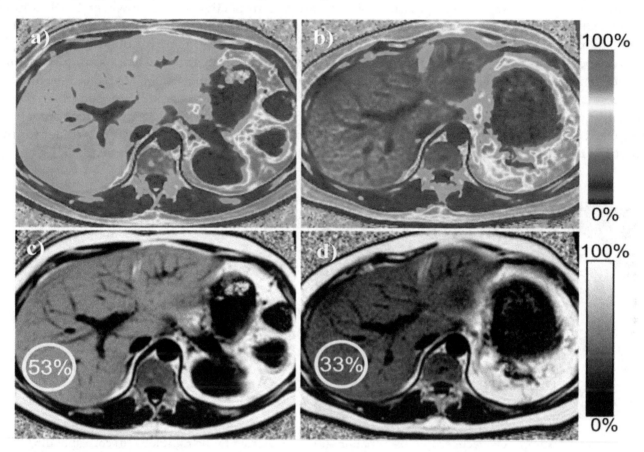

Figure 3. Example of proton density fat fraction liver maps in the same patient before and after treatment. Improvement in the liver steatosis and reduction in liver size is visible. (**a**) pre-treatment color-scale map (**b**) post-treatment color-scale map (**c**) pretreatment gray-scale map (**d**) post-treatment grey-scale map. Figure from Reeder SB, et al. Quantitative Assessment of Liver Fat with Magnetic Resonance Imaging and Spectroscopy. *J. Magn. Reson. Imaging* **2011**, *34*, 729–749 [43].

Although performing very well in terms of analyzing the amount of fat in the liver tissue, MRI-PDFF does not succeed in evaluating other variables that are clinically relevant. A study by Wildman-Tobriner et al. on patients taking part in clinical trials aimed at NAFLD/NASH has shown that the MRI-PDFF values overlap between patients with and without fibrosis, as well as between those with high and low NASH activity scores (NAS ≥ 4). Thus, MRI-PDFF does not seem to allow for discrimination between patients with mild and severe changes in histopathological examination [44]. Importantly, evaluation of steatosis using MRI-PDFF was compromised in case of concomitant fibrosis, with the correlation coefficient for the rate of hepatic steatosis and MRI-PDFF in patients with liver fibrosis of 0.60 as compared to the corresponding R of 0.86 in case of no fibrosis [45]. Therefore, MRI-PDFF should be cautiously interpreted in patients with either imaging or clinical suspicion of liver fibrosis.

Magnetic resonance spectroscopy (MRS) allows us to calculate steatosis by directly measuring chemical composition of tissue in a chosen voxel, basing on the signal strength from each component (protons from water and fat) [46,47]. It is a well-established and accurate method of non-invasive liver fat quantification that has been validated and served as the reference standard in numerous studies [48–54]. A metanalysis performed by Bohte et al. (with histology used as a reference) has shown that the specificity of MRS in terms of detection of mild steatosis is 92% and increases up to

96% for the detection of more advanced fatty accumulation (>25%, >30% or >33%, depending on the study) [15]. These results are in line with a more recent study by Chiang et al., in which the MRS findings were compared to histological examinations in living liver donors with the reported sensitivity and specificity rates of the MR spectroscopy of 95% and 98%, respectively [55]. However, MRS requires sophisticated post-processing methods (spectral analysis), which substantially limits the accessibility to this method, as not every scanner is equipped with this modality. Figure 4 presents an example of liver spectroscopy, with a voxel representing the analyzed region and a corresponding spectrum. Moreover, in contrast to MRI-PDFF, which enables mapping of the whole organ, MRS analyses involve only a small portion of the liver parenchyma. The latter is therefore susceptible for sampling errors, similar to what liver biopsy is criticized for. The MRI-PDFF method is also less dependent on patient compliance. As the acquisition time for MRI-PDFF is shorter than that in the MRS, it is easier for the patient to remain still without breathing and it is also less time consuming in general [36,56].

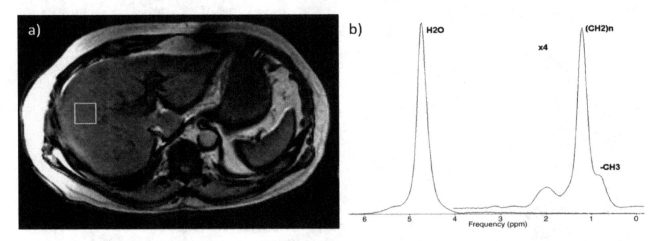

Figure 4. Example of spectroscopic examination: (**a**) voxel located in the right lobe (**b**) corresponding spectrum. Figure from Borra RJ, et al. Nonalcoholic fatty liver disease: rapid evaluation of liver fat content with in-phase and out-of-phase MR imaging. *Radiology* **2009**, *250*, 130–136 [57].

Magnetic resonance elastography (MRE) enables non-invasive assessment of hepatic fibrosis and is currently considered the most accurate non-invasive modality for its assessment, with a very good reproducibility and repeatability [58,59]. In a pooled analysis performed by Singh et al., the mean area under the receiver operating characteristics curve (with 95% confidence interval) values for diagnosing any (≥F1), significant (≥F2) or severe (≥F3) fibrosis and cirrhosis (F4) were 0.86 (0.82–0.90), 0.87 (0.82–0.93), 0.90 (0.84–0.94) and 0.91 (0.76–0.95), respectively [60]. These results were confirmed in another pooled analysis from 2020, by Liang Y. et al., in which the reported corresponding area under the receiver operating characteristics curve values were 0.89, 0.93, 0.93, and 0.95, respectively. The sensitivity rates in that study for of detection mild, significant, and severe liver fibrosis, and liver cirrhosis were 77%, 87%, 89%, and 94%, respectively, with the corresponding specificity rates of 90%, 86%, 84%, and 75%, respectively [61]. MRE also has its major disadvantages, including its high cost and insufficient availability, especially due to the fact that MR scanners are not regularly equipped with the elastography module. Nevertheless, MR elastography provides very good results and corresponds well to the fibrosis stage as assessed by the histopathological examination of liver biopsies. An example of magnetic resonance elastography is presented in Figure 5 [62].

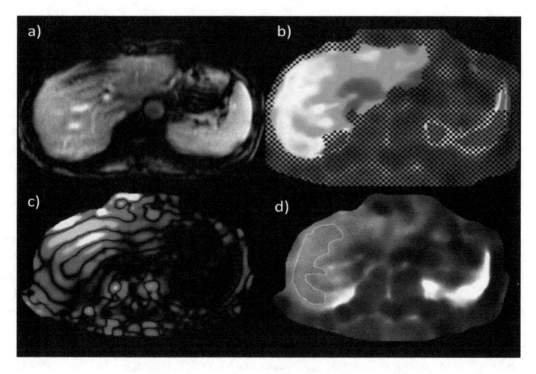

Figure 5. An example of liver stiffness measurement by magnetic resonance elastography (**a**) anatomic images (**b**) confidence map of an elastogram (**c**) wave image data (**d**) elastogram with free drawn region of interest. Figure from Chang, W., et al., Liver Fibrosis Staging with MR Elastography: Comparison of Diagnostic Performance between Patients with Chronic Hepatitis B and Those with Other Etiologic Causes. *Radiology* **2016**, *280*, 88–97 [62].

The stiffness of healthy liver parenchyma in MRE is reported to be between 2.05 to 2.12 kPa [59], and the cut-off for normal liver stiffness is proposed to be set at 2.5 kPa [63]. However, the proposed cut-off values for discriminating between particular stages of fibrosis slightly differ among various studies and authors, with some authors also suggesting that the actual cut-off values may also be dependent upon the type of underlying liver disease. Chang et al., in their study on patients with chronic liver disease and healthy living liver donors, have shown that the MR elastography findings corresponded well with the stage of fibrosis with the areas under the receiver operating characteristics curve values ranging between 0.92 and 0.97. However, the actual liver stiffness value pointing towards the presence of cirrhosis remarkably differed between patients with hepatitis B virus infection (3.67 kPa) and those with other liver diseases (4.65 kPa) [62].

Liver stiffness can also be assessed by magnetic resonance with the use of diffusion weighted imaging (DWI); however, the results are inferior to MR elastography [64–66]. A meta-analysis by Wang et al. has shown that the sensitivity of MRE is 94% in detection of significant (≥F2) and 96% in detection of severe fibrosis (≥F2), remarkably higher than the corresponding values observed for DWI of 77% and 84%, respectively [66]. Some authors try to combine the DWI MR method with serum markers to increase the diagnostic accuracy, and the results show that this may be a reasonable alternative in cases where standard MRE is not available [67]. The authors of that study combined the DWI MR with the aspartate aminotransferase–to–platelet radio index (APRI) [22] and the Fibrosis-4 score, known as the FIB-4 [21]. This increased the diagnostic performance for discrimination between fibrosis grades 0–1 and 2–4: the area under the curve for DWI only was 0.72 and increased to 0.81 and 0.78 after addition of APRI and FIB-4, respectively. The performance to discriminate severe fibrosis (grades 0–2 versus 3–4) also increased −0.79 for DWI only, 0.83 for DWI + APRI, and 0.81 for DWI + FIB-4.

Standard abdominal MR examinations also allows the calculation of the amount of visceral and subcutaneous adipose tissue; however, due to the fact that the scanned area is usually limited to the liver and does not cover the whole abdominal cavity, it might be impossible to calculate all of the volumes (for example whole volume of visceral fat tissue).

4. Ultrasound Based Techniques

Liver steatosis can be detected on a regular B mode ultrasound; however, the diagnostic accuracy is low. Signs of liver steatosis on ultrasound typically comprise hyperechoic, bright liver (the echogenicity of the liver is usually compared to the echogenicity of the kidney), posterior attenuation or impaired visualization of intrahepatic vessels.

Studies have shown that the diagnosis of moderate or severe grades of liver steatosis by ultrasound is characterized by sensitivity and specificity rates of 80–91% and 87–98%, respectively. Nevertheless, these values drop to as low as 53% and 77%, respectively, when detecting steatosis of any grade [68–72].

Controlled attenuation parameter (CAP) is a relatively new method introduced by the Fibro-Scan. It measures liver attenuation to assess the degree of liver steatosis. The results are presented as dB/m (ranging from 100–400) and according to the manufacturers' recommendation reflect the degree of steatosis [73,74]. This method has emerged relatively recently, with the first clinical studies published in 2010 [75], but has gained widespread acceptance and has been validated in numerous studies. Particularly good diagnostic accuracy of CAP was reported in a multicenter prospective study performed on the Chinese population (CAP measurements were compared with biopsy as a reference standard), with areas under the receiver operating characteristics curve of 0.92, 0.92 and 0.88 for detection of steatosis of at least 5%, 34%, and 67%, respectively [76]. These results are in line with another prospective study performed on Korean population, which reported the corresponding values for CAP of 0.885 for the detection of mild steatosis (sensitivity 73.1%, specificity 95.2%), 0.894 for detection of moderate steatosis (sensitivity 82.4%, specificity 86.1%) and 0.800 for detection of severe steatosis (sensitivity 77.8%, specificity 84.1%) [77]. The clinical utility of using CAP as a reference for the assessment of liver steatosis is largely limited by the low positive predictive value. In a study by Ferraioloi et al., the positive predictive values for the detection of mild or moderate steatosis using CAP cut-offs of 219 dB/M and 296 dB/M, respectively, were both below 60% despite relatively large areas under the receiver operating characteristics curve of 0.76 and 0.82, respectively [78]. A meta-analysis performed by Shi KQ et al. has consistently shown that CAP has good sensitivity and specificity, however the authors of the study concluded, that it should not be widely used as a standard method of steatosis assessment due to insufficient accuracy [79]. The positive and negative predictive vales of CAP ranged between 78–80% and 78–84%, depending on the stage of steatosis aimed for detection. Another meta-analysis by Karloas et al. has shown a good accuracy for the diagnosis of any or moderate steatosis with area under the receiver operating characteristics curve for >S0 and >S1 of 0.823 and 0.865, respectively [80]. A metanalysis by Pu et al. from 2019 also provided confirmation of acceptable sensitivity and specificity of CAP in detection of moderate and severe steatosis, yet pointed towards several factors, including age and body mass index, as potentially influencing its accuracy [81].

CAP has been shown to provide inferior diagnostic accuracy in comparison to MRI-PDFF in a study comparing these two methods with a biopsy reference: area under the receiver operating characteristics curve for MRI-PDFF in detection of any steatosis was 0.99 as compared to significantly lower value of 0.85 observed for CAP [82]. These results were also confirmed by another prospective study, which showed even lower value for CAP (0.77 versus 0.99 for MRI-PDFF) [83].

One of the biggest limitations of the use of CAP measurement was the M probe depth, which was not sufficient for obese patients. The manufacturer responded to that problem by introducing the XL probe, allowing for measurement in more overweight patients. The accuracy of measurements with the M and XL probe seem similar [84–86]. Although being an easy and relatively cheap method, CAP has also serious limitations when assessing patients with ascites and obesity, which substantially limits it use in the NAFLD/NASH patients, as vast majority of them is overweight.

Fibroscan device also allows the measurement of the liver stiffness by using the transient elastography technique (TE). There are some reports suggesting that although TE provides very good results, the accuracy in patients with NAFLD/NASH might be decreased. This is because the liver stiffness measurement can be affected by CAP values, particularly with respect to overestimation of the degree of liver fibrosis in the steatotic liver. Therefore, some authors have proposed different cut-off values for NAFLD patients when diagnosing fibrosis in TE [73,87]. In particular, high risk of false positive TE results with respect to detection of significant (F2–F4) and severe (F3–F4) liver fibrosis was noted for the liver stiffness ranges of 8.5–10.5 kPa and 10.1–12.5 kPa, respectively, in case of CAP of 300 to 339 dB/M, and 8.5–11.6 kPa and 10.1–13.6 kPa, respectively, in case of CAP exceeding 340 dB/M [73]. As both liver stiffness measurement by TE and steatosis measurement by CAP are available in the Fibroscan, the adjustment of the cut-off values can be done quickly and easily. However, the results of other studies are conflicting. In a recent study by Eddowes et al. performed on 450 patients with biopsy as reference, the accurate assessment of liver fibrosis and steatosis was reported with no negative influence of steatosis on the measurement of liver stiffness [88]. Although being a cheap, widely available, and easily performed technique, TE has inferior accuracy when comparing to magnetic resonance elastography. The area under the receiver operating characteristics curve for detection of any fibrosis (≥F1) using MRE was 0.82, which was significantly higher than that calculated for TE (0.67) [82]. Figure 6 presents an example of steatosis and fibrosis assessment (Fibroscan) with controlled attenuation parameters and transient elastography.

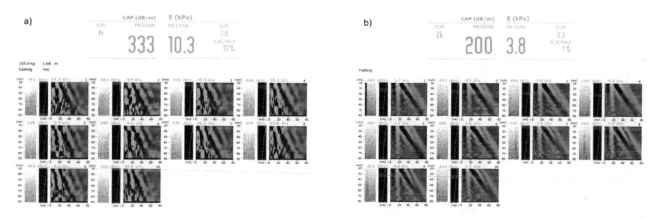

Figure 6. Examples of steatosis assessment by controlled attenuation parameter and liver stiffness assessment by transient elastography (Fibroscan) (**a**) in a patient with severe liver steatosis (grade 3) and severe fibrosis (F3) (**b**) in a patient with no liver steatosis (grade 0) and no liver fibrosis (F0). Images courtesy of Dr. Maciej Janik and Prof. Piotr Milkiewicz from the Liver and Internal Medicine Unit, Medical University of Warsaw.

Another two methods of fibrosis assessment include the shear wave elastography (SWE) and acoustic radiation force impulse (ARFI), both of which can be integrated in regular ultrasound devices. SWE and ARFI have some notable disadvantages, such as the necessity to perform the measurement with patient holding breath. The results may also be influenced by the experience of the performing physician and in case of a recent food intake [89]. All the three methods provide results which are highly correlated with the fibrosis grade and have relatively good accuracy in detecting fibrosis. In a study comparing SWE, TE and ARFI performed by Casinotto et al., all three methods showed very similar diagnostic characteristics for the detection of corresponding grades of liver fibrosis [90]. Similar results were obtained by Lee et al., who also reported the similar ability of TE, SWE and ARFI in the diagnosis of liver fibrosis in a population of Asian NAFLD patients [91]. However, in another study, SWE was shown to provide superior results to TE in the accuracy of detecting any fibrosis, as well as discriminating between different fibrosis grades with areas under the receiver operating characteristics curve for SWE and TE for different fibrosis grades as follows: 0.86 and 0.80, respectively, for any fibrosis (≥F1); 0.88 and 0.78, respectively, for significant (≥F2) fibrosis; 0.93 and 0.83, respectively, for severe (≥F3) fibrosis; and 0.98 and 0.92, respectively, for cirrhosis (F4) [92]. Another study also showed superiority of SWE over TE and ARFI in diagnosing grade F2 or F3 of fibrosis, but without statistical difference regarding diagnosing mild fibrosis (F1) or cirrhosis (F4) [93]. Figure 7 presents an example of liver stiffness measurement by shear-wave elastography.

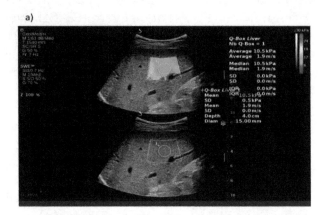
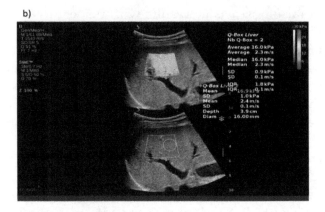

Figure 7. Examples of fibrosis assessment by shear wave elastography (**a**) in a patient with severe liver fibrosis (F3) (**b**) in a patient with cirrhosis (F4). Images courtesy of Dr. Maciej Janik and Prof. Piotr Milkiewicz from the Liver and Internal Medicine Unit, Medical University of Warsaw.

5. Dual-Energy X-ray Absorptiometry

Dual energy X-ray absorptiometry is a quick, relatively inexpensive and safe method of body composition assessment. Due to its clinical usefulness, it has gained wide acceptance and has been proposed in guidelines for the assessment of sarcopenia and obesity in the elderly population (European Working Group on Sarcopenia in Older People Consensus) [94,95]. Interestingly, some authors have proposed the implementation of special algorithms into the DXA examination to assess the liver fat amount. Bazzocchi et al. proposed placing a region of interest (ROI) in the location of the liver to calculate the amount of hepatic fat and have shown good correlation with liver steatosis assessed by biopsy ($\varrho = 0.610$–0.619; $p < 0.001$), with an area under the curve ranging from 0.929 to 0.551 (depending upon sex and BMI category) [96].

6. Predictive Role of Imaging Methods in Patients with NAFLD

Patients with NAFLD are at high risk of developing systemic complications of the disease. This includes, in particular, the development of cardiovascular diseases and occurrence of cardiovascular events in case of underlying pathologies. In a 2014 study based on more than two thousand middle-aged adults without any known liver or heart disease, liver attenuation on computed tomography of less than 40 Hounsfield units, indicative of hepatic steatosis, was associated with approximately 30% more frequent occurrence of coronary artery calcifications and approximately 70% more frequent occurrence of abdominal aortic calcifications [97]. However, this significant association disappeared following adjustment for the amount of visceral fat, pointing towards the pivotal role of the latter as a major contributor to the development of atherosclerosis. Attenuation of the liver under 40 Hounsfield units on computed tomography scans was also found to be associated with subclinical cardiac remodeling and dysfunction in another population-based study, yet this was also largely attributable to increased amount of visceral adipose tissue [98]. These findings were recently supported by the results of the CARDIA study, in which the association between attenuation of the liver under 40 Hounsfield units and several structural and functional heart features lost significance following adjustment for obesity [99]. The same parameter predicted the presence of coronary microvascular dysfunction, which was an independent prognostic factor for the occurrence of a composite cardiovascular event end-point [100]. Notably, hepatic steatosis and fibrosis assessed on TE and CAP were similarly related to the presence of diastolic myocardial dysfunction in a study by Lee et al. [101]. Increased liver stiffness, as indicated by the results of SWE, increased the ability to predict the presence of coronary heart disease [102].

An analysis performed on 50 overweight adolescents revealed that intrahepatic fat content assessed on magnetic resonance spectroscopy was significantly associated with dyslipidemia independently of visceral fat content, as indicated by its positive correlation with plasma triglycerides, triglyceride to high-density lipoprotein ratio, or small dense low-density lipoprotein concentration, among others [103]. Further, the results of large cross-sectional Kangbuk Samsung Health Study comprising more than 100 thousand individuals pointed towards hepatic steatosis assessed on ultrasound as a significant predictor of the presence of coronary artery calcifications [104]. Increased prevalence of coronary artery calcifications in patients with ultrasound evidence for hepatic steatosis was independent of the presence of obesity.

Multiparametric evaluation of MR enabled prediction of the occurrence of liver-related clinical events in a study of 112 patients performed by Pavlides et al. [105]. More specifically, the use of liver inflammation and fibrosis score derived from analysis of T1 and T2 sequences led to the categorization of patients into subgroups based on the risk of developing clinical complications, with score values under 2 being characterized by a 100% negative predictive value. Additional MR analysis of hepatic iron and fat content further increased the predictive capacity of the model. In more than a thousand patients with severe liver fibrosis in the course of NAFLD, the baseline liver stiffness value was strongly associated with the occurrence of both decompensation of liver function and hepatocellular carcinoma, along with liver-related mortality [106]. Subgroup analysis from the same study performed by Petta et al. additionally provided evidence for the prognostic significance of the changes in liver stiffness measurement on TE by at least 20% with respect to those clinical outcomes and, furthermore, overall patient survival. Similarly, MRE-assessed liver stiffness exceeding 6.48 kPa was found to be predictive for the occurrence of liver function decompensation, with higher liver stiffness values also observed in patients with ascites, encephalopathy, and esophageal variceal bleeding [107].

7. Conclusions

Although there are several noninvasive, accurate methods of the assessment of hepatic steatosis or fibrosis, liver biopsy is currently the only method that allows for the precise assessment of both, and moreover also the assessment of the inflammatory process. However, given that the prevalence of obesity, metabolic syndrome and NAFLD is and will be increasing in the upcoming years, alternative, widely accessible and noninvasive methods need to be introduced. Brief summary on the use of imaging techniques on detection of liver steatosis and fibrosis is shown on Figures 8 and 9, respectively. Computed tomography only enables the diagnosis of higher grades of hepatic steatosis; however, new algorithms have been proposed to improve the diagnostic ability. Magnetic resonance spectroscopy provides highly reliable results, but its use is limited due to sophisticated postprocessing.

Proton density fat fraction MRI and the controlled attenuation parameter are the most promising techniques—MRI-PDFF with its ability to reliable quantify the fat percentage and the CAP, with low-cost machines, that can easily be used in outpatient clinics for initial screening purposes. Together with noninvasive methods of liver stiffness measurement, especially the magnetic resonance elastography or TE and SWE, those methods might be of crucial significance in distinguishing patients with moderate or severe changes for further assessment with liver biopsy. Computed tomography, magnetic resonance and transient elastography should be interpreted with respect to predicting patients' clinical outcomes. Tables 1 and 2 present a summary of diagnostic parameters of different methods for steatosis and fibrosis assessment.

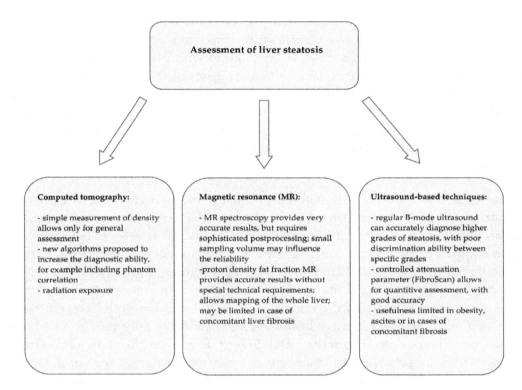

Figure 8. Summary of the imaging techniques for the assessment of liver steatosis.

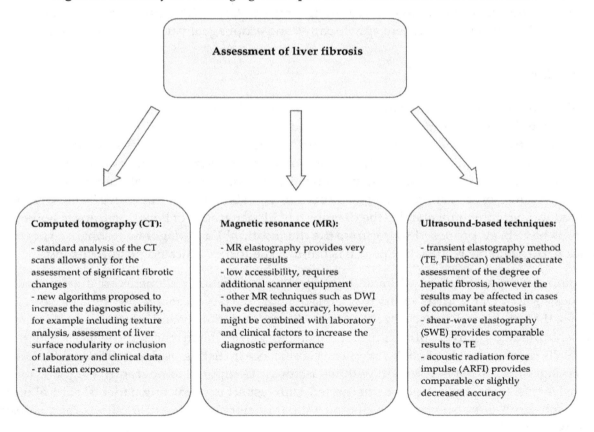

Figure 9. Summary of the imaging techniques for the assessment of liver fibrosis.

Table 1. Summary of the diagnostic parameters of different methods of steatosis assessment.

	Proposed Cut-Off	Sensitivity %	Specificity %
Computed tomography			
simple density measurement			
any steatosis (grade 1–3)	n/a	22–712 [14,15]	86–98 [14,15]
moderate steatosis (grade 2–3)	40 HU	60–82 [14,15]	88–98 [14,15]
phantom calibration [16]			
any steatosis (grade 1–3)	n/a	76% [16]	85% [16]
moderate steatosis (grade 2–3)	n/a	85% [16]	98% [16]
Magnetic resonance			
spectroscopy			
any steatosis (grade 1–3)	n/a	77–95 [15,53,55,56]	81–98 [15,53,55,56]
moderate steatosis (grade 2–3)	n/a	41–91 [15,53,56]	85–99 [15,53,56]
proton density fat fraction			
any steatosis (grade 1–3)	n/a	86–97 [35,36,41–45]	82–100 [35,36,41–45]
moderate steatosis (grade 2–3)	n/a	61–84 [35,36,41–45]	83–96 [35,36,41–45]
Ultrasound based techniques			
simple visual assessment			
any steatosis (grade 1–3)	subjective assessment	53–82 [15,68–72]	76–90 [15,68–72]
moderate steatosis (grade 2–3)		78–91 [15,68–72]	77–98 [15,68–72]
controlled attenuation parameter			
any steatosis	214–289 dB/m [76–80]	66–92 [76–81]	52–96 [76–81]
moderate steatosis	233–311 dB/m [76–80]	60–93 [76–81]	70–92 [76–81]

n/a—Not applicable; HU—Hounsfield Units.

Table 2. Summary of the diagnostic parameters of different methods of fibrosis assessment.

	Proposed Cut-Off	Sensitivity %	Specificity %
Computed tomography			
experimental algorithms			
any fibrosis (≥F1)	n/a	65–78 [18,19]	88–100 [18,19]
significant fibrosis (≥F2)	n/a	68–80 [18,19]	80–97 [18,19]
severe fibrosis (≥F3)	n/a	83–89 [18,19]	84–85 [18,19]
cirrhosis (F4)	n/a	90–98 [18,19]	80–85 [18,19]
Magnetic resonance			
elastography			
any fibrosis (≥F1)	1.77–5.02 kPa [60–62]	75–81 [60–62]	77–100 [60–62]
significant fibrosis (≥F2)	2.38–5.37 kPa [60–62,64]	79–97 [60–62,64]	81–100 [60–62,64]
severe fibrosis (≥F3)	2.43–5.97 kPa [60–62,64]	83–100 [60–62,64]	84–95 [60–62,64]
cirrhosis (F4)	2.74–6.7 kPa [60–62,64]	88–100 [60–62,64]	75–95 [60–62,64]
diffusion weighted imaging			
any fibrosis (≥F1)	n/a	75–86 [64–66]	71–94 [64–66]
significant fibrosis (≥F2)	n/a	67–92 [64–66]	61–91 [64–66]
severe fibrosis (≥F3)	n/a	48–90 [64–66]	65–100 [64–66]
cirrhosis (F4)	n/a	75–100 [64–66]	60–72 [64–66]
Ultrasound based techniques			
acoustic radiation force impulse			
any fibrosis (≥F1)	1.35 m/s [93]	61 [93]	96 [93]
significant fibrosis (≥F2)	0.95–1.38 m/s [90,91,93]	46–90 [90,91,93]	36–91 [90,91,93]
severe fibrosis (≥F3)	1.15–1.53 m/s [90,91,93]	59–90 [90,91,93]	63–90 [90,91,93]
cirrhosis (F4)	1.3–2.04 m/s [90,91,93]	44–90 [90,91,93]	67–90 [90,91,93]
transient elastography			
any fibrosis (≥F1)	6.7–8 kPa [92,93]	65–83 [92,93]	83–91 [92,93]
significant fibrosis (≥F2)	6.2–9.8 kPa [90–93]	60–90 [90–93]	45–92 [90–93]
severe fibrosis (≥F3)	8–12.5 kPa [90–93]	57–90 [90–93]	61–92 [90–93]
cirrhosis (F4)	9.5–16.1 kPa [90–93]	65–92 [90–93]	62–92 [90–93]
shear wave elastography			
any fibrosis (≥F1)	6.5–7.8 kPa [92,93]	68–84 [92,93]	91–100 [92,93]
significant fibrosis (≥F2)	6.3–8.7 kPa [90–93]	71–90 [90–93]	50–92 [90–93]
severe fibrosis (≥F3)	8.3–10.7 kPa [90–93]	71–91 [90–93]	71–90 [90–93]
cirrhosis (F4)	10.1–15.1 kPa [90–93]	58–97 [90–93]	72–93 [90–93]

n/a—Not applicable.

Author Contributions: All authors have read and agreed to the published version of the manuscript.

Acknowledgments: The authors would like to express their gratitude for Maciej Janik and Piotr Milkiewicz from the Liver and Internal Medicine Unit, Medical University of Warsaw, for providing pictures presented in Figures 6 and 7. Michał Grąt received a stipend for outstanding young scientists from the Ministry of Science and Higher Education of the Republic of Poland (571/STYP/14/2019).

Abbreviations

NAFLD	non-alcoholic fatty liver disease
NASH	non-alcoholic steatohepatitis
MRS	magnetic resonance spectroscopy
MRI-PDFF	magnetic resonance imaging proton density fat fraction
CAP	controlled attenuation parameter
MRE	magnetic resonance imaging
TE	transient elastography
SWE	shear wave elastography
ARFI	acoustic radiation force impulse
CT	computed tomography
BMI	body mass index
HCC	hepatocellular carcinoma
NAS	NASH activity score
DWI	diffusion weighted imaging
APRI	aminotransferase-to-platelet ratio index
FIB-4	Fibrosis-4 score

References

1. Chalasani, N.; Younossi, Z.; Lavine, J.E.; Diehl, A.M.; Brunt, E.M.; Cusi, K.; Charlton, M.; Sanyal, A.J. The diagnosis and management of non-alcoholic fatty liver disease: Practice Guideline by the American Association for the Study of Liver Diseases, American College of Gastroenterology, and the American Gastroenterological Association. *Hepatology* **2012**, *55*, 2005–2023. [CrossRef] [PubMed]

2. Vernon, G.; Baranova, A.; Younossi, Z.M. Systematic review: The epidemiology and natural history of non-alcoholic fatty liver disease and non-alcoholic steatohepatitis in adults. *Aliment. Pharmacol. Ther.* **2011**, *34*, 274–285. [CrossRef] [PubMed]

3. Oda, K.; Uto, H.; Mawatari, S.; Ido, A. Clinical features of hepatocellular carcinoma associated with nonalcoholic fatty liver disease: A review of human studies. *Clin. J. Gastroenterol.* **2015**, *8*, 1–9. [CrossRef] [PubMed]

4. Arulanandan, A.; Ang, B.; Bettencourt, R.; Hooker, J.; Behling, C.; Lin, G.Y.; Valasek, M.A.; Ix, J.H.; Schnabl, B.; Sirlin, C.B.; et al. Association between quantity of liver fat and cardiovascular risk in patients with nonalcoholic fatty liver disease independent of nonalcoholic steatohepatitis. *Clin. Gastroenterol. Hepatol.* **2015**, *13*, 1513–1520.e1. [CrossRef]

5. Jennings, J.; Faselis, C.; Yao, M.D. NAFLD-NASH: An under-recognized epidemic. *Curr. Vasc. Pharmacol.* **2018**, *16*, 209–213. [CrossRef]

6. Motamed, N.; Rabiee, B.; Poustchi, H.; Dehestani, B.; Hemasi, G.R.; Khonsari, M.R.; Maadi, M.; Saeedian, F.S.; Zamani, F. Non-alcoholic fatty liver disease (NAFLD) and 10-year risk of cardiovascular diseases. *Clin. Res. Hepatol. Gastroenterol.* **2017**, *41*, 31–38. [CrossRef]

7. Athyros, V.G.; Tziomalos, K.; Katsiki, N.; Doumas, M.; Karagiannis, A.; Mikhailidis, D.P. Cardiovascular risk across the histological spectrum and the clinical manifestations of non-alcoholic fatty liver disease: An update. *World J. Gastroenterol.* **2015**, *21*, 6820–6834. [CrossRef]

8. Younossi, Z.M.; Koenig, A.B.; Abdelatif, D.; Fazel, Y.; Henry, L.; Wymer, M. Global epidemiology of nonalcoholic fatty liver disease-Meta-analytic assessment of prevalence, incidence, and outcomes. *Hepatology* **2016**, *64*, 73–84. [CrossRef]

9.   Estes, C.; Razavi, H.; Loomba, R.; Younossi, Z.; Sanyal, A.J. Modeling the epidemic of nonalcoholic fatty liver disease demonstrates an exponential increase in burden of disease. *Hepatology* **2018**, *67*, 123–133. [CrossRef]

10.   Agopian, V.G.; Kaldas, F.M.; Hong, J.C.; Whittaker, M.; Holt, C.; Rana, A.; Zarrinpar, A.; Petrowsky, H.; Farmer, D.; Yersiz, H.; et al. Liver transplantation for nonalcoholic steatohepatitis: The new epidemic. *Ann. Surg.* **2012**, *256*, 624–633. [CrossRef]

11.   Spengler, E.K.; Loomba, R. Recommendations for diagnosis, referral for liver biopsy, and treatment of nonalcoholic fatty liver disease and nonalcoholic steatohepatitis. *Mayo Clin. Proc.* **2015**, *90*, 1233–1246. [CrossRef] [PubMed]

12.   Leoni, S.; Tovoli, F.; Napoli, L.; Serio, I.; Ferri, S.; Bolondi, L. Current guidelines for the management of non-alcoholic fatty liver disease: A systematic review with comparative analysis. *World J. Gastroenterol.* **2018**, *24*, 3361–3373. [CrossRef] [PubMed]

13.   Chalasani, N.; Younossi, Z.; Lavine, J.E.; Charlton, M.; Cusi, K.; Rinella, M.; Harrison, S.A.; Brunt, E.M.; Sanyal, A.J. The diagnosis and management of nonalcoholic fatty liver disease: Practice guidance from the American Association for the Study of Liver Diseases. *Hepatology* **2018**, *67*, 328–357. [CrossRef] [PubMed]

14.   Piekarski, J.; Goldberg, H.I.; Royal, S.A.; Axel, L.; Moss, A.A. Difference between liver and spleen CT numbers in the normal adult: Its usefulness in predicting the presence of diffuse liver disease. *Radiology* **1980**, *137*, 727–729. [CrossRef] [PubMed]

15.   Bohte, A.E.; van Werven, J.R.; Bipat, S.; Stoker, J. The diagnostic accuracy of US, CT, MRI and 1H-MRS for the evaluation of hepatic steatosis compared with liver biopsy: A meta-analysis. *Eur. Radiol.* **2011**, *21*, 87–97. [CrossRef] [PubMed]

16.   Guo, Z.; Blake, G.M.; Li, K.; Liang, W.; Zhang, W.; Zhang, Y.; Xu, L.; Wang, L.; Brown, J.K.; Cheng, X.; et al. Liver fat content measurement with quantitative CT validated against MRI Proton density fat fraction: A prospective study of 400 healthy volunteers. *Radiology* **2020**, *294*, 89–97. [CrossRef] [PubMed]

17.   Lubner, M.G.; Jones, D.; Kloke, J.; Said, A.; Pickhardt, P.J. CT texture analysis of the liver for assessing hepatic fibrosis in patients with hepatitis C virus. *Br. J. Radiol.* **2019**, *92*, 20180153. [CrossRef]

18.   Pickhardt, P.J.; Malecki, K.; Kloke, J.; Lubner, M.G. Accuracy of liver surface nodularity quantification on MDCT as a noninvasive biomarker for staging hepatic fibrosis. *AJR Am. J. Roentgenol.* **2016**, *207*, 1194–1199. [CrossRef]

19.   Lubner, M.G.; Jones, D.; Said, A.; Kloke, J.; Lee, S.; Pickhardt, P.J. Accuracy of liver surface nodularity quantification on MDCT for staging hepatic fibrosis in patients with hepatitis C virus. *Abdom. Radiol. (N. Y.)* **2018**, *43*, 2980–2986. [CrossRef]

20.   Pickhardt, P.J.; Graffy, P.M.; Said, A.; Jones, D.; Welsh, B.; Zea, R.; Lubner, M.G. Multiparametric CT for noninvasive staging of hepatitis C virus-related liver fibrosis: Correlation with the histopathologic fibrosis score. *AJR Am. J. Roentgenol.* **2019**, *212*, 547–553. [CrossRef]

21.   Sterling, R.K.; Lissen, E.; Clumeck, N.; Sola, R.; Correa, M.C.; Montaner, J.; Mark, S.S.; Torriani, F.J.; Dieterich, D.T.; Thomas, D.L.; et al. Development of a simple noninvasive index to predict significant fibrosis in patients with HIV/HCV coinfection. *Hepatology* **2006**, *43*, 1317–1325. [CrossRef] [PubMed]

22.   Wai, C.T.; Greenson, J.K.; Fontana, R.J.; Kalbfleisch, J.D.; Marrero, J.A.; Conjeevaram, H.S.; Lok, A.S. A simple noninvasive index can predict both significant fibrosis and cirrhosis in patients with chronic hepatitis C. *Hepatology* **2003**, *38*, 518–526. [CrossRef] [PubMed]

23.   Strulov Shachar, S.; Williams, G.R. The obesity paradox in cancer-moving beyond BMI. *Cancer Epidemiol. Biomark. Prev.* **2017**, *26*, 13–16. [CrossRef] [PubMed]

24.   Grąt, K.; Pacho, R.; Grąt, M.; Krawczyk, M.; Zieniewicz, K.; Rowiński, O. Impact of body composition on the risk of hepatocellular carcinoma recurrence after liver transplantation. *J. Clin. Med.* **2019**, *8*, 1672. [CrossRef]

25.   Kim, H.I.; Kim, J.T.; Yu, S.H.; Kwak, S.H.; Jang, H.C.; Park, K.S.; Kim, S.Y.; Lee, H.K.; Cho, Y.M. Gender differences in diagnostic values of visceral fat area and waist circumference for predicting metabolic syndrome in Koreans. *J. Korean Med. Sci.* **2011**, *26*, 906–913. [CrossRef]

26.   Lim, S.; Kim, J.H.; Yoon, J.W.; Kang, S.M.; Choi, S.H.; Park, Y.J.; Kim, K.W.; Cho, N.H.; Shin, H.; Park, K.S.; et al. Optimal cut points of waist circumference (WC) and visceral fat area (VFA) predicting for metabolic syndrome (MetS) in elderly population in the Korean Longitudinal Study on Health and Aging (KLoSHA). *Arch. Gerontol. Geriatr.* **2012**, *54*, e29–e34. [CrossRef]

27. Hyun, Y.J.; Kim, O.Y.; Jang, Y.; Ha, J.W.; Chae, J.S.; Kim, J.Y.; Yeo, H.Y.; Paik, J.K.; Lee, J.H. Evaluation of metabolic syndrome risk in Korean premenopausal women: Not waist circumference but visceral fat. *Circ. J.* **2008**, *72*, 1308–1315. [CrossRef]

28. Zhou, C.J.; Cheng, Y.F.; Xie, L.Z.; Hu, W.L.; Chen, B.; Xu, L.; Huang, C.J.; Cai, M.; Shen, X.; Liu, C.B. Metabolic syndrome, as defined based on parameters including visceral fat area, predicts complications After surgery for rectal cancer. *Obes. Surg.* **2020**, *30*, 319–326. [CrossRef]

29. Seo, J.A.; Kim, B.G.; Cho, H.; Kim, H.S.; Park, J.; Baik, S.H.; Choi, D.S.; Park, M.H.; Jo, S.A.; Koh, Y.H.; et al. The cutoff values of visceral fat area and waist circumference for identifying subjects at risk for metabolic syndrome in elderly Korean: Ansan Geriatric (AGE) cohort study. *BMC Public Health* **2009**, *9*, 443. [CrossRef]

30. Weston, A.D.; Korfiatis, P.; Kline, T.L.; Philbrick, K.A.; Kostandy, P.; Sakinis, T.; Sugimoto, M.; Takahashi, N.; Erickson, B.J. Automated abdominal segmentation of CT scans for body composition analysis using deep learning. *Radiology* **2019**, *290*, 669–679. [CrossRef]

31. Lee, S.J.; Liu, J.; Yao, J.; Kanarek, A.; Summers, R.M.; Pickhardt, P.J. Fully automated segmentation and quantification of visceral and subcutaneous fat at abdominal CT: Application to a longitudinal adult screening cohort. *Br. J. Radiol.* **2018**, *91*, 20170968. [CrossRef] [PubMed]

32. Montano-Loza, A.J.; Mazurak, V.C.; Ebadi, M.; Meza-Junco, J.; Sawyer, M.B.; Baracos, V.E.; Kneteman, N. Visceral adiposity increases risk for hepatocellular carcinoma in male patients with cirrhosis and recurrence after liver transplant. *Hepatology* **2018**, *67*, 914–923. [CrossRef] [PubMed]

33. Kang, G.H.; Cruite, I.; Shiehmorteza, M.; Wolfson, T.; Gamst, A.C.; Hamilton, G.; Bydder, M.; Middleton, M.S.; Sirlin, C.B. Reproducibility of MRI-determined proton density fat fraction across two different MR scanner platforms. *J. Magn. Reson. Imaging* **2011**, *34*, 928–934. [CrossRef] [PubMed]

34. Yokoo, T.; Shiehmorteza, M.; Hamilton, G.; Wolfson, T.; Schroeder, M.E.; Middleton, M.S.; Bydder, M.; Gamst, A.C.; Kono, Y.; Kuo, A.; et al. Estimation of hepatic proton-density fat fraction by using MR imaging at 3.0 T. *Radiology* **2011**, *258*, 749–759. [CrossRef] [PubMed]

35. Kang, B.K.; Yu, E.S.; Lee, S.S.; Lee, Y.; Kim, N.; Sirlin, C.B.; Cho, E.Y.; Yeom, S.K.; Byun, J.H.; Park, S.H.; et al. Hepatic fat quantification: A prospective comparison of magnetic resonance spectroscopy and analysis methods for chemical-shift gradient echo magnetic resonance imaging with histologic assessment as the reference standard. *Invest. Radiol.* **2012**, *47*, 368–375. [CrossRef]

36. Di Martino, M.; Pacifico, L.; Bezzi, M.; Di Miscio, R.; Sacconi, B.; Chiesa, C.; Catalano, C. Comparison of magnetic resonance spectroscopy, proton density fat fraction and histological analysis in the quantification of liver steatosis in children and adolescents. *World J. Gastroenterol.* **2016**, *22*, 8812–8819. [CrossRef]

37. Noureddin, M.; Lam, J.; Peterson, M.R.; Middleton, M.; Hamilton, G.; Le, T.A.; Bettencourt, R.; Changchien, C.; Brenner, D.A.; Sirlin, C.; et al. Utility of magnetic resonance imaging versus histology for quantifying changes in liver fat in nonalcoholic fatty liver disease trials. *Hepatology* **2013**, *58*, 1930–1940. [CrossRef]

38. Hines, C.D.; Frydrychowicz, A.; Hamilton, G.; Tudorascu, D.L.; Vigen, K.K.; Yu, H.; McKenzie, C.A.; Sirlin, C.B.; Brittain, J.H.; Reeder, S.B. T(1) independent, T(2) (*) corrected chemical shift based fat-water separation with multi-peak fat spectral modeling is an accurate and precise measure of hepatic steatosis. *J. Magn. Reson. Imaging* **2011**, *33*, 873–881. [CrossRef]

39. Negrete, L.M.; Middleton, M.S.; Clark, L.; Wolfson, T.; Gamst, A.C.; Lam, J.; Changchien, C.; Deyoung-Dominguez, I.M.; Hamilton, G.; Loomba, R.; et al. Inter-examination precision of magnitude-based MRI for estimation of segmental hepatic proton density fat fraction in obese subjects. *J. Magn. Reson. Imaging* **2014**, *39*, 1265–1271. [CrossRef]

40. Yokoo, T.; Serai, S.D.; Pirasteh, A.; Bashir, M.R.; Hamilton, G.; Hernando, D.; Hu, H.H.; Hetterich, H.; Kühn, J.P.; Kukuk, G.M.; et al. Linearity, bias, and precision of hepatic proton density fat fraction measurements by using MR imaging: A meta-analysis. *Radiology* **2018**, *286*, 486–498. [CrossRef]

41. Gu, J.; Liu, S.; Du, S.; Zhang, Q.; Xiao, J.; Dong, Q.; Xin, Y. Diagnostic value of MRI-PDFF for hepatic steatosis in patients with non-alcoholic fatty liver disease: A meta-analysis. *Eur. Radiol.* **2019**, *29*, 3564–3573. [CrossRef] [PubMed]

42. Middleton, M.S.; Heba, E.R.; Hooker, C.A.; Bashir, M.R.; Fowler, K.J.; Sandrasegaran, K.; Brunt, E.M.; Kleiner, D.E.; Doo, E.; Van Natta, M.L.; et al. Agreement between magnetic resonance imaging proton density fat fraction measurements and pathologist-assigned steatosis grades of liver biopsies from adults with nonalcoholic steatohepatitis. *Gastroenterology* **2017**, *153*, 753–761. [CrossRef] [PubMed]

43. Reeder, S.B.; Cruite, I.; Hamilton, G.; Sirlin, C.B. Quantitative assessment of liver fat with magnetic resonance imaging and spectroscopy. *J. Magn. Reson. Imaging* **2011**, *34*, 729–749. [CrossRef] [PubMed]

44. Wildman-Tobriner, B.; Middleton, M.M.; Moylan, C.A.; Rossi, S.; Flores, O.; Chang, Z.A.; Abdelmalek, M.F.; Sirlin, C.B.; Bashir, M.R. Association between magnetic resonance imaging-proton density fat fraction and liver histology features in patients with nonalcoholic fatty liver disease or nonalcoholic steatohepatitis. *Gastroenterology* **2018**, *155*, 1428–1435.e2. [CrossRef]

45. Idilman, I.S.; Aniktar, H.; Idilman, R.; Kabacam, G.; Savas, B.; Elhan, A.; Celik, A.; Bahar, K.; Karcaaltincaba, M. Hepatic steatosis: Quantification by proton density fat fraction with MR imaging versus liver biopsy. *Radiology* **2013**, *267*, 767–775. [CrossRef]

46. Thomsen, C.; Becker, U.; Winkler, K.; Christoffersen, P.; Jensen, M.; Henriksen, O. Quantification of liver fat using magnetic resonance spectroscopy. *Magn. Reson. Imaging* **1994**, *12*, 487–495. [CrossRef]

47. Chang, J.S.; Taouli, B.; Salibi, N.; Hecht, E.M.; Chin, D.G.; Lee, V.S. Opposed-phase MRI for fat quantification in fat-water phantoms with 1H MR spectroscopy to resolve ambiguity of fat or water dominance. *AJR Am. J. Roentgenol.* **2006**, *187*, W103–W106. [CrossRef]

48. Wei, J.L.; Leung, J.C.; Loong, T.C.; Wong, G.L.; Yeung, D.K.; Chan, R.S.; Chan, H.L.; Chim, A.M.; Woo, J.; Chu, W.C.; et al. Prevalence and severity of nonalcoholic fatty liver disease in non-obese patients: A population study using proton-magnetic resonance spectroscopy. *Am. J. Gastroenterol.* **2015**, *110*, 1306–1314. [CrossRef]

49. Longo, R.; Pollesello, P.; Ricci, C.; Masutti, F.; Kvam, B.J.; Bercich, L.; Crocè, L.S.; Grigolato, P.; Paoletti, S.; de Bernard, B.; et al. Proton MR spectroscopy in quantitative in vivo determination of fat content in human liver steatosis. *J. Magn. Reson. Imaging* **1995**, *5*, 281–285. [CrossRef]

50. Zhang, H.J.; He, J.; Pan, L.L.; Ma, Z.M.; Han, C.K.; Chen, C.S.; Chen, Z.; Han, H.W.; Chen, S.; Sun, Q.; et al. Effects of moderate and vigorous exercise on nonalcoholic fatty liver disease: A randomized clinical trial. *JAMA Intern. Med.* **2016**, *176*, 1074–1082. [CrossRef]

51. Kramer, H.; Pickhardt, P.J.; Kliewer, M.A.; Hernando, D.; Chen, G.H.; Zagzebski, J.A.; Reeder, S.B. Accuracy of liver fat quantification with advanced CT, MRI, and ultrasound techniques: Prospective comparison with MR spectroscopy. *AJR Am. J. Roentgenol.* **2017**, *208*, 92–100. [CrossRef]

52. Heger, M.; Marsman, H.A.; Bezemer, R.; Cloos, M.A.; van Golen, R.F.; van Gulik, T.M. Non-invasive quantification of triglyceride content in steatotic rat livers by (1)H-MRS: When water meets (too much) fat. *Acad. Radiol.* **2011**, *18*, 1582–1592. [CrossRef] [PubMed]

53. Zheng, D.; Guo, Z.; Schroder, P.M.; Zheng, Z.; Lu, Y.; Gu, J.; He, X. Accuracy of MR imaging and MR spectroscopy for detection and quantification of hepatic steatosis in living liver donors: A meta-analysis. *Radiology* **2017**, *282*, 92–102. [CrossRef] [PubMed]

54. Raptis, D.A.; Fischer, M.A.; Graf, R.; Nanz, D.; Weber, A.; Moritz, W.; Tian, Y.; Oberkofler, C.E.; Clavien, P.A. MRI: The new reference standard in quantifying hepatic steatosis? *Gut* **2012**, *61*, 117–127. [CrossRef]

55. Chiang, H.J.; Chang, W.P.; Chiang, H.W.; Lazo, M.Z.; Chen, T.Y.; Ou, H.Y.; Tsang, L.L.; Huang, T.L.; Chen, C.L.; Cheng, Y.F. Magnetic resonance spectroscopy in living-donor liver transplantation. *Transplant. Proc.* **2016**, *48*, 1003–1006. [CrossRef] [PubMed]

56. Cassidy, F.H.; Yokoo, T.; Aganovic, L.; Hanna, R.F.; Bydder, M.; Middleton, M.S.; Hamilton, G.; Chavez, A.D.; Schwimmer, J.B.; Sirlin, C.B. Fatty liver disease. MR imaging techniques for the detection and quantification of liver steatosis. *Radiographics* **2009**, *29*, 231–260. [CrossRef]

57. Borra, R.J.; Salo, S.; Dean, K.; Lautamäki, R.; Nuutila, P.; Komu, M.; Parkkola, R. Nonalcoholic fatty liver disease: Rapid evaluation of liver fat content with in-phase and out-of-phase MR imaging. *Radiology* **2009**, *250*, 130–136. [CrossRef]

58. Lee, Y.; Lee, J.M.; Lee, J.E.; Lee, K.B.; Lee, E.S.; Yoon, J.H.; Yu, M.H.; Baek, J.H.; Shin, C.I.; Han, J.K.; et al. MR elastography for noninvasive assessment of hepatic fibrosis: Reproducibility of the examination and reproducibility and repeatability of the liver stiffness value measurement. *J. Magn. Reson. Imaging* **2014**, *39*, 326–331. [CrossRef]

59. Lee, D.H.; Lee, J.M.; Han, J.K.; Choi, B.I. MR elastography of healthy liver parenchyma: Normal value and reliability of the liver stiffness value measurement. *J. Magn. Reson. Imaging* **2013**, *38*, 1215–1223. [CrossRef]

60. Singh, S.; Venkatesh, S.K.; Loomba, R.; Wang, Z.; Sirlin, C.; Chen, J.; Yin, M.; Miller, F.H.; Low, R.N.; Hassanein, T.; et al. Magnetic resonance elastography for staging liver fibrosis in non-alcoholic fatty liver disease: A diagnostic accuracy systematic review and individual participant data pooled analysis. *Eur. Radiol.* **2016**, *26*, 1431–1440. [CrossRef]

61.   Liang, Y.; Li, D. Magnetic resonance elastography in staging liver fibrosis in non-alcoholic fatty liver disease: A pooled analysis of the diagnostic accuracy. *BMC Gastroenterol.* **2020**, *20*, 89. [CrossRef] [PubMed]

62.   Chang, W.; Lee, J.M.; Yoon, J.H.; Han, J.K.; Choi, B.I.; Yoon, J.H.; Lee, K.B.; Lee, K.W.; Yi, N.J.; Suh, K.S. Liver fibrosis staging with MR elastography: Comparison of diagnostic performance between patients with chronic hepatitis B and those with other etiologic causes. *Radiology* **2016**, *280*, 88–97. [CrossRef] [PubMed]

63.   Srinivasa Babu, A.; Wells, M.L.; Teytelboym, O.M.; Mackey, J.E.; Miller, F.H.; Yeh, B.M.; Ehman, R.L.; Venkatesh, S.K. Elastography in chronic liver disease: Modalities, techniques, limitations, and future directions. *Radiographics* **2016**, *36*, 1987–2006. [CrossRef] [PubMed]

64.   Hennedige, T.P.; Wang, G.; Leung, F.P.; Alsaif, H.S.; Teo, L.L.; Lim, S.G.; Wee, A.; Venkatesh, S.K. Magnetic resonance elastography and diffusion weighted imaging in the evaluation of hepatic fibrosis in chronic hepatitis B. *Gut Liver* **2017**, *11*, 401–408. [CrossRef]

65.   Wang, Y.; Ganger, D.R.; Levitsky, J.; Sternick, L.A.; McCarthy, R.J.; Chen, Z.E.; Fasanati, C.W.; Bolster, B.; Shah, S.; Zuehlsdorff, S.; et al. Assessment of chronic hepatitis and fibrosis: Comparison of MR elastography and diffusion-weighted imaging. *AJR Am. J. Roentgenol.* **2011**, *196*, 553–561. [CrossRef]

66.   Wang, Q.B.; Zhu, H.; Liu, H.L.; Zhang, B. Performance of magnetic resonance elastography and diffusion-weighted imaging for the staging of hepatic fibrosis: A meta-analysis. *Hepatology* **2012**, *56*, 239–247. [CrossRef]

67.   Kromrey, M.L.; Le Bihan, D.; Ichikawa, S.; Motosugi, U. Diffusion-weighted MRI-based virtual elastography for the assessment of liver fibrosis. *Radiology* **2020**, *295*, 127–135. [CrossRef]

68.   Palmentieri, B.; de Sio, I.; La Mura, V.; Masarone, M.; Vecchione, R.; Bruno, S.; Torella, R.; Persico, M. The role of bright liver echo pattern on ultrasound B-mode examination in the diagnosis of liver steatosis. *Dig. Liver Dis.* **2006**, *38*, 485–489. [CrossRef]

69.   Van Werven, J.R.; Marsman, H.A.; Nederveen, A.J.; Smits, N.J.; ten Kate, F.J.; van Gulik, T.M.; Stoker, J. Assessment of hepatic steatosis in patients undergoing liver resection: Comparison of US, CT, T1-weighted dual-echo MR imaging, and point-resolved 1H MR spectroscopy. *Radiology* **2010**, *256*, 159–168. [CrossRef]

70.   Petzold, G.; Lasser, J.; Rühl, J.; Bremer, S.C.B.; Knoop, R.F.; Ellenrieder, V.; Kunsch, S.; Neesse, A. Diagnostic accuracy of B-Mode ultrasound and Hepatorenal Index for graduation of hepatic steatosis in patients with chronic liver disease. *PLoS ONE* **2020**, *15*, e0231044. [CrossRef]

71.   Hernaez, R.; Lazo, M.; Bonekamp, S.; Kamel, I.; Brancati, F.L.; Guallar, E.; Clark, J.M. Diagnostic accuracy and reliability of ultrasonography for the detection of fatty liver: A meta-analysis. *Hepatology* **2011**, *54*, 1082–1090. [CrossRef] [PubMed]

72.   Lee, S.S.; Park, S.H.; Kim, H.J.; Kim, S.Y.; Kim, M.Y.; Kim, D.Y.; Suh, D.J.; Kim, K.M.; Bae, M.H.; Lee, J.Y.; et al. Non-invasive assessment of hepatic steatosis: Prospective comparison of the accuracy of imaging examinations. *J. Hepatol.* **2010**, *52*, 579–585. [CrossRef] [PubMed]

73.   Petta, S.; Wong, V.W.; Cammà, C.; Hiriart, J.B.; Wong, G.L.; Marra, F.; Vergniol, J.; Chan, A.W.; Di Marco, V.; Merrouche, W.; et al. Improved noninvasive prediction of liver fibrosis by liver stiffness measurement in patients with nonalcoholic fatty liver disease accounting for controlled attenuation parameter values. *Hepatology* **2017**, *65*, 1145–1155. [CrossRef] [PubMed]

74.   Sasso, M.; Miette, V.; Sandrin, L.; Beaugrand, M. The controlled attenuation parameter (CAP): A novel tool for the non-invasive evaluation of steatosis using Fibroscan. *Clin. Res. Hepatol. Gastroenterol.* **2012**, *36*, 13–20. [CrossRef] [PubMed]

75.   Sasso, M.; Beaugrand, M.; de Ledinghen, V.; Douvin, C.; Marcellin, P.; Poupon, R.; Sandrin, L.; Miette, V. Controlled attenuation parameter (CAP): A novel VCTE™ guided ultrasonic attenuation measurement for the evaluation of hepatic steatosis: Preliminary study and validation in a cohort of patients with chronic liver disease from various causes. *Ultrasound Med. Biol.* **2010**, *36*, 1825–1835. [CrossRef]

76.   Shen, F.; Zheng, R.D.; Mi, Y.Q.; Wang, X.Y.; Pan, Q.; Chen, G.Y.; Cao, H.X.; Chen, M.L.; Xu, L.; Chen, J.N.; et al. Controlled attenuation parameter for non-invasive assessment of hepatic steatosis in Chinese patients. *World J. Gastroenterol.* **2014**, *20*, 4702–4711. [CrossRef]

77.   Chon, Y.E.; Jung, K.S.; Kim, S.U.; Park, J.Y.; Park, Y.N.; Kim, D.Y.; Ahn, S.H.; Chon, C.Y.; Lee, H.W.; Park, Y.; et al. Controlled attenuation parameter (CAP) for detection of hepatic steatosis in patients with chronic liver diseases: A prospective study of a native Korean population. *Liver Int.* **2014**, *34*, 102–109. [CrossRef]

78. Ferraioli, G.; Tinelli, C.; Lissandrin, R.; Zicchetti, M.; Dal Bello, B.; Filice, G.; Filice, C. Controlled attenuation parameter for evaluating liver steatosis in chronic viral hepatitis. *World J. Gastroenterol.* **2014**, *20*, 6626–6631. [CrossRef]

79. Shi, K.Q.; Tang, J.Z.; Zhu, X.L.; Ying, L.; Li, D.W.; Gao, J.; Fang, Y.X.; Li, G.L.; Song, Y.J.; Deng, Z.J.; et al. Controlled attenuation parameter for the detection of steatosis severity in chronic liver disease: A meta-analysis of diagnostic accuracy. *J. Gastroenterol. Hepatol.* **2014**, *29*, 1149–1158. [CrossRef]

80. Karlas, T.; Petroff, D.; Sasso, M.; Fan, J.G.; Mi, Y.Q.; de Lédinghen, V.; Kumar, M.; Lupsor-Platon, M.; Han, K.H.; Cardoso, A.C.; et al. Individual patient data meta-analysis of controlled attenuation parameter (CAP) technology for assessing steatosis. *J. Hepatol.* **2017**, *66*, 1022–1030. [CrossRef]

81. Pu, K.; Wang, Y.; Bai, S.; Wei, H.; Zhou, Y.; Fan, J.; Qiao, L. Diagnostic accuracy of controlled attenuation parameter (CAP) as a non-invasive test for steatosis in suspected non-alcoholic fatty liver disease: A systematic review and meta-analysis. *BMC Gastroenterol.* **2019**, *19*, 51. [CrossRef] [PubMed]

82. Park, C.C.; Nguyen, P.; Hernandez, C.; Bettencourt, R.; Ramirez, K.; Fortney, L.; Hooker, J.; Sy, E.; Savides, M.T.; Alquiraish, M.H.; et al. Magnetic resonance elastography vs. transient elastography in detection of fibrosis and noninvasive measurement of steatosis in patients with biopsy-proven nonalcoholic fatty liver disease. *Gastroenterology* **2017**, *152*, 598–607.e2. [CrossRef] [PubMed]

83. Runge, J.H.; Smits, L.P.; Verheij, J.; Depla, A.; Kuiken, S.D.; Baak, B.C.; Nederveen, A.J.; Beuers, U.; Stoker, J. MR Spectroscopy-derived proton density fat fraction is superior to controlled attenuation parameter for detecting and grading hepatic steatosis. *Radiology* **2018**, *286*, 547–556. [CrossRef] [PubMed]

84. Chan, W.K.; Nik Mustapha, N.R.; Wong, G.L.; Wong, V.W.; Mahadeva, S. Controlled attenuation parameter using the FibroScan® XL probe for quantification of hepatic steatosis for non-alcoholic fatty liver disease in an Asian population. *United Eur. Gastroenterol. J.* **2017**, *5*, 76–85. [CrossRef]

85. Oeda, S.; Takahashi, H.; Imajo, K.; Seko, Y.; Ogawa, Y.; Moriguchi, M.; Yoneda, M.; Anzai, K.; Aishima, S.; Kage, M.; et al. Accuracy of liver stiffness measurement and controlled attenuation parameter using FibroScan® M/XL probes to diagnose liver fibrosis and steatosis in patients with nonalcoholic fatty liver disease: A multicenter prospective study. *J. Gastroenterol.* **2020**, *55*, 428–440. [CrossRef]

86. Cardoso, A.C.; Cravo, C.; Calçado, F.L.; Rezende, G.; Campos, C.F.F.; Neto, J.M.A.; Luz, R.P.; Soares, J.A.S.; Moraes-Coelho, H.S.; Leite, N.C.; et al. The performance of M and XL probes of FibroScan for the diagnosis of steatosis and fibrosis on a Brazilian nonalcoholic fatty liver disease cohort. *Eur. J. Gastroenterol. Hepatol.* **2020**, *32*, 231–238. [CrossRef]

87. Lee, J.I.; Lee, H.W.; Lee, K.S. Value of controlled attenuation parameter in fibrosis prediction in nonalcoholic steatohepatitis. *World J. Gastroenterol.* **2019**, *25*, 4959–4969. [CrossRef]

88. Eddowes, P.J.; Sasso, M.; Allison, M.; Tsochatzis, E.; Anstee, Q.M.; Sheridan, D.; Guha, I.N.; Cobbold, J.F.; Deeks, J.J.; Paradis, V.; et al. Accuracy of fibroscan controlled attenuation parameter and liver stiffness measurement in assessing steatosis and fibrosis in patients with nonalcoholic fatty liver disease. *Gastroenterology* **2019**, *156*, 1717–1730. [CrossRef]

89. Popescu, A.; Bota, S.; Sporea, I.; Sirli, R.; Danila, M.; Racean, S.; Suseanu, D.; Gradinaru, O.; Ivascu Siegfried, C. The influence of food intake on liver stiffness values assessed by acoustic radiation force impulse elastography-preliminary results. *Ultrasound Med. Biol.* **2013**, *39*, 579–584. [CrossRef]

90. Cassinotto, C.; Boursier, J.; de Lédinghen, V.; Lebigot, J.; Lapuyade, B.; Cales, P.; Hiriart, J.B.; Michalak, S.; Bail, B.L.; Cartier, V.; et al. Liver stiffness in nonalcoholic fatty liver disease: A comparison of supersonic shear imaging, FibroScan, and ARFI with liver biopsy. *Hepatology* **2016**, *63*, 1817–1827. [CrossRef]

91. Lee, M.S.; Bae, J.M.; Joo, S.K.; Woo, H.; Lee, D.H.; Jung, Y.J.; Kim, B.G.; Lee, K.L.; Kim, W. Prospective comparison among transient elastography, supersonic shear imaging, and ARFI imaging for predicting fibrosis in nonalcoholic fatty liver disease. *PLoS ONE* **2017**, *12*, e0188321. [CrossRef] [PubMed]

92. Leung, V.Y.; Shen, J.; Wong, V.W.; Abrigo, J.; Wong, G.L.; Chim, A.M.; Chu, S.H.; Chan, A.W.; Choi, P.C.; Ahuja, A.T.; et al. Quantitative elastography of liver fibrosis and spleen stiffness in chronic hepatitis B carriers: Comparison of shear-wave elastography and transient elastography with liver biopsy correlation. *Radiology* **2013**, *269*, 910–918. [CrossRef] [PubMed]

93. Cassinotto, C.; Lapuyade, B.; Mouries, A.; Hiriart, J.B.; Vergniol, J.; Gaye, D.; Castain, C.; Le Bail, B.; Chermak, F.; Foucher, J.; et al. Non-invasive assessment of liver fibrosis with impulse elastography: Comparison of Supersonic Shear Imaging with ARFI and FibroScan®. *J. Hepatol.* **2014**, *61*, 550–557. [CrossRef] [PubMed]

94. Cruz-Jentoft, A.J.; Baeyens, J.P.; Bauer, J.M.; Boirie, Y.; Cederholm, T.; Landi, F.; Martin, F.C.; Michel, J.P.; Rolland, Y.; Schneider, S.M.; et al. Sarcopenia: European consensus on definition and diagnosis: Report of the European Working Group on Sarcopenia in Older People. *Age Ageing* **2010**, *39*, 412–423. [CrossRef]

95. Cruz-Jentoft, A.J.; Bahat, G.; Bauer, J.; Boirie, Y.; Bruyère, O.; Cederholm, T.; Cooper, C.; Landi, F.; Rolland, Y.; Sayer, A.A.; et al. Sarcopenia: Revised European consensus on definition and diagnosis. *Age Ageing* **2019**, *48*, 16–31. [CrossRef]

96. Bazzocchi, A.; Diano, D.; Albisinni, U.; Marchesini, G.; Battista, G.; Guglielmi, G. Liver in the analysis of body composition by dual-energy X-ray absorptiometry. *Br. J. Radiol.* **2014**, *87*, 20140232. [CrossRef]

97. Van Wagner, L.B.; Ning, H.; Lewis, C.E.; Shay, C.M.; Wilkins, J.; Carr, J.J.; Terry, J.G.; Lloyd-Jones, D.M.; Jacobs, D.R., Jr.; Carnethon, M.R. Associations between nonalcoholic fatty liver disease and subclinical atherosclerosis in middle-aged adults: The coronary artery risk development in young adults study. *Atherosclerosis* **2014**, *235*, 599–605. [CrossRef]

98. VanWagner, L.B.; Wilcox, J.E.; Colangelo, L.A.; Lloyd-Jones, D.M.; Carr, J.J.; Lima, J.A.; Lewis, C.E.; Rinella, M.E.; Shah, S.J. Association of nonalcoholic fatty liver disease with subclinical myocardial remodeling and dysfunction: A population-based study. *Hepatology* **2015**, *62*, 773–783. [CrossRef]

99. Van Wagner, L.B.; Wilcox, J.E.; Ning, H.; Lewis, C.E.; Carr, J.J.; Rinella, M.E.; Shah, S.J.; Lima, J.A.C.; Lloyd-Jones, D.M. Longitudinal association of non-alcoholic fatty liver disease with changes in myocardial structure and function: The CARDIA study. *J. Am. Heart Assoc.* **2020**, *9*, e014279.

100. Vita, T.; Murphy, D.J.; Osborne, M.T.; Bajaj, N.S.; Keraliya, A.; Jacob, S.; Diaz Martinez, A.J.; Nodoushani, A.; Bravo, P.; Hainer, J.; et al. Association between nonalcoholic fatty liver disease at ct and coronary microvascular dysfunction at myocardial perfusion PET/CT. *Radiology* **2019**, *291*, 330–337. [CrossRef]

101. Lee, Y.H.; Kim, K.J.; Yoo, M.E.; Kim, G.; Yoon, H.J.; Jo, K.; Youn, J.C.; Yun, M.; Park, J.Y.; Shim, C.Y.; et al. Association of non-alcoholic steatohepatitis with subclinical myocardial dysfunction in non-cirrhotic patients. *J. Hepatol.* **2018**, *68*, 764–772. [CrossRef] [PubMed]

102. Song, Y.; Dang, Y.; Wang, P.; Tian, G.; Ruan, L. CHD is associated with higher grades of NAFLD predicted by liver stiffness. *J. Clin. Gastroenterol.* **2020**, *54*, 271–277. [CrossRef] [PubMed]

103. Jin, R.; Le, N.A.; Cleeton, R.; Sun, X.; Cruz Muños, J.; Otvos, J.; Vos, M.B. Amount of hepatic fat predicts cardiovascular risk independent of insulin resistance among Hispanic-American adolescents. *Lipids Health Dis.* **2015**, *14*, 39. [CrossRef] [PubMed]

104. Chang, Y.; Ryu, S.; Sung, K.C.; Cho, Y.K.; Sung, E.; Kim, H.N.; Jung, H.S.; Yun, K.E.; Ahn, J.; Shin, H.; et al. Alcoholic and non-alcoholic fatty liver disease and associations with coronary artery calcification: Evidence from the Kangbuk Samsung Health Study. *Gut* **2019**, *68*, 1667–1675. [CrossRef] [PubMed]

105. Pavlides, M.; Banerjee, R.; Sellwood, J.; Kelly, C.J.; Robson, M.D.; Booth, J.C.; Collier, J.; Neubauer, S.; Barnes, E. Multiparametric magnetic resonance imaging predicts clinical outcomes in patients with chronic liver disease. *J. Hepatol.* **2016**, *64*, 308–315. [CrossRef] [PubMed]

106. Petta, S.; Sebastiani, G.; Viganò, M.; Ampuero, J.; Wai-Sun Wong, V.; Boursier, J.; Berzigotti, A.; Bugianesi, E.; Fracanzani, A.L.; Cammà, C.; et al. Monitoring occurrence of liver-related events and survival by transient elastography in patients with nonalcoholic fatty liver disease and compensated advanced chronic liver disease. *Clin. Gastroenterol. Hepatol.* **2020**. [CrossRef]

107. Han, M.A.T.; Vipani, A.; Noureddin, N.; Ramirez, K.; Gornbein, J.; Saouaf, R.; Baniesh, N.; Cummings-John, O.; Okubote, T.; Setiawan, V.W.; et al. MR elastography-based liver fibrosis correlates with liver events in nonalcoholic fatty liver patients: A multi-center study. *Liver Int.* **2020**. [CrossRef]

3

Mitochondrial Transfer by Human Mesenchymal Stromal Cells Ameliorates Hepatocyte Lipid Load in a Mouse Model of NASH

Mei-Ju Hsu [1,†], Isabel Karkossa [2,†], Ingo Schäfer [3], Madlen Christ [1], Hagen Kühne [1], Kristin Schubert [2], Ulrike E. Rolle-Kampczyk [2], Stefan Kalkhof [2,4,5], Sandra Nickel [1], Peter Seibel [3], Martin von Bergen [2,6] and Bruno Christ [1,*]

[1] Applied Molecular Hepatology Laboratory, Department of Visceral, Transplant, Thoracic and Vascular Surgery, University of Leipzig Medical Center, 04103 Leipzig, Germany; hsumeiju@gmail.com (M.-J.H.); madlen.christ@medizin.uni-leipzig.de (M.C.); hagen.kuehne@freenet.de (H.K.); sandra.brueckner@medizin.uni-leipzig.de (S.N.)

[2] Department of Molecular Systems Biology, Helmholtz Centre for Environmental Research (UFZ), 04318 Leipzig, Germany; isabel.karkossa@ufz.de (I.K.); kristin.schubert@ufz.de (K.S.); ulrike.rolle-kampczyk@ufz.de (U.E.R.-K.); stefan.kalkhof@hs-coburg.de (S.K.); martin.vonbergen@ufz.de (M.v.B.)

[3] Molecular Cell Therapy, Center for Biotechnology and Biomedicine, Leipzig University, 04103 Leipzig, Germany; ingo.schaefer@bbz.uni-leipzig.de (I.S.); peter.seibel@bbz.uni-leipzig.de (P.S.)

[4] Institute for Bioanalysis, University of Applied Sciences Coburg, 96450 Coburg, Germany

[5] Department of Therapy Validation, Fraunhofer Institute for Cell Therapy and Immunology, 04103 Leipzig, Germany

[6] Institute of Biochemistry, Leipzig University, 04103 Leipzig, Germany

* Correspondence: bruno.christ@medizin.uni-leipzig.de

† These authors contributed equally to this work.

Abstract: Mesenchymal stromal cell (MSC) transplantation ameliorated hepatic lipid load; tissue inflammation; and fibrosis in rodent animal models of non-alcoholic steatohepatitis (NASH) by as yet largely unknown mechanism(s). In a mouse model of NASH; we transplanted bone marrow-derived MSCs into the livers; which were analyzed one week thereafter. Combined metabolomic and proteomic data were applied to weighted gene correlation network analysis (WGCNA) and subsequent identification of key drivers. Livers were analyzed histologically and biochemically. The mechanisms of MSC action on hepatocyte lipid accumulation were studied in co-cultures of hepatocytes and MSCs by quantitative image analysis and immunocytochemistry. WGCNA and key driver analysis revealed that NASH caused the impairment of central carbon; amino acid; and lipid metabolism associated with mitochondrial and peroxisomal dysfunction; which was reversed by MSC treatment. MSC improved hepatic lipid metabolism and tissue homeostasis. In co-cultures of hepatocytes and MSCs; the decrease of lipid load was associated with the transfer of mitochondria from the MSCs to the hepatocytes via tunneling nanotubes (TNTs). Hence; MSCs may ameliorate lipid load and tissue perturbance by the donation of mitochondria to the hepatocytes. Thereby; they may provide oxidative capacity for lipid breakdown and thus promote recovery from NASH-induced metabolic impairment and tissue injury.

Keywords: non-alcoholic steatohepatitis (NASH); tunneling nanotubes (TNTs); primary hepatocytes; organelle transfer; mesenchymal stromal cells

1. Introduction

Obesity is a prevalent health problem worldwide, which has been attributed mainly to Western-style diets in combination with reduced physical activity. It is often associated with metabolic co-morbidities, such as diabetes type 2 and non-alcoholic fatty liver diseases (NAFLD), the latter of which has a global prevalence of 24% and is currently the leading cause of chronic liver disease in Europe and in the USA [1]. NAFLD may progress from simple steatosis to chronically inflammatory diseases like non-alcoholic steatohepatitis (NASH), cirrhosis, and hepatocellular carcinoma (HCC) [2,3]. On the cellular level, hepatocyte mitochondrial, peroxisomal and microsomal oxidation of fatty acids, and basal lipophagy [4] are involved in the utilization of hepatic lipids. However, impairment of lipid metabolism may cause an imbalance of utilization and storage, eventually contributing to hepatocyte lipid overload. Lipotoxicity induces endoplasmic reticulum (ER) stress, leading to calcium release from the ER, thus raising cytosolic calcium levels, which in turn interferes with protective autophagy and inhibits the breakdown of lipids, thus aggravating cellular lipid overload [5]. In addition, mitochondrial dysfunction is contributing to the pathogenesis of NAFLD by favoring hepatic lipid storage, and by promoting the production of reactive oxygen species (ROS) as well as lipid peroxidation [6–8]. Besides mitochondrial β-oxidation, peroxisomes are involved in long-chain fatty acid β-oxidation and microsomes in ω-oxidation of fatty acids. Like mitochondrial impairment, dysfunction of peroxisomal and microsomal fatty acid metabolism contributes to the pathogenesis of NASH by favoring lipid storage and production of ROS, respectively [9,10].

Pharmacological therapy may address NASH-associated co-morbidities like diabetes [11], yet, liver transplantation in NASH patients has been shown to reduce the risk of progression into HCC [12,13]. Indeed, NASH features the second most common indication for liver transplantation in the USA [1,14]. However, the invasiveness of organ transplantation, lifelong immune suppression, the shortage of donor livers, and eventually the high costs altogether fostered the search for alternative therapy approaches [15,16]. Mesenchymal stromal cells (MSCs) have been demonstrated to ameliorate NASH in rodent animal models [17–19]. Transplantation of hepatocyte-like cells derived from human bone marrow mesenchymal stromal cells (MSCs) alleviated lipid load, ameliorated hepatic inflammation as well as fibrosis, and enhanced proliferation of host hepatocytes in an experimental model of NASH in the immunodeficient mouse [20]. In line, transplantation of MSCs decreased fibrosis and activation of hepatic stellate cells in mouse and rat liver cirrhosis triggered by carbon tetrachloride (CCl_4) [21,22]. MSC restored ammonia and purine metabolism in a mouse model of acute liver failure [23], improved acute liver injury caused by acetaminophen [24], and enhanced liver regeneration in mice and rats after extended hepatectomy [25,26]. Clinically, the application of MSC ameliorated inborn errors of liver metabolism, such as ornithine carbamoyltransferase deficiency [27], decreased the severe bleeding complications in a hemophilia A patient [28], and improved liver function in cirrhotic patients [29–31]. However, some studies revealed only transient or even negligible effects of MSC treatment of liver diseases [32,33]. Thus, the identification of the mechanisms involved in MSC action is crucial to improve the therapeutic potential of MSCs.

Here, we showed in a mouse model of NASH and in co-cultures of fat-laden hepatocytes and MSCs that MSCs shifted pathological lipid storage to utilization likely by the transfer of MSC-derived functional mitochondria to the hepatocytes.

2. Experimental Section

2.1. Experimental Design

Xenotransplantation of human bone marrow-derived mesenchymal stromal cells was performed in immunodeficient Pfp/Rag2$^{-/-}$ mice (C57BL6, B6.129S6-Rag2(tm1Fwa)Prf1(tm1Clrk)N12. Taconic; Ejby, Denmark). At the age of 12 weeks, male mice were either fed a NASH–inducing methionine-choline-deficient diet (MP Biomedicals, Eschwege, Germany), or kept on a standard rodent chow. After five weeks of feeding, all mice underwent 1/3 partial hepatectomy and received 1.5×10^6 human MSCs (differentiated into the hepatocytic lineage) via splenic injection as described before [34]. PBS served as the vehicle control. The four resulting groups represented +NASH+MSC, +NASH-MSC, -NASH+MSC, and -NASH-MSC. The procedures for the isolation and hepatocytic differentiation of MSCs from human bone marrow have been described in detail previously [35], and were approved by the Institutional Ethics Review Board Leipzig (Ethik-Kommission an der Medizinischen Fakultät der Universität Leipzig; file no. 282/11-lk; 1 December 2016). After surgery, respective feeding regimes were continued for another week until mice were sacrificed, and livers harvested. Mice were housed under controlled conditions at a 12-h light/dark cycle, at an ambient temperature of $22 \pm 2\,°C$, and humidity of 50%–60%. All experimental procedures involving animals were approved by the federal authorities of Saxony (Saxon State Directorate Chemnitz; file no. TVV_54_16; 2 May 2017) and followed the guidelines of the animal welfare act.

2.2. Proteome and Metabolome Analyses

2.2.1. Liver Metabolite and Protein Extraction and Preparation for Protein Quantification by Stable Isotope Labeling of Mammals (SILAM)

Frozen liver tissue samples (100–200 mg) were homogenized with a ball mill in 500 µL of lysis buffer A (40 mM Tris base, 7 M urea, 4% CHAPS, 100 mM dithiothreitol (DTT), 0.5% (v/v) biolyte). Benzonase was added and the homogenates were incubated at room temperature for 20 min and afterwards centrifuged at $12.000\times g$ for 20 min at 30 °C. The resulting supernatant was collected, and the pellet was again extracted using 500 µL of lysis buffer B (40 mM Tris base, 5 M urea, 2 M thiourea, 4% CHAPS, 100 mM DTT, 0.5% (v/v) biolyte). After centrifugation, the supernatants of the first and the second extraction were combined. Then, 50 µL of the combined supernatants were desalted to 50 mM ammonium bicarbonate by centrifugal filtration using filtration units (molecular weight cutoff of 10 kDa, Vivacon 500, Sartorius Group, Göttingen, Germany). The permeate was applied for metabolomics analyses. The protein concentrations in the retentate were determined using a detergent-compatible colorimetric protein assay (660 nm Protein Assay, Thermo Scientific–Pierce, Dreieich, Germany). Analogously, a protein extract of a liver of a $^{13}C_6$-lysine-labeled black6 mouse ($^{13}C_6$-lysine, 97%, Cambridge Isotope Laboratories, Inc., Tewksbury, MA, USA) was prepared as an isotope-labeled standard.

2.2.2. In-Gel Tryptic Digestion and Liquid Chromatography-Tandem Mass Spectrometry (GeLC-MS/MS)

Protein mixtures were mixed with 0.5 M Tris-HCl buffer (pH 6.8) containing 40% (v/v) SDS, 20% (v/v) glycerol, 2% (v/v) bromophenol-blue, and 10% (v/v) 2-mercaptoethanol. After heating for 5 min at 95 °C, a 1-D-SDS-PAGE was carried out using Laemmli's protocol. Proteins were stained with Coomassie Brillant Blue G-250 and each lane was cut into 10 pieces of equal size. Gel pieces were washed twice in 200 µL of ACN/50 mM ABC (ammonium bicarbonate, Fluka (Thermo Fisher Scientific, Dreieich, Germany), 1:1, (v/v)) for 10 min at room temperature (RT). Reduction and alkylation of disulfide bonds were performed by adding 10 mM dithiothreitol/10 mM ABC (Thermo Fisher Scientific, Dreieich, Germany) for 30 min at RT followed by incubation in 100 mM iodacetamide/10 mM ABC (Sigma-Aldrich, Taufkirchen, Germany) for 30 min at RT in the dark. After another washing step in 10 mM ABC for 10 min at RT, proteins were digested by incubating each gel slice with 300 ng of trypsin (Promega, Mannheim, Germany) in 50 mM ABC at 37 °C overnight. Proteolysis was quenched by 10% formic acid and proteolytic peptides were extracted. Samples were dried by vacuum centrifugation and resuspended in 20 µL of 0.1% formic acid. Extracted peptides were analyzed by online reversed-phase nanoscale liquid chromatography tandem mass spectrometry on a NanoAcquity UPLC system (Waters Corporation, Milford, MA, USA) connected to an LTQ-Orbitrap XL ETD (Thermo Fisher Scientific, Waltham, MA, USA) and equipped with a chip-based nano ESI source (TriVersaNanoMate, Advion, Ithaca, NY, USA) as described previously [36]. Protein identification and relative quantification were performed using Proteome Discoverer (version 1.4, Thermo Scientific,

Bremen, Germany). Oxidation (methionine) and acetylation (protein N-termini) were used as variable modifications, while carbamidomethylation (cysteine) was set as a fixed modification. A database search was carried out by the search engine MASCOT against the UniProt mouse reference proteome (www.uniprot.org, 05-2014). Relative protein quantification was performed based on the measured ratios (treated mouse vs. isotopically labeled mouse standard) of all lysine-containing peptides. Fold changes (FCs) between different groups were calculated in reference to the internal control.

2.2.3. Metabolome

Targeted metabolomics was conducted using the AbsoluteIDQ p150 kit (BIOCRATES Life Sciences AG, Innsbruck, Austria) as described before [26]. In brief, metabolites were extracted from the livers as descripted above, and prepared according to the manufacturer's protocol [37]. Multiple reaction monitoring was carried out on an Agilent 1100 series binary HPLC system (Agilent Technologies, Waldbronn, Germany) coupled to a 4000 QTRAP (AB Sciex, Darmstadt, Germany) via a TurboIon spray source. The data evaluation for the quantification of metabolite concentrations was performed with the MetIQ software package.

2.3. Combined Analysis and Visualization of Proteome and Metabolome Data

2.3.1. Weighted Gene Correlation Network Analysis (WGCNA)

FCs of proteins and metabolites were analyzed in R-3.5.0 with the use of several packages [38–46]. Hierarchical clustering was conducted with Euclidean distance measure. To unravel changes for single proteins and metabolites, the data were filtered for analytes that were quantified at least in duplicate for the particular comparison, and the Student's t-test was performed for analytes that were identified at least in triplicate (Supplementary Material file 1, FCs and p-values proteomics, FCs and p-values metabolomics). For WGCNA, the average log2-transformed FCs of proteins and metabolites that were quantified at least in duplicate over all data sets (406 proteins and 148 metabolites) were scaled to integer values between 0 and 100 (Supplementary Material file 1, WGCNA data). The networks were constructed across all the measured samples with the R package WGCNA [47] as described before [48]. The used trait matrix, containing the different comparisons, may be found in the Supplementary Material file 1, WGCNA trait matrix. The soft power threshold for WGCNA was set to 18 to arrive at the network adjacency. The Topology Overlap Matrix (TOM) was created using a cut height of 0.15 and a minimum module size of 25. The analysis identified 11 modules of co-expressed analytes, identified with different colors. A summary of the analytes that were assigned to each module can be found in the Supplementary Material file 1, WGCNA module contents. Finally, for each of the obtained modules, significantly enriched KEGG (Kyoto Encyclopedia of Genes and Genomes) pathways were determined using R-3.5.0 [49–51] without defining a p-value threshold. For this purpose, the mouse database was used as background [52]. Lists of all enriched pathways for each module can be found in the Supplementary Material file 1, WGCNA KEGG results.

2.3.2. Identification of Key Drivers

Identification of trait-specific key drivers was performed based on the WGCNA results as described before [48]. Therefore, module- and trait-specific gene significances and module memberships were calculated for each analyte. Key drivers were assumed to be analytes with absolute gene significance ≥0.75 and absolute module membership ≥0.75 (Supplementary Material file 1, WGCNA key drivers). Gene names (Supplementary Material file 1, FCs and p-values proteomics) and KEGG pathways (Supplementary Material file 1, KEGG pathway mapping) were assigned to proteins using the DAVID Bioinformatics Resources 6.8 [53]. Thus, key drivers for the observed effects were identified. From the whole proteome, proteins that are related to mmu03320: PPAR signaling pathway, mmu04975: Fat digestion and absorption, mmu04610: Complement and coagulation cascades, mmu00190: Oxidative phosphorylation, mmu00480: Glutathione metabolism, mmu04932:

Non-alcoholic fatty liver disease (NAFLD), mmu04146: Peroxisome, mmu00061: Fatty acid biosynthesis, mmu00062: Fatty acid elongation, mmu01212: Fatty acid metabolism, and mmu00071: Fatty acid degradation were extracted for deeper insights into effects (Supplementary Material file 2, Figure S1).

2.4. Immunohistochemistry

A comprehensive list of antibodies used throughout this study is given in Supplementary Material file 2, Table S1. Mouse livers were fixed in 4% paraformaldehyde overnight and embedded in paraffin. Slices of 1 μm were dewaxed and rehydrated by standard procedures. Heat-mediated epitope retrieval was done in either citrate buffer (pH 6.0) or Tris-EDTA buffer (pH 9.0) for 30 min. Endogenous peroxidases were blocked with 3% hydrogen peroxide/methanol for 20 min followed by a 60-min blocking step in 5% BSA/0.5% Tween20, and additionally a 15-min avidin and 15-min biotin block (SP-2001, Avidin-Biotin Blocking Kit, Vectorlabs, Eching, Germany). Primary antibodies against Cyp2e1 (1:200, ab28146, abcam, Cambridge, UK) and 4-HNE (1:500, HNE11-S, Alpha Diagnostic International, San Antonio, TX, USA) were applied overnight at 4 °C, subsequently coupled to biotin-labelled secondary goat anti-rabbit antibody (1:200, 111-065-003, Dianova, Hamburg, Germany), and visualized by the Vectastain Elite ABC Kit (PK-6100, Vectorlabs, Eching, Germany) followed by DAB chromogen (Thermo Fisher Scientific, Dreieich, Germany) incubation. Hematoxylin was used as a nuclei counterstain. For immunofluorescence, slices were blocked in 5% goat serum/PBS (ccpro, Oberdorla, Germany) for 20 min and in 5% BSA/0.5% Tween20 for 60 min. Sections were subsequently incubated with primary antibodies against CD36 (1:100, NB400-144, Novusbio, Wiesbaden-Nordenstadt, Germany), E-cadherin (1:200, BD 610182, eBioscience, Heidelberg, Germany), and β-catenin (1:500, BD 610154, eBioscience, Heidelberg, Germany) overnight at 4 °C. Corresponding secondary antibodies, i.e., goat anti-rabbit AlexaFlour 568 (1:200, A11036, Life Technologies, Ober-Olm, Germany) to CD36, goat-anti-mouse Cy3 (1: 300, 115-165-003, Dianova, Hamburg, Germany) to E-cadherin, and goat anti-mouse AlexaFlour 488 (1:300, 115-545-003, Dianova, Hamburg, Germany) to β-catenin, were applied for 1 h at room temperature followed by nuclear staining with DAPI (1:1000, Carl Roth GmbH + Co. KG, Karlsruhe, Germany) for 5 min, respectively. Slides were mounted with 50% glycerol solution and lacquer, and images taken using the Zeiss Axio Observer.Z1 microscope. For the co-stain of human mitochondria in mouse hepatocytes, antigen retrieval using dewaxed slices was performed by heating for 30 min in citrate buffer (14,746, SignalStain unmasking solution, Cell Signaling Technology, Frankfurt/Main, Germany) and subsequent cooling on ice for 30 min. After two washings in PBS, slices were blocked for 80 min using 5% goat serum and 0.3% TritonX-100 in PBS. Primary antibodies against mouse cyclophilin A (1:100, 2175, Cell Signaling Technology, Frankfurt/Main, Germany) and anti-human mitochondria (1:200, MAB 1273, Millipore, Darmstadt, Germany) were added overnight at 4 °C, and slices washed 3 times with PBS thereafter. The first secondary antibody (1:200 goat anti-mouse Cy3; 115-165-003, Dianova, Hamburg, Germany) was added for 60 min at room temperature and slices were washed 2 times for 10 min each with PBS. The second secondary antibody (1:500 goat anti-rabbit AlexaFluor 488, 4412, Cell Signaling Technology, Frankfurt/Main, Germany) was added for 60 min at room temperature. After 3 washings for 5 min each with PBS, nuclei were stained with DAPI and slides finally mounted with 50% glycerol solution and lacquer. Images were taken using the Zeiss Axio Observer.Z1 microscope equipped with ApoTome.2 at 40× magnification.

2.5. Western Blotting

In total, 30–40 mg of liver tissue were lysed in RIPA buffer (50 mM Tris, 150 mM NaCl, 0.1% SDS, 1% Triton X-100, 1 mM EDTA+EGTA, 0.5% Na-deoxycholate, pH 7.5) supplemented with protease inhibitors (Roche, Mannheim, Germany). Crude lysates were centrifuged at 13,000 rpm for 15 min and the clear supernatant was collected. The protein concentration was determined by the bicinchoninic acid assay. Then, 50 μg of protein were subjected to standard SDS gel electrophoresis and blotted onto PVDF membranes. Non-specific binding was blocked with 5% skim milk (vinculin), or 5% BSA (PPARα, CD36) in Tris-buffered saline Tween-20 (TBS-T) for two hours. The primary and secondary antibodies used were as follows: anti-PPARα (1:1000, MAI-822 Thermo Fischer Scientific, Dreieich, Germany), anti-CD36 (1:1000, NB400-144, Novusbio, Wiesbaden-Nordenstadt, Germany), anti-Vinculin (1:3000, 05-386, Merck, Darmstadt, Germany), anti-rabbit-HRP (1:7500, BD 554021, eBioscience, Heidelberg, Germany), and anti-mouse-HRP (1:7500, BD 554002, eBioscience, Heidelberg, Germany). Blots were developed using the enhanced chemiluminescence Prime reagent kit (GE Healthcare, Buckinghamshire, UK). Vinculin was used for the normalization and calculation of the relative abundances.

2.6. Quantification of Liver Triglyceride Content

In total, 100 mg of liver tissue were homogenized in 1 mL of 5% Igepal (I3021, Sigma-Aldrich, Taufkirchen, Germany) using a pestle and mortar. Samples were heated for 4 min at 95 °C in a thermomixer, cooled at room temperature, heated again, and then centrifuged using a microcentrifuge at maximal speed. Supernatants were collected and diluted 1:10 with distilled water. Then, 25 μL of the samples were pre-warmed at 37 °C for 1–5 min and subjected to the Triglyceride Assay Kit-Quantification (ab65336, Abcam, Berlin, Germany), essentially as described by the supplier.

2.7. Isolation of Primary Mouse Hepatocytes and Co-Culture with Hepatocytic Differentiated MSCs

Primary hepatocytes (HCs) were isolated from male Pfp/Rag2$^{-/-}$ mouse livers by the two-step liver perfusion with collagenase (NB4G, Serva Electrophoresis GmbH, Heidelberg, Germany) as described [54]. HCs and hepatocytic differentiated MSCs at the cell number ratios as indicated were initially seeded onto collagen-coated dishes at a total cell density of 40,000 cells/cm^2 and grown for 3 h in minimal essential medium (MEM) (Merck, Darmstadt, Germany) containing 2% fetal calf serum (FCS) (Gibco, Darmstadt, Germany) to allow for attachment. The medium was replaced by either standard hepatocyte growth medium (HGM, [55]) supplemented with EGF and HGF (20 ng/mL each) serving as the control, or two different steatosis-inducing media: methionine-choline-deficient (MCD, c.c.pro Oberdorla, Germany) or HGM supplemented with 0.5 mM palmitic acid (C16:0). To identify potential paracrine effects mediated by the MSCs, conditioned media were collected from MSCs, hepatocytes, and co-cultures of both after 2 days of culture, centrifuged at 270× g to remove cell debris, and subsequently used to treat hepatocytes under control (HGM) and treatment conditions (MCD or C16:0) for an additional 1 and 2 days. Phase contrast pictures were captured with a Primovert inverted microscope with the Zen software (Zeiss, Jena, Germany).

2.8. Cell Labeling with Fluorescent Vital Dyes

To highlight MSCs in co-culture with hepatocytes using a fluorescence microscope, MSCs in suspension were pre-labeled prior to seeding with either 5-(and 6)-carboxyfluorescein diacetate succinimidyl ester (CFSE; Ex/Em: 494/521) or CellTrace Yellow (Ex/Em: 546/579) at a final concentration of 5 μM by shaking in the dark at 37 °C for 30 min. Cells were subsequently washed with PBS containing 20% of FCS, followed by two washes with 5% FCS [56]. Fluorescent dyes as mentioned above were from Thermo Fisher Scientific, Dreieich, Germany. To label mitochondria, MSCs in suspension were stained with 500 nM of MitoTracker Deep Red (Ex/Em: 644/665) or 150 nM of MitoTracker Red CMXRos (Ex/Em: 579/599) in PBS at 37 °C for 45 min with gentle shaking, followed by 3 washes with PBS. MitoTracker dyes were kindly provided by Prof. Dr. Lea Ann Dailey and Dr. Lysann Tietze, Institute of Pharmacy, University of Halle-Wittenberg, Halle, Germany. Labeled cells in suspension were kept in the dark on ice prior to further use.

2.9. Fluorescence Staining after Cell Fixation

Cells grown on coverslips were fixed with 3.7% formaldehyde at room temperature for 15 min, followed by 3 washings with PBS. Neutral triglycerides and lipids were labeled with Oil red O (ORO) as previously described [57]. For immunostaining, fixed cells were permeabilized with 0.1% Triton X-100 for 5 min at RT, followed by blocking with PBS containing 5% BSA for 1 h and additional blocking with 5% normal goat serum for 1 h. Cells were further stained with the mouse anti-human mitochondria antibody (1:400, MAB1273, Millipore, Darmstadt, Germany), or the rabbit anti-apoptosis-inducing factor (AIF) antibody (1:400, Rabbit mAb 5318, Cell Signaling Technology, Frankfurt/Main, Germany, kindly provided by Prof. Dr. Gabriela Aust, Department of Visceral, Transplant, Thoracic and Vascular Surgery, University of Leipzig Medical Center, Leipzig, Germany) in 1% BSA overnight at 4 °C. The following day, cells were incubated with goat anti-mouse antibodies conjugated with Cy3 (115-165-003, Dianova, Hamburg, Germany) or goat anti-rabbit antibodies conjugated with Alexa Fluor 488 (A11008, Thermo Fisher Scientific, Dreieich, Germany). To visualize cell morphology and discriminate between MSCs and hepatocytes, cells were stained with 0.1% CytoPainter Phalloidin-iFlour405 (ab176752, Abcam, Berlin, Germany) in 1% BSA in PBS for 1.5 h at RT to label F-actin. Where indicated, nuclei were counterstained with 1 µg/mL of 4,6-diamidino-2-phenylindole (DAPI).

2.10. Image Capture and Analysis

Images were taken using the Zeiss Axio Observer.Z1 inverted microscope at 20× magnification, or with ApoTome.2 at 40×. Lipid content was quantified by image analysis using the ImageJ software (ImageJ 1.42, National Institutes of Health, Bethesda, MD, USA). Results were normalized as the percentage amount of stain/100 HCs out of 6-10 microscopic visual fields per group. Results from 4 independent experiments are expressed as mean ± standard deviation (SD). Pictures of time-lapse live cell imaging were captured at an interval of 15 min using a laser scanning confocal microscope (Leica Microsystems, Wetzlar, Germany) at a magnification of 20×. One-µm-thick sections were acquired with a total z volume of 25 µm, and the maximum intensity projections are presented (cf. Figure 5B,C, and Supplementary Material file 2, Figure S6A–C).

2.11. Morphological Subtyping of Mitochondria

The cells were stained with 150 nM of MitoTracker Red CMXRos as described under 'Cell labeling with fluorescent vital dyes', followed by fixation. Pictures were captured using the Zeiss Axio Observer.Z1 inverted microscope equipped with ApoTome.2 with a 40× objective. Intact cells were cropped using Adobe Photoshop CS6 (v. 13.0, München, Germany). On average, the mitochondrial morphology of 18.31 hepatocytes and 12.58 MSC per group was analyzed by the automatic subtyping and quantification software MicroP, as developed and described by Peng et al. [58].

2.12. RNA Isolation, cDNA Synthesis and PCR

RNA was isolated using the QIAzol Lysis Reagent (Qiagen, Hilden, Germany). The cDNA was synthesized using the Maxima H Minus First Strand cDNA Synthesis Kit (Thermo Fischer Scientific, Dreieich, Germany). PCR was carried out using the PCR Master Mix (2×) (Thermo Fischer Scientific, Dreieich, Germany) and appropriate primer pairs as listed in Supplementary Material file 2, Table S2. PCR products were separated in Tris/borate/EDTA (TBE) agarose gels and quantified with ImageJ. Beta-2-microglobulin (B2M) was used for normalization.

2.13. Statistical Analysis

Results are shown as means ± standard deviation (SD) from 3–7 livers in each group run in analytical duplicates unless otherwise indicated. Statistical comparisons, if not otherwise indicated, were made using either the paired t-test or two-way ANOVA. Differences between groups were considered significant at a p value of ≤0.05.

3. Results

We and others have shown that the transplantation of mesenchymal stromal cells into mice suffering from NASH attenuated the lipid load, reduced inflammation, and resolved fibrosis [18,34,59,60]. Yet, the mechanism behind remained mainly elusive. Here, we aimed by omics approaches in combination with network analyses to identify pathways and key players in NASH, which were affected by MSC treatment. Potential mechanisms of MSC action as deduced from the WGNCA were investigated in co-cultures of hepatocytes and MSCs.

3.1. WGCNA Suggests a Shift from Lipid Storage to Utilization by MSCs

Based on the protein and metabolite intensities, which were obtained by applying untargeted proteomics and targeted metabolomics to mouse livers, ratios were calculated for the following comparisons to get insights into the mechanisms of the MSC treatment: +NASH-MSC vs. -NASH-MSC, +NASH+MSC vs. -NASH-MSC, -NASH+MSC vs. -NASH-MSC, +NASH+MSC vs. +NASH-MSC, +NASH-MSC vs. -NASH+MSC, and +NASH+MSC vs. -NASH+MSC. Those values were used for further analyses.

By WGCNA, co-expressed proteins and metabolites were summarized into modules, followed by correlation of the obtained module eigengenes (modules first principal component) with traits. In total, 11 modules were identified and the results of the correlation with selected traits are shown in Figure 1A, while the complete module–trait correlation can be found in Supplementary Material file 2, Figure S2. For each of the obtained modules, significantly enriched pathways were determined using KEGG (Kyoto Encyclopedia of Genes and Genomes, Supplementary Material file 1, WGCNA KEGG results). Anti-correlations for NASH and MSCs are observable for the magenta, turquoise, black, and blue module, showing significant (p-value ≤ 0.05) enrichment of KEGG pathways related to amino acid biosynthesis and central carbon metabolism (Supplementary Material file 2, Figure S2). Additionally, in the case of +NASH-MSC vs. -NASH-MSC and +NASH+MSC vs. +NASH-MSC, the described anti-correlation was observable but for the red, brown, green, green-yellow, yellow, and purple module that also showed significant enrichment of pathways connected to amino acid metabolism and central carbon metabolism, and in addition also to fatty acid degradation and metabolism as well as peroxisome proliferator-activated receptor (PPAR) signaling. The PPAR signaling showed the highest enrichment in the brown module, which positively correlated with +NASH-MSC vs. -NSH-MSC and negatively with +NASH+MSC vs. +NASH-MSC. This indicates that proteins that are assigned to this pathway in KEGG tended to show increased abundances upon NASH and decreased abundances upon MSC treatment. Interestingly, the comparison of +NASH+MSC vs. -NASH-MSC did not lead to high correlations, neither in the brown module containing PPAR signaling pathway-related proteins, nor in most of the other modules, indicating that the MSCs were successfully used to treat NASH, resulting in expression profiles similar to what was observable in the control group (Figure 1A).

Furthermore, a key driver analysis was conducted for the traits NASH and +NASH+MSC vs. +NASH-MSC based on the WGCNA results (Supplementary Material file 1, WGCNA key drivers). This analysis allowed the identification of analytes that were highly connected to the particular modules and traits, suggesting their critical role as mediators for the observed effects (Supplementary Material file 2, Figure S3). KEGG pathways were assigned to all, within this study, identified proteins (Supplementary Material file 1, KEGG pathway mapping) to identify the functions of the selected key drivers. Thereby, we focused on the following KEGG pathways: Non-alcoholic fatty liver disease (NAFLD), PPAR signaling pathway, fat digestion and absorption, complement and coagulation cascades, oxidative phosphorylation, glutathione metabolism, peroxisome, fatty acid biosynthesis, fatty acid elongation, fatty acid metabolism, and fatty acid degradation (Supplementary Material file 2, Figure S1). Figure 1B shows Log2(FCs) and p-values for a selection of the obtained key drivers. Apparently, metabolites gave information about NASH effects and more importantly also about effects upon MSC treatment. This was also true for the identified key driver proteins that furthermore gave insights into affected pathways. Proteins that were identified to be key drivers were mainly related to cellular stress (e.g., Sod2, Gstm2, Mgst1, Gstp1), as indicated by their contribution to the KEGG pathways glutathione metabolism and peroxisome. Furthermore, lipid metabolism was affected (e.g., Apob, Fasn), with an assignment of key drivers to fat digestion and absorption as well as fatty acid biosynthesis and metabolism. Interestingly, several of the identified key drivers showed opposite Log2(FCs) for +NASH+MSC vs. +NASH-MSC compared to the other investigated ratios, indicating that the MSC treatment of NASH compensated the NASH effects. In summary, the WGCNA showed an anti-correlation of NASH effects and effects upon MSC treatment as well as only minor effects for the MSC-treated NASH as compared to the control group. This indicated that MSCs reversed NASH effects, which was also confirmed by the expression profiles of the identified key drivers.

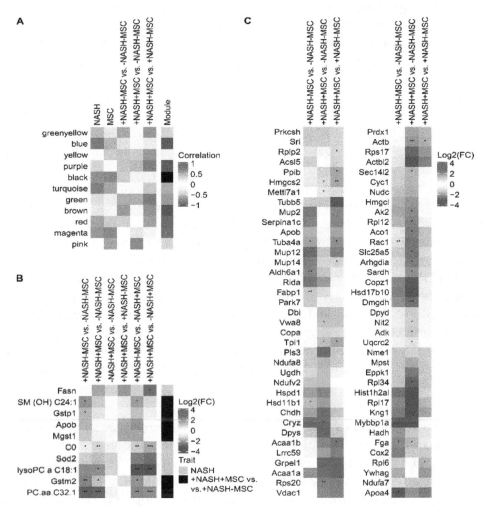

Figure 1. Integrative analysis of proteome and metabolome. (**A**) Correlations of WGCNA-created modules with relevant traits. Based on this, key drivers for the traits NASH and +NASH+MSC vs. +NASH-MSC were identified; (**B**) Log2(FCs) and *p*-values for selected key drivers; (**C**) Log2(FCs) and *p*-values are presented for selected candidates, which showed differences, albeit not significant throughout, between +NASH-MSC and +NASH+MSC. Significances are indicated with asterisks (*p*-value ≤ 0.05: *, *p*-value ≤ 0.01: **, *p*-value ≤ 0.001: ***). Euclidean clustering was applied to all heatmaps shown.

The hepatic acute-phase reaction is the defense response of the liver to injury, trauma, or inflammation [61]. It is associated with an increase of the expression of 'positive' acute-phase proteins (APP) on the expense of the 'negative' APPs [61]. The proteome analysis showed that the APPs Serpina1c (alpha-1-antitrypsin), which can be assigned to complement and coagulation cascades in KEGG, and several Mup (major urinary proteins) were significantly increased in +NASH-MSC livers as compared to control livers (Figure 1C). This increase was ameliorated in NASH livers receiving MSCs to levels comparable to the control group. Moreover, analysis of differentially expressed proteins revealed that compared to healthy (-NASH-MSC) control livers, +NASH-MSC livers showed a marked decrease in the expression of mitochondrial proteins Ndufa7 (NADH dehydrogenase 1 alpha subunit 7, KEGG: Oxidative phosphorylation, NAFLD), Cox2 (cytochrome c oxidase subunit 2, KEGG: Oxidative phosphorylation, NAFLD), and Hadh (hydroxyacyl-CoA dehydrogenase, KEGG: Fatty acid elongation, degradation, and metabolism). Ndufa7 and Cox2, as parts of complexes I and IV of the respiratory chain, and Hadh, as a key factor in the metabolism of short-chain fatty acids, are directly involved in mitochondrial β-oxidation and energy production. In addition, cytosolic proteins Acsl5 (long-chain fatty acid-CoA (Coenzyme A) ligase 5, KEGG: Fatty acid biosynthesis, degradation, and metabolism, PPAR signaling pathway, peroxisome) and Fabp1 (liver-specific fatty acid-binding protein 1, KEGG: PPAR signaling pathway, fat digestion and absorption) were increased in +NASH-MSC livers, indicating the stimulation of fatty acid activation towards triglyceride synthesis. Furthermore, the peroxisomal Acaa1a (acetyl-coenzyme A acyltransferase 1, KEGG: Fatty acid degradation and metabolism, PPAR signaling pathway) showed decreased abundances in NASH livers, which might be associated with the reduction of peroxisomal lipid oxidation. In addition, the fat digestion and absorption-related proteins Apoa4 (apolipoprotein A4) and Apob (apolipoprotein B100) showed the opposite behavior in +NASH-MSC livers compared to MSC-treated NASH livers, with Apoa4 being decreased in NASH livers compared to controls, whilst Apob was increased. This indicates an impairment of lipoprotein secretion (Figure 1C). Taken together, in the NASH livers, lipid metabolism seemed to be shifted from utilization to storage. As a hallmark of NASH, liver lipid deposition is increased due to the excess provision of fatty acids from the adipose tissue in conjunction with the impairment of hepatocyte mitochondrial β-oxidation, involving a decrease in respiratory chain activity [62], and impairment of the secretion of triglycerides via very low density lipoproteins (VLDL). The latter has been shown to be hampered due to decreased expression of the microsomal triglyceride transfer protein (MTTP), a chaperone involved in VLDL assembly [63]. The proteomic changes as described above and the decrease in serum and increase in liver triglycerides, respectively, as shown in our previous study in this NASH model [34], may suggest that the impairment of fatty acid oxidation and triglyceride secretion contributed, at least in part, to hepatosteatosis and inflammation in livers of the MCD diet-fed mice and amelioration by MSC treatment. Since mitochondrial impairment might be a major cause of lipid accumulation, we anticipated that MSC treatment might improve mitochondrial function.

Since MSCs, besides others, reversed the NASH-induced decrease of Acaa1a, and PPAR signaling was among the significantly enriched pathways in the modules that showed an anti-correlation between +NASH-MSC vs. -NASH-MSC and +NASH+MSC vs. +NASH-MSC, we speculated that this pathway could play a role in the attenuation of pathological lipid storage in NASH livers. Thus, we analyzed the expression of the peroxisome proliferator-activated receptor alpha (PPARα), the key regulator of peroxisomes and liver lipid metabolism [64]. Semi-quantitative Western blot analysis revealed that PPARα was suppressed to low levels in +NASH-MSC livers. Upon MSC transplantation, PPARα was re-expressed, albeit to a significantly lower extent than in controls (-NASH-MSC), corroborating that peroxisomal lipid metabolism may potentially contribute to MSC-mediated lipid clearance (Figure 2A). In addition to the uptake by Fatp1, fatty acids are transported into hepatocytes by the fatty acid translocase CD36. Semi-quantitative Western blot analysis of CD36 revealed that expression was upregulated in +NASH-MSC as compared to -NASH-MSC livers, which was not impacted by MSC treatment (Figure 2A). As verified by fluorescence immunohistochemistry, it seemed that predominant peripheral, presumably membranous localization of CD36 in +NASH-MSC livers changed to predominant cytoplasmic localization in +NASH+MSC-livers (Figure 2B). Since translocase activity of CD36 is associated with membrane localization [65], the cytoplasmic shift by MSC treatment might indicate the attenuation of fatty acid uptake.

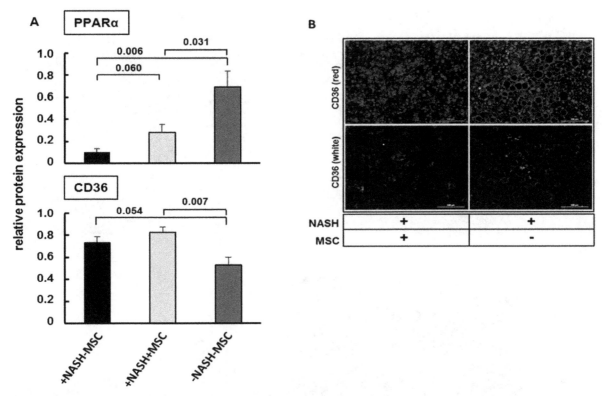

Figure 2. Expression of CD36 and PPARα in MCD-treated mice with and without MSC application. (**A**) Upregulation of CD36 expression and downregulation of PPARα in NASH livers and partial reversal by MSCs as shown by semiquantitative Western blot analysis of liver cytosolic extracts from 6 different animals in each group. Vinculin was used for normalization. Values represent means ± SEM and significant differences as indicated by the *p*-values over the horizontal lines were identified by applying the Student's *t*-test for unpaired values; (**B**) fluorescent immunohistochemical detection of CD36 in representative liver slices of +NASH-MSC livers and after treatment with MSC (+NASH+MSC). Scale bar 100 μm.

In summary, we reason that MSC alleviated the lipid burden in NASH livers by the improvement of lipid utilization by mitochondria in conjunction with the mutual balance of fatty acid import and lipid export.

3.2. Improvement of Tissue Homeostasis by MSCs

NASH is associated with an increased expression of Cyp2e1, a cytochrome P450 family member involved in the metabolism of polyunsaturated fatty acids [66]. The enzyme produces reactive oxygen species, leading to lipid peroxidation and formation of the byproduct 4-hydroxynonenal (4-HNE) [67]. To evaluate, whether oxidative stress was increased in NASH livers, we analyzed 4-hydroxynonenal (4-HNE) and Cyp2e1 by immunohistochemistry. In control livers, Cyp2e1 was zonally expressed in pericentral hepatocytes both untreated (-NASH-MSC) and treated with MSCs (-NASH+MSC), which was paralleled by weak zonal detection of 4-HNE. In NASH livers, both Cyp2e1 and 4-HNE were increased particularly in perivenous regions displaying a high fat content. Treatment with MSCs lowered both again to levels comparable to controls (Figure 3A), suggesting that MSCs ameliorated oxidative stress associated with enhanced lipid oxidation in NASH livers.

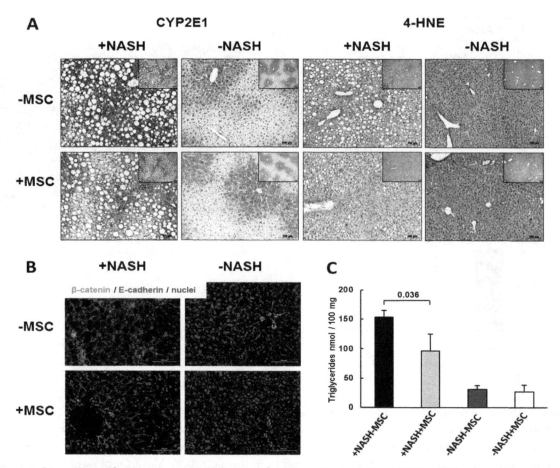

Figure 3. Liver tissue deterioration in MCD-treated mice and reversal by MSCs. (**A**) Immunohistochemical detection of Cyp2e1 and 4-HNE reveals an increase in perivenous localization in NASH livers, and restoration of zonation to nearly normal by MSC treatment. Pictures are representative for 3 different animals out of each group. White "holes" represent lipid droplets in NASH livers (original magnification 10×). The insets show lower magnifications for an overview impression (original magnification 5×). (**B**) luorescent immunohistochemical detection of adherens junction proteins β-catenin (green fluorescence) and E-cadherin (red, yellow in the overlay) indicates periportal zonation of E-cadherin, which is lost in NASH livers and restored by treatment with MSCs. Pictures are representative for 3 different animals out of each group. Scale bar 100 μm. (**C**) Hepatic triglycerides in control (-NASH) and in MCD diet-fed (+NASH) mice either treated without (-MSC) or with (+MSC) human bone marrow-derived MSCs. Values are means ± SD from 5 animals in each group. The horizontal line indicates the significant difference between the +NASH-MSC and the +NASH+MSC group at $p = 0.036$. In addition to Johnson transformation, an ANOVA was performed $p = 0.0001$, post-hoc Dunett T $p = 0.024$.

Liver function is strongly dependent on the polar orientation of hepatocytes along the sinusoids, i.e., facing the bile canaliculi with their apical and the sinusoids with their basolateral side. Chronic liver damage induces hepatocyte epithelial-mesenchymal transitions (EMTs) with a loss of hepatocyte polarity and eventually functionality [68]. The periportal expression of E-cadherin (E-cad), indicative for the epithelial organization of the hepatic parenchyma, was abrogated in NASH mouse livers as shown before [69]. Here, we confirmed this finding by immunohistochemical detection of E-cad and β-catenin (β-cat) co-localizing in the cell membrane at adherens junctions. In -NASH-MSC livers, both proteins were co-localized in periportal hepatocytes, indicating intact adherens junctions and hepatocyte polarity. In +NASH-MSC livers, however, periportal enrichment of E-cad was abrogated. Treatment with MSCs restored cell–cell contacts, and periportal expression of E-cad re-appeared co-localizing with β-catenin, comparable to -NASH-MSC control livers (Figure 3B). Consistent with the improvement of tissue homeostasis, MSC treatment lowered hepatic triglycerides significantly by about 40% (Figure 3C).

Taken together, MSCs thus supported restoration of tissue homeostasis by the alleviation of NASH-associated pathomechanisms like lipid load, oxidative stress, acute damage response, and EMT, corroborating results shown previously [34]. Since the WGNCA and key driver analysis suggested that the metabolic overload might be due to mitochondrial impairment, these data might corroborate the hypothesis that the MSCs might restore mitochondrial function.

3.3. MSCs Decreased Hepatocyte Lipid Load In Vitro

In order to study MSCs' effects on fat-laden hepatocytes (HCs) in more detail, we established an in vitro model of hepatocyte steatosis by growing primary mouse HCs in steatosis-inducing medium, i.e., methionine-choline-deficient medium (MCD) or hepatocyte growth medium (HGM) supplemented with palmitic acid (C16:0). HGM served as a control. The mouse hepatocyte cultures in HGM and MCD medium were initially characterized in terms of the functional maintenance of hepatocyte-specific metabolism. No differences of urea synthesis were observed between the culture of cells in HGM or MCD medium. As expected [70,71], the synthesis rate decreased after one day of culture and then remained stable until 5 days of culture. The expression of selected lipid metabolism genes did not show obvious differences between culture in HGM or MCD medium. Changes over time were similar under all conditions tested. The expression of albumin was equal at each point in time, and under both culture conditions, indicating that the MCD medium did not affect hepatocyte-specific functions (Supplementary Material file 2, Figure S4A,B). Lipid content was quantified after 3 days of culture by image analysis of lipids after staining with Oilred O (ORO) (Figure 4A). Compared with the HGM group, MCD and C16:0 triggered a significant increase in the accumulation of lipids by 1.71- and 2.28-fold, respectively (Figure 4B). To gain further insight into the mechanisms involved in the amelioration of lipid load in livers of NASH mice by MSC treatment, HCs were co-cultured with MSCs at ratios of HCs to MSCs of 1:0, 10:1, 5:1, 1:1, or 0:1, and grown in HGM (Figure 4C), MCD (Figure 4D), or C16:0 (Figure 4E) for an additional 3 days. To note, the morphology of nuclei featured differences between HCs and MSCs, with the former displaying round-shaped and mostly binuclear with intensive DAPI staining and prominent nucleoli, and the latter presenting with oval-shaped nuclei and weaker DAPI staining. This clear distinction allowed us to readily discriminate between HCs and MSCs using fluorescence microscopy. Furthermore, the ORO staining in MSCs was undetectable under all treatment conditions (Figure 4C–E(e)), indicating that the MSCs did not accumulate lipids. When HCs were co-cultured at decreasing HC to MSC ratios, a decrease in ORO staining was observed (Figure 4C–E(a–d)). Co-culture of HCs and MSCs at a ratio of 1:1 significantly decreased the lipid load in HC from 12.56% ± 2.7 to 6.51% ± 2.39 when cultured in HGM, from 24.46 % ± 8.75 to 7.62% ± 4.18 in MCD medium, and from 28.67% ± 6.66 to 17.00% ± 2.65 in C16:0 (Figure 4F), suggesting that the MSCs supported lipid degradation in the hepatocytes. The expression of the mRNAs of Acaa1a, Acaa1b, and PPARα was higher in co-cultures in MCD medium as compared to hepatocytes alone (Supplementary Material file 2, Figure S4C), indicating that the MSCs also improved functional features in the mouse hepatocytes. This corroborated data in vivo showing a correction of lipid metabolism by MSC treatment.

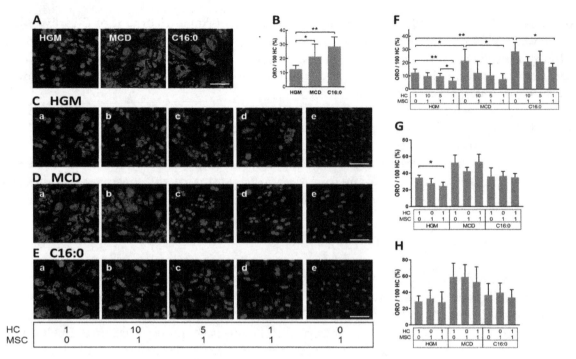

Figure 4. Induction of lipid droplet formation in cultured hepatocytes (HCs) by steatosis-inducing medium and reversal by MSCs in co-culture. Primary HCs were either cultured in HGM medium or treated with steatosis-inducing MCD medium or HGM supplemented with 0.5 mM palmitic acid (C16:0) for 3 days. (**A**) Visualization of hepatocyte lipids with Oil red O (red) and (**B**) quantification. HCs cultured (**a**) alone or together with MSCs at ratios of HCs to MSCs of (**b**) 10:1, (**c**) 5:1, (**d**) 1:1, or (**e**) 0:1 were grown for 3 days either in (**C**) HGM, or in (**D**) MCD, or in (**E**) HGM supplemented with C16:0. (**C–E**) lipid stain and (**F**) quantification. Nuclei were counterstained with DAPI (blue). Conditioned media were collected from either HC (1:0) or MSC (0:1) mono-cultures, or co-culture (ratio 1:1) and transferred to HCs grown for an additional (**G**) 1 or (**H**) 2 days in either HGM, MCD medium, or HGM supplemented with C16:0. The lipid stain with Oil red O was quantified by image analysis and the results from 3 independent cell cultures were normalized as the percentage amount of stain/100 hepatocytes and expressed as mean ± SD. Statistical comparisons were made using unpaired t-tests, and differences between groups were considered significant if the p-value was ≤0.05. *: $p ≤ 0.05$; **: $p ≤ 0.01$. Scale bar 100 µm. MSCs: human bone marrow-derived mesenchymal stromal cells; HCs: mouse primary hepatocytes; HGM: hepatocyte growth medium; MCD: methionine-choline-deficient medium.

MSCs may exert their effects via paracrine mechanisms involving soluble factors [72,73], or via extracellular vesicles [74]. Therefore, conditioned media (HGM, MCD, or C16:0) were collected separately from HCs, MSCs, and co-cultures of both after 48 h of culture. The media were subsequently added to HCs grown for 2 days in corresponding media and hepatocyte lipid load was determined after another 1 (Figure 4G) or 2 days (Figure 4H) by image analysis of ORO-stained lipid droplets.

A significant decrease in lipid accumulation in HCs was observed only when HCs were grown in HGM and treated with conditioned medium from co-cultures for one additional day (Figure 4G). The effect was no longer observed the day after (Figure 4H). No other condition revealed a lipid-reducing effect of the conditioned media, implicating that the lipolytic effect of MSCs in HCs was largely not mediated by soluble factors derived from MSCs, suggesting that direct cell-to-cell communication was required.

3.4. MSCs Communicated with Hepatocytes via Tunneling Nanotubes in a Microtubule-Dependent Manner

Irrespective of the growth in different media, MSCs communicated directly with hepatocytes in co-cultures via long filopodium-like tubes originating from the MSCs and touching the HCs or other MSCs (Figure 5A). These tubes were enriched in F-actin (cf. Figure 6A), one of the indispensable features of tunneling nanotubes (TNTs), thus potentially classifying them as TNTs. Using a live cell analysis system, we observed that the formation of TNTs was achieved by cell–cell contact between the MSCs and the targeted cell, followed by subsequent moving of the MSCs apart and leaving a tubular structure behind (Supplementary Material file 2, Figure S5). TNTs are known to exchange molecular and corpuscular messages between cells, and mitochondria are common cargos of TNTs [75–77]. To understand the direction of communication between HCs and MSCs, the MSCs were pre-labeled with MitoTracker Deep Red FM and CellTrace™ Yellow prior to co-culture. The pre-labeling procedure was toxic to the HCs. Therefore, pre-labeled MSCs were co-cultured with HCs and the whole culture was stained with CellTrace™ CFSE the next day to serve as a counterstain (Figure 5B,C). The results unraveled a bi-directional cargo exchange between HCs and MSCs. The net speed of cargo transportation from HCs to MSCs (Figure 5B) and from MSCs to HCs (Figure 5C) was 627 and 1656 nm/min, respectively.

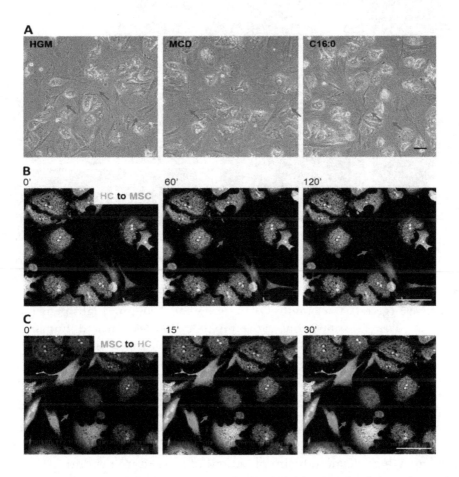

Figure 5. TNT-mediated cargo exchange between HCs and MSCs. (**A**) On day 1 of co-culture, the TNT structures (red arrows) derived from MSCs were readily detectable by phase contrast microscopy in cultures grown under all tested conditions. Scale bar 100 μm. Corresponding movies may be opened in Supplementary Material file 3; (**B**) The delivery of cargos from HCs to MSCs and (**C**) from MSCs to HCs was monitored by co-culture of HCs and MSCs pre-labeled with CellTrace™ Yellow and MitoTracker™ Deep Red FM (pseudo-colored green and red, respectively). The whole culture was stained with CellTrace™ CFSE (pseudo-colored white) and the pictures were captured using time-lapse confocal imaging. When the first picture was taken, this time point was designated as time 0, to which the other time points refer. The direction of movement of cargos in the TNTs is indicated by the red arrows. Scale bar 100 μm. Higher magnification images are available in Supplementary Material file 2, Figure S6A–C. Corresponding movies may be opened in Supplementary Material file 4.

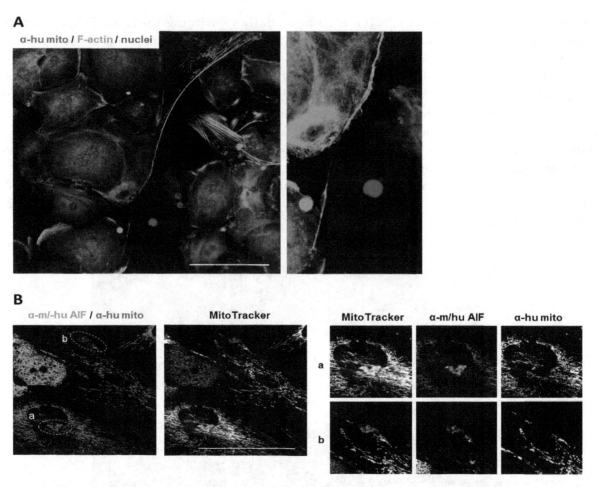

Figure 6. TNTs between HCs and MSCs are used to transport mitochondria. (**A**) Human MSC-derived mitochondria, stained in red with the anti-human-specific antibody against human mitochondria, are delivered to co-cultured mouse hepatocytes (mostly bi-nucleated). F-actin was stained with Phalloidin-iFluor 488 (green), nuclei with DAPI. Scale bar; 100 μm. Right panel: Computational enlargement of an area as shown on the left panel; (**B**) Mouse and human mitochondrial apoptosis-inducing factor (AIF) (green) and human mitochondria (red) were detected by fluorescent immunocytochemistry using species-specific antibodies, and cells were further stained with MitoTracker™ Deep Red FM (white). (**a**) and (**b**) show higher magnification pictures (computational enlargements) of circled areas shown in the panels on the left. Scale bar 100 μm.

To note, though the MSCs were pre-labeled with MitoTracker to visualize the potential movement of mitochondria in TNTs, the observability was limited by the magnification and the photostability of the fluorophore. Therefore, we confirmed the involvement of human mitochondria in TNT transportation by using the anti-human mitochondria antibody, clearly indicating the transport of MSC-derived human mitochondria into the mouse hepatocytes via TNTs (Figure 6A; Supplementary Material file 2, Figure S7A). In addition, our preliminary data also show that human peroxisomes were delivered towards HCs via the TNTs (Supplementary Material file 2, Figure S7B).

The anti-AIF (anti-apoptosis-inducing factor) monoclonal antibody detects the mitochondrial antigen AIF of both mouse and human origin. AIF does not necessarily locate in the mitochondria; it is also released to the cytoplasm in response to mitochondrial membrane permeabilization [78]. In the co-culture of human MSCs and mouse hepatocytes, AIF staining was mainly enriched in HCs. Yet, also in the MSCs, AIF was detectable in patches and a weaker staining in the MSC mitochondrial network (Figure 6B). The origin and nature of the AIF in the MSCs was further confirmed by using the anti-human mitochondria antibody and MitoTracker. The patchy AIF in the MSCs co-localized with MitoTracker but was negative for anti-human mitochondria staining (Figure 6B(a,b)), suggesting that these structures were derivatives of mitochondria of mouse origin. At present, we cannot say that mouse mitochondria in the MSCs were delivered via the TNTs, but the results corroborate the assumption of a bi-directional exchange between HCs and MSCs. The functional meaning, however, remains elusive and needs further investigations.

To further confirm the character of the TNTs and unravel potential functional consequences, we examined the expression of relevant molecular motors or proteins by RT-PCR using human-specific primers in association with the two most studied cytoskeleton proteins related to TNT delivery, tubulin (representing microtubule-based transport) and actin (representing actin-based transport). Compared with MSC mono-cultures, the mRNA expression of human microtubule-associated proteins, namely Ras homolog family member T1 (Rhot1, also known as mitochondrial Rho GTPase 1; MIRO1) and kinesin family member 5B (KIF5B), were upregulated in co-cultures (Figure 7A). However, neither inducers of actin-based TNTs, RAS like proto-oncogene A (RALA) and TNFα-induced protein 2 (TNFAIP2), were altered. The results implied that in the co-culture with mouse hepatocytes, human MSCs may facilitate the expression of the microtubule-related but not actin-related gene expression to foster human MSC-derived TNT-dependent cargo transport.

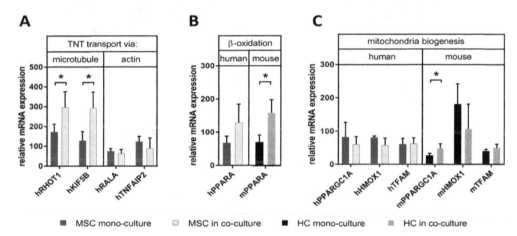

Figure 7. Expression of factors involved in (**A**) microtubule- and actin-based tubular transport, (**B**) hepatocyte lipid utilization, and (**C**) mitochondria biogenesis. Expression levels were analyzed by RT-PCR using species-specific primer pairs (blue/light blue columns for the use of human (h) primers, black/grey columns for the use of mouse (m) primers) and mRNA levels normalized with beta-2-microglobulin. Results are expressed as mean ± SD. Statistical comparisons from 3-5 independent cell cultures were made using the 2-way ANOVA test after log transformation, and differences between groups were considered significant if the p value was ≤0.05 (*). h: human; m: mouse; RHOT: Ras Homolog Family Member T1, also known as mitochondrial Rho GTPase 1 (MIRO1); KIF5B: kinesin family member 5B; RALA: RAS like proto-oncogene A; TNFAIP2: TNFα-induced protein 2; PPARGC1A: PPARα coactivator 1α, also known as PGC1α; HMOX1: heme oxygenase-1; TFAM: mitochondrial transcription factor A; PPARA: peroxisome proliferator-activated receptor α.

3.5. MSCs May Have Enhanced Lipid Utilization in HCs by Eliciting Oxidative Capacity

We hypothesized that the transportation of organelles from MSCs to HCs may promote lipid utilization in HCs in two ways: 1) By the activation of the key regulators of lipid utilization, like, e.g., peroxisome proliferator-activated receptor α (PPARA), and/or 2) by increasing the lipid-oxidizing capacity in HCs by the increase in the amount of MSC-derived mitochondria. To discriminate between human and mouse effects, we used species-specific primer pairs in RT-PCR experiments. The expression of mouse PPARA, but not human PPARA, was significantly higher in co-culture than in HC mono-culture (Figure 7B), corroborating the gene array results as shown above (Supplementary Material file 2, Figure S4C) and further suggesting that MSCs may elicit the utilization of lipids and fatty acids in HCs. Next, we analyzed the expression of markers involved in mitochondria biogenesis like PGC1α, mitochondrial transcription factor A (TFAM), and heme oxygenase-1 (HMOX1) by species-specific RT-PCR to discriminate between mouse and human effects. Only the expression of mouse PGC1α (PPARGC1A; PPARγ coactivator 1 α), a regulator of mitochondria biogenesis, was significantly enhanced in co-cultures with MSCs as compared with HCs alone (Figure 7C). Albeit not significantly, there was a trend of higher expression of mTFAM, while mHMOX1 was even decreased if affected at all. No human markers of mitochondria biogenesis were changed in co- vs. mono-cultures (Figure 7C). Therefore, also taking the results as shown in Figure 8A,B into account, it may be suggested that the MSCs might promote mitochondria biogenesis in the mouse hepatocytes. This, however, needs further confirmation.

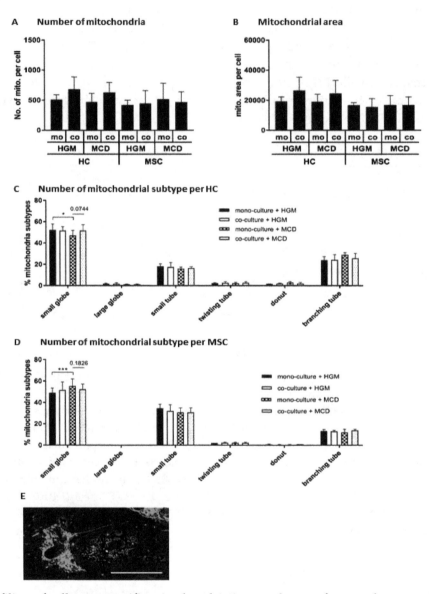

Figure 8. Profiling of cell-type-specific mitochondria in co-cultures of mouse hepatocytes and human MSCs. On day 1 of co-culture, fluorescence images of cells stained with MitoTracker Red CMXRos were analyzed for the (**A**) number and (**B**) area of mitochondria and percentages of mitochondria subtypes (**C**) in HCs and (**D**) in MSCs using the software MicroP. The statistical comparisons from 4 independent cell cultures were made using the 2-way ANOVA test. Results are expressed as mean ± SD. Statistical comparisons were made using unpaired t-tests, and differences between groups were considered significant for the p-values *: $p \leq 0.05$; ***: $p \leq 0.001$. (**E**) The globular morphology of MSC mitochondria was confirmed (cf. also Supplementary Material file 2, Figure S7) in MSCs co-cultured with HCs in HGM or MCD medium. The mitochondria were stained (pseudo-colored in green) and the picture was merged with the light microscopy image. Scale bar 50 μm. mo: mono-culture; co: co-culture.

Neither the number (Figure 8A) nor the area (Figure 8B) of mitochondria in MSCs and HCs were altered by any treatment. Yet, albeit not significant, there was a trend of higher mitochondria numbers in HCs when co-cultured with MSCs, both in HGM and in MCD medium, suggesting that MSCs might increase the number of mitochondria in HCs, in line with data shown in Figure 7C. The percentage of one of the mitochondrial subtypes, small globules, was significantly decreased in HCs when cultured in MCD medium, which was reversed in part in co-cultures with MSCs (Figure 8C). When cultured in MCD medium, the percentage of small globules was significantly increased in MSCs, suggesting that this condition might increase specific subtypes of mitochondria in MSCs (Figure 8D). Taking into consideration the mitochondrial globular shape as shown in Figure 6A in co-cultures of HCs and MSCs, it was very obvious that preferentially small dotted (small globules) MSC-derived mitochondria were detectable in TNT bridging to HCs (Figure 8E).

Taken together, these results show that MSCs may deliver mitochondria (and bona fide peroxisomes) to HCs, which might support lipid breakdown both by providing oxidative capacity and by support of the hepatocytes' own capacity of lipid utilization potentially by the support of mitochondria biogenesis. However, the mutual interactions between recipient and donor mitochondria and the impact on the recipient lipid metabolism remains to be further elucidated.

3.6. Human BM-MSCs Delivered Mitochondria to Mouse Hepatocytes In Vivo

In order to show that human mitochondria from transplanted MSCs were delivered to mouse hepatocytes after hepatic transplantation in vivo, liver slices were co-stained with an anti-mouse-specific cyclophilin and the anti-human-specific mitochondria antibody. Image analysis using the Zeiss Axio Observer.Z1 microscope equipped with ApoTome.2 showed that human mitochondria were only detectable in livers, which received human MSC transplants (Figure 9A). Signals co-localized with cyclophilin (Figure 9B), clearly indicating that donor human MSC-derived mitochondria were delivered to the host mouse hepatocytes. At this point in time, these results would be in line with the hypothesis that the delivery could involve TNTs as demonstrated in vitro (cf. Figure 6A).

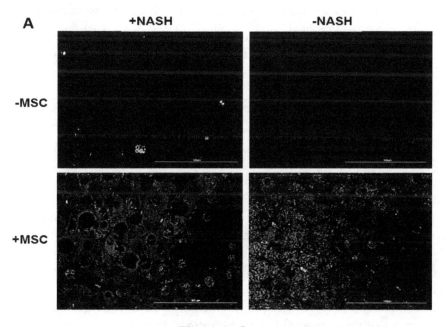

Figure 9. *Cont.*

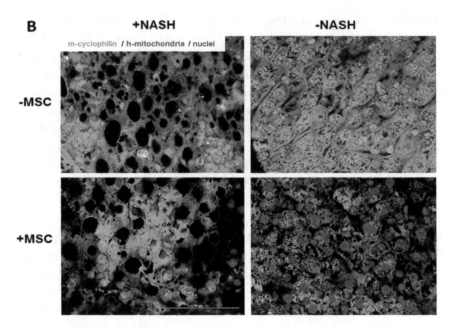

Figure 9. Human MSC-derived mitochondria in mouse hepatocytes of animals receiving MSC transplants. Here, 2-μm slices of mouse livers either fed the control (-NASH) or the MCD diet (+NASH) and treated without (-MSC) or with (+MSC) human bone marrow-derived MSC were co-stained with the anti-mouse cyclophilin or the anti-human mitochondria antibody and images captured using the Zeiss Axio Observer.Z1 microscope equipped with ApoTome.2 with a 40× objective. (**A**) Black and white images of pictures shown in (B) indicate human mitochondria (lower panels) in livers, which were transplanted with human MSCs. Non-transplanted livers (upper panels) were void of signals; (**B**) Immuno-fluorescent co-stain of mouse cyclophilin (green channel), and human mitochondria (red channel) indicating human mitochondria in mouse hepatocytes; nuclei were stained with DAPI (blue).

4. Discussion

4.1. Pathobiochemical Consequences of Changes in Metabolic Protein Expression and Correction by MSCs

Based on the proteomics and metabolomics data, the WGCNA predicted a MCD diet-induced deregulation of central carbon and amino acid metabolism likely associated with mitochondrial dysfunction, which were reversed by MSC treatment, rendering most of the affected metabolic pathways not significantly different from controls.

NASH is characterized by the accumulation of triglycerides in hepatocytes, a predominant sign of metabolic impairment. In the MCD model of NASH, it has been shown that VLDL secretion is inhibited due to the attenuated expression of the chaperone microsomal triglyceride transfer protein (MTP), which is essential for the proper folding of apolipoprotein B (ApoB) [79]. Here, we showed that ApoB was slightly increased, likely due to the accumulation of the non-functional protein, while the expression of ApoA4, involved in VLDL secretion [80], was downregulated. The increased expression of hepatocyte fatty acid transporters Fatp1 and CD36 fostered fatty acid uptake and together with the perturbance of lipid (lipoprotein) secretion likely caused an imbalance of lipid metabolism favoring storage over secretion. In addition to the attenuation of triglyceride secretion, the utilization of fatty acids by mitochondrial β-oxidation seemed to be impaired by the downregulation of proteins of the respiratory chain as obvious from the key driver analysis. Further, at the individual level of expressed genes, Acaa1a and b, involved in peroxisomal fatty acid oxidation, were downregulated, indicating an additional impairment of peroxisomal lipid utilization. In total, these findings are consistent with NASH-induced changes in central carbon and amino acid metabolism (as side reactions associated with glycolysis and the tricarboxylic acid cycle [81]) promoting lipid storage due to failure of lipid utilization and secretion as commonly observed in rodent NASH models and in humans [82–84].

Taken together, the pathobiochemical changes in the mouse liver upon MCD diet feeding are in line with major features of NASH as described [85,86]. In the study presented here, MSCs ameliorated the hepatic lipid load consistent with the improvement of NASH-induced metabolic changes as unraveled by WGCNA. To our knowledge, this is the first study to show the impact of MSCs on key metabolic pathways involved in the pathogenesis of NASH. However, the molecular and/or cellular mechanism(s) engaged remain open. Since it is conceivable that the MSCs did not impact on each individual biochemical pathway separately, or even by different mechanisms, it may be assumed that the MSCs primarily attenuated the hepatocyte lipid load by a unique mechanism, and consecutively improved overall metabolic homeostasis.

4.2. Histopathological Consequences of Hepatocyte Lipid Load and Improvement by MSCs

The accumulation of lipids in hepatocytes is associated with an overproduction of reactive oxygen species (ROS) that progressively exceeds the cellular detoxification capabilities. Microsomal Cyp2e1 is a major site of fatty acid metabolism, which has been found to be elevated in fatty liver diseases in humans and rodents [66]. Cyp2e1 plays a critical part in the pathogenesis of NASH by the production of ROS, which foster protein and lipid peroxidation associated with cellular stress and damage [67]. This is in line with our findings of increased Cyp2e1 and elevated 4-HNE as a byproduct of lipid peroxidation in the NASH livers. As identified by the key driver analysis in the NASH livers, the upregulation of proteins involved in protection from oxidative stress like Mgst1 and Gstp1 [87] may be interpreted as an adaptive response to increased oxidative stress, while downregulation of proteins like Sod2 involved in mitochondrial superoxide detoxification may even aggravate oxidative stress and mitochondrial impairment [88].

Alpha-1-antitrypsin and major urinary proteins increased in the NASH livers, indicative for the onset of the acute-phase reaction, the hepatic defense response to injury and inflammation. Likewise, the expression and localization of the cell adhesion proteins E-cadherin and β-catenin changed in the NASH as compared to control livers, indicative for the perturbation of the epithelial organization of the hepatic parenchyma. Epithelial-mesenchymal transitions in the liver have been attributed to be essential in regeneration of the liver after injury [89]. Hence, tissue deterioration in the NASH livers may indicate regeneration due to hepatocellular death.

MSC ameliorated oxidative stress, inflammation, and tissue damage, corroborating our previous results showing regression of fibrosis and cell death as well as attenuation of inflammatory pathways [20], consistent with findings demonstrating resolution of inflammation, fibrosis, and lipid load in rodent models of NASH [90,91]. The mechanisms behind, however, remain elusive. Again, it is unlikely that the MSCs impacted on single individual pathways involved in the perturbation of tissue homeostasis by different modes of action. Therefore, we hypothesize that the overall improvement of tissue homeostasis secondarily followed the attenuation of the hepatocyte lipid load. This implies that metabolic improvement preceded the restoration of tissue architecture, which was likely to be achieved by the regenerative capacity of the liver itself.

4.3. Mitochondrial Transfer by MSCs May Attenuate Hepatocyte Lipid Load

Previous reports including mouse datasets into WGCNA approaches identified mitochondrial dysfunction as a key event in the pathogenesis of NASH [92], consistent with our data that aberrant expression of mitochondrial proteins may drive mitochondrial dysfunction. Indeed, in consequence of insulin resistance, the increased flux of free fatty acids from the adipose tissue to the liver has long been suggested as a major cause of the metabolic overload and eventually dysfunction of mitochondria in the pathogenesis of NASH [7,8,93]. Based on these facts, we hypothesized that the improvement of mitochondrial function in the host liver by transplanted MSCs may play a central role in the amelioration of lipid load in the NASH livers. In the in vitro experiments, we observed a physical long-distance connection between MSCs and hepatocytes. These protrusions contained filamentous actin and carried whole organelles, features that have been specifically attributed to phenomena called tunneling nanotubes (TNTs) [94,95]. TNTs are thin membranous structures mediating direct intercellular communication between non-adjacent cells. They have been shown to transport subcellular components, e.g., mitochondria and lysosomes as well as plasma membrane components, mRNA, electrical signals, and calcium ions [96]. Our in vitro data present evidence for a transfer of mitochondria from MSCs to the hepatocytes via TNTs. Since the steatosis-inducing media used here is known to cause mitochondrial dysfunction associated with excess lipid storage, ROS generation, and cytotoxicity [97,98], the donation of functional mitochondria by the MSCs might contribute to the attenuation of lipid load in the hepatocytes. Hence, we suggest that the transferred mitochondria may compensate for a lack of oxidative phosphorylation capacity and thereby improve lipid utilization, which is in line with the lipid-lowering effect of MSCs as shown both in vitro and in vivo. Our work does not provide direct evidence that the delivery of mitochondria is involved in the reduction of triglycerides in hepatocytes. We used inhibitors of the respiratory chain and microtubule assembly in order to demonstrate correction of hepatocyte metabolism by MSC-derived donor mitochondria. Yet, most of the inhibitors were toxic to the hepatocytes, thus not allowing to discriminate between toxicity and specific effects on targets to be inhibited. It may not be excluded that part of the hepatocyte lipid resources may be metabolized by the MSC transplants. This would require the transfer of lipids to the MSCs, which we neither observed in vitro nor in vivo. Additionally, MSCs may have stimulated lipid breakdown in the host hepatocytes to release free fatty acids, which then could be metabolized by the MSCs. This would require some paracrine mechanisms, which, however, we may exclude, because MSC-derived conditioned medium was not effective. In addition, MSCs did not accumulate lipids in vitro, indicating that their lipid metabolism might be different from the hepatocytes. Indeed, in their niche, MSC energy metabolism may primarily rely on anaerobic glycolysis rather than oxidative phosphorylation [99]. Our results are consistent with data shown in a high-fat diet-fed mouse model, in which MSC transplants improved mitochondrial morphology and metabolic performance in the host liver [100]. This may describe a general mechanism of MSC action, since stem cell-derived donor mitochondria increased oxidative phosphorylation and ATP generation, and reduced ROS production in host cells like, e.g., myeloma cells [101], macrophages [102], cardiomyocytes [103], and airway epithelial cells [104]. Thus, the concept of MSC-derived mitochondrial transfer to improve recipient cell oxidative metabolism is now well established [105]. However, in our model of NASH, mechanistic questions remain open: How are diseased mitochondria cleared from the hepatocytes (e.g., by mitophagy)? Which are the mechanisms protecting the donated healthy mitochondria? How is the pool of donor mitochondria replenished in donating MSC? These questions are topics of our current work.

In our mouse model, we saw that MSC transplants entered the liver parenchyma primarily at the periportal area of the liver sinusoid, resulting in zonal enrichment of the MSCs [20]. For this animal model, we calculated that a 1% repopulation of the hepatic parenchyma by transplanted MSCs may be achieved, i.e., 6.6×10^5 transplanted cells in the host liver [106]. Assuming that a cell on average may contain 1500 mitochondria [107], this cell number corresponds to 9.9×10^8 donor mitochondria. A mouse liver contains 66×10^6 hepatocytes [108] corresponding to 9.9×10^{10} mitochondria. In conclusion, 1% on average of all mitochondria in a mouse hepatocyte ought to be of human MSC donor origin. This is in the same order of magnitude as shown in a co-culture model of human bone marrow-derived MSCs and myeloma cells, which improved cellular respiration in the range of 10–50% depending on the cell line under investigation [101]. If we assume in a simple approximation that this increase would solely contribute to lipid degradation and oxidation, this would account for the decrease in hepatocyte lipid content as shown here in vivo and in vitro of roughly 40%.

5. Conclusions

Metabolically, the diet-induced NASH was characterized by an impairment of the central carbon metabolism likely due to mitochondrial and peroxisomal dysfunction. The enhancement of membrane transporters of fatty acids may have increased fatty acid uptake. In association with the impairment of utilization and lipoprotein secretion, the enhancement of triglyceride synthesis and storage may follow. MSCs, transplanted into a mouse host liver, ameliorated lipid storage and associated perturbance of tissue homeostasis likely by the donation of healthy mitochondria to the hepatocytes via TNTs, thus providing oxidative capacity for lipid breakdown and eventually restoration of tissue homeostasis.

Author Contributions: Conceptualization, M.-J.H., I.K., S.K., M.v.B., P.S. and B.C.; methodology, M.-J.H., I.K., I.S., M.C., H.K., K.S., U.E.R.-K., S.K. and S.N.; software, I.S., I.K., K.S. and U.E.R.-K.; validation, H.K., M.C., S.K. and S.N.; formal analysis, M.-J.H., I.K., M.C., I.S., H.K., S.K. and S.N.; investigation, M.-J.H., I.K., S.K., I.S., M.C., H.K., S.K. and S.N.; resources, M.C., K.S., U.E.R.-K., P.S., M.v.B. and B.C.; data curation, M.-J.H., I.K., M.C. and B.C.; writing—original draft preparation, M.-J.H., I.K., H.K. and B.C.; writing—review and editing, M.-J.H., I.K., M.C., S.K., S.N., P.S., M.v.B. and B.C.; visualization, M.-J.H., I.K., M.C., H.K., S.K., S.N. and B.C.; supervision, K.S., U.E.R.-K., P.S., M.v.B. and B.C.; project administration, M.v.B. and B.C.; funding acquisition, M.-J.H. and B.C. All authors have read and agreed to the published version of the manuscript.

Acknowledgments: The authors are deeply thankful for the valuable contributions to this study made by Sandra Winkler and Sven Baumann. The authors greatly appreciate the technical support by Jacqueline Kobelt. We acknowledge support from Leipzig University for Open Access Publishing.

References

1.   Younossi, Z.; Anstee, Q.M.; Marietti, M.; Hardy, T.; Henry, L.; Eslam, M.; George, J.; Bugianesi, E. Global burden of nafld and nash: Trends, predictions, risk factors and prevention. *Nat. Rev. Gastroenterol. Hepatol.* **2018**, *15*, 11–20. [CrossRef]

2.   Tilg, H.; Moschen, A.R. Mechanisms behind the link between obesity and gastrointestinal cancers. *Best Pract. Res. Clin. Gastroenterol.* **2014**, *28*, 599–610. [CrossRef] [PubMed]

3.   Calle, E.E.; Rodriguez, C.; Walker-Thurmond, K.; Thun, M.J. Overweight, obesity, and mortality from cancer in a prospectively studied cohort of U.S. Adults. *N. Engl. J. Med.* **2003**, *348*, 1625–1638. [CrossRef] [PubMed]

4.   Singh, R.; Kaushik, S.; Wang, Y.; Xiang, Y.; Novak, I.; Komatsu, M.; Tanaka, K.; Cuervo, A.M.; Czaja, M.J. Autophagy regulates lipid metabolism. *Nature* **2009**, *458*, 1131–1135. [CrossRef]

5.   Park, H.W.; Park, H.; Semple, I.A.; Jang, I.; Ro, S.H.; Kim, M.; Cazares, V.A.; Stuenkel, E.L.; Kim, J.J.; Kim, J.S.; et al. Pharmacological correction of obesity-induced autophagy arrest using calcium channel blockers. *Nat. Commun.* **2014**, *5*, 4834. [CrossRef] [PubMed]

6.   Nassir, F.; Ibdah, J.A. Role of mitochondria in nonalcoholic fatty liver disease. *Int. J. Mol. Sci.* **2014**, *15*, 8713–8742. [CrossRef]

7.   Pessayre, D.; Fromenty, B. Nash: A mitochondrial disease. *J. Hepatol.* **2005**, *42*, 928–940. [CrossRef] [PubMed]

8.   Begriche, K.; Igoudjil, A.; Pessayre, D.; Fromenty, B. Mitochondrial dysfunction in nash: Causes, consequences and possible means to prevent it. *Mitochondrion* **2006**, *6*, 1–28. [CrossRef] [PubMed]

9.   Hall, D.; Poussin, C.; Velagapudi, V.R.; Empsen, C.; Joffraud, M.; Beckmann, J.S.; Geerts, A.E.; Ravussin, Y.; Ibberson, M.; Oresic, M.; et al. Peroxisomal and microsomal lipid pathways associated with resistance to hepatic steatosis and reduced pro-inflammatory state. *J. Biol. Chem.* **2010**, *285*, 31011–31023. [CrossRef]

10. Wu, Z.; Yang, F.; Jiang, S.; Sun, X.; Xu, J. Induction of liver steatosis in bap31-deficient mice burdened with tunicamycin-induced endoplasmic reticulum stress. *Int. J. Mol. Sci.* **2018**, *19*, 2291. [CrossRef]

11. Sumida, Y.; Yoneda, M. Current and future pharmacological therapies for nafld/nash. *J. Gastroenterol.* **2018**, *53*, 362–376. [CrossRef] [PubMed]

12. Lewin, S.M.; Mehta, N.; Kelley, R.K.; Roberts, J.P.; Yao, F.Y.; Brandman, D. Liver transplantation recipients with nonalcoholic steatohepatitis have lower risk hepatocellular carcinoma. *Liver Transplant. Off. Publ. Am. Assoc. Study Liver Dis. Int. Liver Transplant. Soc.* **2017** *23*, 1015–1022. [CrossRef]

13. Cholankeril, G.; Wong, R.J.; Hu, M.; Perumpail, R.B.; Yoo, E.R.; Puri, P.; Younossi, Z.M.; Harrison, S.A.; Ahmed, A. Liver transplantation for nonalcoholic steatohepatitis in the us: Temporal trends and outcomes. *Dig. Dis. Sci.* **2017**, *62*, 2915–2922. [CrossRef] [PubMed]

14. Noureddin, M.; Vipani, A.; Bresee, C.; Todo, T.; Kim, I.K.; Alkhouri, N.; Setiawan, V.W.; Tran, T.; Ayoub, W.S.; Lu, S.C.; et al. Nash leading cause of liver transplant in women: Updated analysis of indications for liver transplant and ethnic and gender variances. *Am. J. Gastroenterol.* **2018**, *113*, 1649–1659. [CrossRef] [PubMed]

15. Alfaifi, M.; Eom, Y.W.; Newsome, P.N.; Baik, S.K. Mesenchymal stromal cell therapy for liver diseases. *J. Hepatol.* **2018**, *68*, 1272–1285. [CrossRef]

16. Christ, B.; Bruckner, S.; Winkler, S. The therapeutic promise of mesenchymal stem cells for liver restoration. *Trends Mol. Med.* **2015**, *21*, 673–686. [CrossRef]

17. Rinella, M.E.; Elias, M.S.; Smolak, R.R.; Fu, T.; Borensztajn, J.; Green, R.M. Mechanisms of hepatic steatosis in mice fed a lipogenic methionine choline-deficient diet. *J. Lipid Res.* **2008**, *49*, 1068–1076. [CrossRef]

18. Pelz, S.; Stock, P.; Bruckner, S.; Christ, B. A methionine-choline-deficient diet elicits nash in the immunodeficient mouse featuring a model for hepatic cell transplantation. *Exp. Cell Res.* **2012**, *318*, 276–287. [CrossRef]

19. Wang, H.; Wang, D.; Yang, L.; Wang, Y.; Jia, J.; Na, D.; Chen, H.; Luo, Y.; Liu, C. Compact bone-derived mesenchymal stem cells attenuate nonalcoholic steatohepatitis in a mouse model by modulation of cd4 cells differentiation. *Int. Immunopharmacol.* **2017**, *42*, 67–73. [CrossRef]

20. Winkler, S.; Christ, B. Treatment of nash with human mesenchymal stem cells in the immunodeficient mouse. *Methods Mol. Biol.* **2014**, *1213*, 51–56.

21. Tanimoto, H.; Terai, S.; Taro, T.; Murata, Y.; Fujisawa, K.; Yamamoto, N.; Sakaida, I. Improvement of liver fibrosis by infusion of cultured cells derived from human bone marrow. *Cell Tissue Res.* **2013**, *354*, 717–728. [CrossRef] [PubMed]

22. Bruckner, S.; Zipprich, A.; Hempel, M.; Thonig, A.; Schwill, F.; Roderfeld, M.; Roeb, E.; Christ, B. Improvement of portal venous pressure in cirrhotic rat livers by systemic treatment with adipose tissue-derived mesenchymal stromal cells. *Cytotherapy* **2017**, *19*, 1462–1473. [CrossRef] [PubMed]

23. Banas, A.; Teratani, T.; Yamamoto, Y.; Tokuhara, M.; Takeshita, F.; Osaki, M.; Kato, T.; Okochi, H.; Ochiya, T. Rapid hepatic fate specification of adipose-derived stem cells and their therapeutic potential for liver failure. *J. Gastroenterol. Hepatol.* **2009**, *24*, 70–77. [CrossRef]

24. Stock, P.; Bruckner, S.; Winkler, S.; Dollinger, M.M.; Christ, B. Human bone marrow mesenchymal stem cell-derived hepatocytes improve the mouse liver after acute acetaminophen intoxication by preventing progress of injury. *Int. J. Mol. Sci.* **2014**, *15*, 7004–7028. [CrossRef] [PubMed]

25. Herrero, A.; Prigent, J.; Lombard, C.; Rosseels, V.; Daujat-Chavanieu, M.; Breckpot, K.; Najimi, M.; Deblandre, G.; Sokal, E.M. Adult-derived human liver stem/progenitor cells infused 3 days postsurgery improve liver regeneration in a mouse model of extended hepatectomy. *Cell Transplant.* **2017**, *26*, 351–364. [CrossRef]

26. Tautenhahn, H.M.; Bruckner, S.; Baumann, S.; Winkler, S.; Otto, W.; von Bergen, M.; Bartels, M.; Christ, B. Attenuation of postoperative acute liver failure by mesenchymal stem cell treatment due to metabolic implications. *Ann. Surg.* **2016**, *263*, 546–556. [CrossRef]

27. Sokal, E.M.; Stephenne, X.; Ottolenghi, C.; Jazouli, N.; Clapuyt, P.; Lacaille, F.; Najimi, M.; de Lonlay, P.; Smets, F. Liver engraftment and repopulation by in vitro expanded adult derived human liver stem cells in a child with ornithine carbamoyltransferase deficiency. *Jimd Rep.* **2014**, *13*, 65–72.

28. Sokal, E.M.; Lombard, C.A.; Roelants, V.; Najimi, M.; Varma, S.; Sargiacomo, C.; Ravau, J.; Mazza, G.; Jamar, F.; Versavau, J.; et al. Biodistribution of liver-derived mesenchymal stem cells after peripheral injection in a hemophilia a patient. *Transplantation* **2017**, *101*, 1845–1851. [CrossRef]

29. Kharaziha, P.; Hellstrom, P.M.; Noorinayer, B.; Farzaneh, F.; Aghajani, K.; Jafari, F.; Telkabadi, M.; Atashi, A.; Honardoost, M.; Zali, M.R.; et al. Improvement of liver function in liver cirrhosis patients after autologous mesenchymal stem cell injection: A phase i-ii clinical trial. *Eur. J. Gastroenterol. Hepatol.* **2009**, *21*, 1199–1205. [CrossRef]

30. Jang, Y.O.; Kim, Y.J.; Baik, S.K.; Kim, M.Y.; Eom, Y.W.; Cho, M.Y.; Park, H.J.; Park, S.Y.; Kim, B.R.; Kim, J.W.; et al. Histological improvement following administration of autologous bone marrow-derived mesenchymal stem cells for alcoholic cirrhosis: A pilot study. *Liver Int. Off. J. Int. Assoc. Study Liver* **2014**, *34*, 33–41. [CrossRef]

31. Suk, K.T.; Yoon, J.H.; Kim, M.Y.; Kim, C.W.; Kim, J.K.; Park, H.; Hwang, S.G.; Kim, D.J.; Lee, B.S.; Lee, S.H.; et al. Transplantation with autologous bone marrow-derived mesenchymal stem cells for alcoholic cirrhosis: Phase 2 trial. *Hepatology* **2016**, *64*, 2185–2197. [CrossRef] [PubMed]

32. Kanazawa, Y.; Verma, I.M. Little evidence of bone marrow-derived hepatocytes in the replacement of injured liver. *Proc. Natl. Acad. Sci. USA* **2003**, *100* (Suppl. 1), 11850–11853. [CrossRef] [PubMed]

33. Higashiyama, R.; Moro, T.; Nakao, S.; Mikami, K.; Fukumitsu, H.; Ueda, Y.; Ikeda, K.; Adachi, E.; Bou-Gharios, G.; Okazaki, I.; et al. Negligible contribution of bone marrow-derived cells to collagen production during hepatic fibrogenesis in mice. *Gastroenterology* **2009**, *137*, 1459–1466.e1451. [CrossRef] [PubMed]

34. Winkler, S.; Borkham-Kamphorst, E.; Stock, P.; Bruckner, S.; Dollinger, M.; Weiskirchen, R.; Christ, B. Human mesenchymal stem cells towards non-alcoholic steatohepatitis in an immunodeficient mouse model. *Exp. Cell Res.* **2014**, *326*, 230–239. [CrossRef] [PubMed]

35. Stock, P.; Bruckner, S.; Ebensing, S.; Hempel, M.; Dollinger, M.M.; Christ, B. The generation of hepatocytes from mesenchymal stem cells and engraftment into murine liver. *Nat. Protoc.* **2010**, *5*, 617–627. [CrossRef] [PubMed]

36. Müller, S.A.; Kohajda, T.; Findeiss, S.; Stadler, P.F.; Washietl, S.; Kellis, M.; von Bergen, M.; Kalkhof, S. Optimization of parameters for coverage of low molecular weight proteins. *Anal. Bioanal. Chem.* **2010**, *398*, 2867–2881. [CrossRef] [PubMed]

37. Römisch-Margl, W.; Prehn, C.; Bogumil, R.; Röhring, C.; Suhre, K.; Adamski, J. Procedure for tissue sample preparation and metabolite extraction for high-throughput targeted metabolomics. *Metabolomics* **2012**, *8*, 133–142. [CrossRef]

38. Wickham, H.; Bryan, J. Readxl: Read Excel Files. Available online: https://CRAN.R-project.org/package=readxl (accessed on 10 September 2020).

39. Spiess, A.N. Qpcr: Modelling and Analysis of Real-Time pcr Data. R Package v. 1.4-1. Available online: https://CRAN.R-project.org/package=qpcR (accessed on 10 September 2020).

40. Wickham, H.; Henry, L. Tidyr: EASILY tidy Data with "Spread ()" and "Gather ()" Functions. R Package Version 0.8. 0. Available online: https://CRAN.R-project.org/package=tidyr (accessed on 10 September 2020).

41. Wickham, H. The split-apply-combine strategy for data analysis. *J. Stat. Softw.* **2011**, *40*, 1–29. [CrossRef]

42. Mahto, A. Splitstackshape: Stack and Reshape Datasets after Splitting Concatenated Values. Available online: https://CRAN.R-project.org/package=splitstackshape (accessed on 10 September 2020).

43. Love, M.I.; Huber, W.; Anders, S. Moderated estimation of fold change and dispersion for rna-seq data with deseq2. *Genome Biol.* **2014**, *15*, 550. [CrossRef]

44. Gu, Z.; Eils, R.; Schlesner, M. Complex heatmaps reveal patterns and correlations in multidimensional genomic data. *Bioinformatics* **2016**, *32*, 2847–2849. [CrossRef]

45. Sakai, R. Dendsort: Modular Leaf Ordering Methods for Dendrogram Nodes. R Package Version 0.3. 3. *F1000 Res.* **2015**, *3*, 177. [CrossRef] [PubMed]

46. Xiao, N. Ggsci: Scientific Journal and Sci-fi Themed Color Palettes For'ggplot2'. R Package Version 2. 2018. Available online: https://CRAN.R-project.org/package=ggsci (accessed on 10 September 2020).

47. Langfelder, P.; Horvath, S. Wgcna: An r package for weighted correlation network analysis. *BMC Biolnform.* **2008**, *9*, 559. [CrossRef] [PubMed]

48. Karkossa, I.; Bannuscher, A.; Hellack, B.; Bahl, A.; Buhs, S.; Nollau, P.; Luch, A.; Schubert, K.; von Bergen, M.; Haase, A. An in-depth multi-omics analysis in rle-6tn rat alveolar epithelial cells allows for nanomaterial categorization. *Part Fibre Toxicol* **2019**, *16*, 38. [CrossRef] [PubMed]

49. Yu, G.; Wang, L.G.; Han, Y.; He, Q.Y. Clusterprofiler: An r package for comparing biological themes among gene clusters. *Omics A J. Integr. Biol.* **2012**, *16*, 284–287. [CrossRef] [PubMed]

50. Durinck, S.; Spellman, P.T.; Birney, E.; Huber, W. Mapping identifiers for the integration of genomic datasets with the r/bioconductor package biomart. *Nat. Protoc.* **2009**, *4*, 1184–1191. [CrossRef]

51. Durinck, S.; Moreau, Y.; Kasprzyk, A.; Davis, S.; De Moor, B.; Brazma, A.; Huber, W. Biomart and bioconductor: A powerful link between biological databases and microarray data analysis. *Bioinformatics* **2005**, *21*, 3439–3440. [CrossRef]

52. Carlson, M. Org.Mm.Eg.Db: Genome Wide Annotation for Mouse. 2018. Available online: https://bioconductor.org/packages/release/data/annotation/html/org.Mm.eg.db.html (accessed on 10 September 2020). [CrossRef]

53. Huang, D.W.; Sherman, B.T.; Lempicki, R.A. Systematic and integrative analysis of large gene lists using david bioinformatics resources. *Nat. Protoc.* **2009**, *4*, 44–57. [CrossRef]

54. Winkler, S.; Hempel, M.; Bruckner, S.; Mallek, F.; Weise, A.; Liehr, T.; Tautenhahn, H.M.; Bartels, M.; Christ, B. Mouse white adipose tissue-derived mesenchymal stem cells gain pericentral and periportal hepatocyte features after differentiation in vitro, which are preserved in vivo after hepatic transplantation. *Acta Physiol.* **2015**, *215*, 89–104. [CrossRef]

55. Block, G.D.; Locker, J.; Bowen, W.C.; Petersen, B.E.; Katyal, S.; Strom, S.C.; Riley, T.; Howard, T.A.; Michalopoulos, G.K. Population expansion, clonal growth, and specific differentiation patterns in primary cultures of hepatocytes induced by hgf/sf, egf and tgf alpha in a chemically defined (hgm) medium. *J. Cell Biol.* **1996**, *132*, 1133–1149. [CrossRef]

56. Quah, B.J.; Warren, H.S.; Parish, C.R. Monitoring lymphocyte proliferation in vitro and in vivo with the intracellular fluorescent dye carboxyfluorescein diacetate succinimidyl ester. *Nat. Protoc.* **2007**, *2*, 2049–2056. [CrossRef]

57. Winkler, S.; Hempel, M.; Hsu, M.J.; Gericke, M.; Kuhne, H.; Bruckner, S.; Erler, S.; Burkhardt, R.; Christ, B. Immune-deficient pfp/rag2(-/-) mice featured higher adipose tissue mass and liver lipid accumulation with growing age than wildtype c57bl/6n mice. *Cells* **2019**, *8*, 775. [CrossRef] [PubMed]

58. Peng, J.Y.; Lin, C.C.; Chen, Y.J.; Kao, L.S.; Liu, Y.C.; Chou, C.C.; Huang, Y.H.; Chang, F.R.; Wu, Y.C.; Tsai, Y.S.; et al. Automatic morphological subtyping reveals new roles of caspases in mitochondrial dynamics. *PLoS Comput. Biol.* **2011**, *7*, e1002212. [CrossRef] [PubMed]

59. Lee, C.W.; Hsiao, W.T.; Lee, O.K. Mesenchymal stromal cell-based therapies reduce obesity and metabolic syndromes induced by a high-fat diet. *Transl. Res. J. Lab. Clin. Med.* **2017**, *182*, 61–74.e68. [CrossRef] [PubMed]

60. Seki, A.; Sakai, Y.; Komura, T.; Nasti, A.; Yoshida, K.; Higashimoto, M.; Honda, M.; Usui, S.; Takamura, M.; Takamura, T.; et al. Adipose tissue-derived stem cells as a regenerative therapy for a mouse steatohepatitis-induced cirrhosis model. *Hepatology* **2013**, *58*, 1133–1142. [CrossRef]

61. Ramadori, G.; Christ, B. Cytokines and the hepatic acute-phase response. *Semin. Liver Dis.* **1999**, *19*, 141–155. [CrossRef] [PubMed]

62. Lee, J.; Park, J.S.; Roh, Y.S. Molecular insights into the role of mitochondria in non-alcoholic fatty liver disease. *Arch. Pharmacal Res.* **2019**, *42*, 935–946. [CrossRef]

63. Musso, G.; Gambino, R.; Cassader, M. Recent insights into hepatic lipid metabolism in non-alcoholic fatty liver disease (nafld). *Prog. Lipid Res.* **2009**, *48*, 1–26. [CrossRef] [PubMed]

64. Pawlak, M.; Lefebvre, P.; Staels, B. Molecular mechanism of pparalpha action and its impact on lipid metabolism, inflammation and fibrosis in non-alcoholic fatty liver disease. *J. Hepatol.* **2015**, *62*, 720–733. [CrossRef]

65. Bonen, A.; Campbell, S.E.; Benton, C.R.; Chabowski, A.; Coort, S.L.; Han, X.X.; Koonen, D.P.; Glatz, J.F.; Luiken, J.J. Regulation of fatty acid transport by fatty acid translocase/cd36. *Proc. Nutr. Soc.* **2004**, *63*, 245–249. [CrossRef]

66. Aubert, J.; Begriche, K.; Knockaert, L.; Robin, M.A.; Fromenty, B. Increased expression of cytochrome p450 2e1 in nonalcoholic fatty liver disease: Mechanisms and pathophysiological role. *Clin. Res. Hepatol. Gastroenterol.* **2011**, *35*, 630–637. [CrossRef]

67. Leung, T.M.; Nieto, N. Cyp2e1 and oxidant stress in alcoholic and non-alcoholic fatty liver disease. *J. Hepatol.* **2013**, *58*, 395–398. [CrossRef] [PubMed]

68. Xie, G.; Diehl, A.M. Evidence for and against epithelial-to-mesenchymal transition in the liver. *Am. J. Physiol. Gastrointest. Liver Physiol.* **2013**, *305*, G881–G890. [CrossRef]

69. Hempel, M.; Schmitz, A.; Winkler, S.; Kucukoglu, O.; Bruckner, S.; Niessen, C.; Christ, B. Pathological implications of cadherin zonation in mouse liver. *Cell. Mol. Life Sci. Cmls* **2015**, *72*, 2599–2612. [CrossRef] [PubMed]

70. Aurich, H.; Koenig, S.; Schneider, C.; Walldorf, J.; Krause, P.; Fleig, W.E.; Christ, B. Functional characterization of serum-free cultured rat hepatocytes for downstream transplantation applications. *Cell Transplant.* **2005**, *14*, 497–506. [CrossRef] [PubMed]

71. Schneider, C.; Aurich, H.; Wenkel, R.; Christ, B. Propagation and functional characterization of serum-free cultured porcine hepatocytes for downstream applications. *Cell Tissue Res.* **2006**, *323*, 433–442. [CrossRef]

72. Winkler, S.; Hempel, M.; Bruckner, S.; Tautenhahn, H.M.; Kaufmann, R.; Christ, B. Identification of pathways in liver repair potentially targeted by secretory proteins from human mesenchymal stem cells. *Int. J. Mol. Sci.* **2016**, *17*, 1099. [CrossRef]

73. van Poll, D.; Parekkadan, B.; Cho, C.H.; Berthiaume, F.; Nahmias, Y.; Tilles, A.W.; Yarmush, M.L. Mesenchymal stem cell-derived molecules directly modulate hepatocellular death and regeneration in vitro and in vivo. *Hepatology* **2008**, *47*, 1634–1643. [CrossRef]

74. Varderidou-Minasian, S.; Lorenowicz, M.J. Mesenchymal stromal/stem cell-derived extracellular vesicles in tissue repair: Challenges and opportunities. *Theranostics* **2020**, *10*, 5979–5997. [CrossRef]

75. Shen, J.; Zhang, J.H.; Xiao, H.; Wu, J.M.; He, K.M.; Lv, Z.Z.; Li, Z.J.; Xu, M.; Zhang, Y.Y. Mitochondria are transported along microtubules in membrane nanotubes to rescue distressed cardiomyocytes from apoptosis. *Cell Death Dis.* **2018**, *9*, 81. [CrossRef]

76. Vignais, M.L.; Caicedo, A.; Brondello, J.M.; Jorgensen, C. Cell connections by tunneling nanotubes: Effects of mitochondrial trafficking on target cell metabolism, homeostasis, and response to therapy. *Stem Cells Int.* **2017**, *2017*, 6917941. [CrossRef]

77. Lu, J.; Zheng, X.; Li, F.; Yu, Y.; Chen, Z.; Liu, Z.; Wang, Z.; Xu, H.; Yang, W. Tunneling nanotubes promote intercellular mitochondria transfer followed by increased invasiveness in bladder cancer cells. *Oncotarget* **2017**, *8*, 15539–15552. [CrossRef] [PubMed]

78. Ravagnan, L.; Roumier, T.; Kroemer, G. Mitochondria, the killer organelles and their weapons. *J. Cell. Physiol.* **2002**, *192*, 131–137. [CrossRef] [PubMed]

79. Sparks, J.D.; Sparks, C.E. Overindulgence and metabolic syndrome: Is foxo1 a missing link? *J. Clin. Investig.* **2008**, *118*, 2012–2015. [CrossRef] [PubMed]

80. Hoover-Plow, J.; Huang, M. Lipoprotein(a) metabolism: Potential sites for therapeutic targets. *Metab. Clin. Exp.* **2013**, *62*, 479–491. [CrossRef] [PubMed]

81. Mazat, J.P.; Ransac, S. The fate of glutamine in human metabolism. The interplay with glucose in proliferating cells. *Metabolites* **2019**, *9*, 81. [CrossRef]

82. Cazanave, S.; Podtelezhnikov, A.; Jensen, K.; Seneshaw, M.; Kumar, D.P.; Min, H.K.; Santhekadur, P.K.; Banini, B.; Mauro, A.G.; Oseini, A.M.; et al. The transcriptomic signature of disease development and progression of nonalcoholic fatty liver disease. *Sci. Rep.* **2017**, *7*, 17193. [CrossRef]

83. Teufel, A.; Itzel, T.; Erhart, W.; Brosch, M.; Wang, X.Y.; Kim, Y.O.; von Schonfels, W.; Herrmann, A.; Bruckner, S.; Stickel, F.; et al. Comparison of gene expression patterns between mouse models of nonalcoholic fatty liver disease and liver tissues from patients. *Gastroenterology* **2016**, *151*, 513–525.e510. [CrossRef]

84. Bessone, F.; Razori, M.V.; Roma, M.G. Molecular pathways of nonalcoholic fatty liver disease development and progression. *Cell. Mol. Life Sci. Cmls* **2019**, *76*, 99–128. [CrossRef]

85. Lambert, J.E.; Ramos-Roman, M.A.; Browning, J.D.; Parks, E.J. Increased de novo lipogenesis is a distinct characteristic of individuals with nonalcoholic fatty liver disease. *Gastroenterology* **2014**, *146*, 726–735. [CrossRef]

86. Hyotylainen, T.; Jerby, L.; Petaja, E.M.; Mattila, I.; Jantti, S.; Auvinen, P.; Gastaldelli, A.; Yki-Jarvinen, H.; Ruppin, E.; Oresic, M. Genome-scale study reveals reduced metabolic adaptability in patients with non-alcoholic fatty liver disease. *Nat. Commun.* **2016**, *7*, 8994. [CrossRef]

87. Hardwick, R.N.; Fisher, C.D.; Canet, M.J.; Lake, A.D.; Cherrington, N.J. Diversity in antioxidant response enzymes in progressive stages of human nonalcoholic fatty liver disease. *Drug Metab. Dispos. Biol. Fate Chem.* **2010**, *38*, 2293–2301. [CrossRef] [PubMed]

88. Velarde, M.C.; Flynn, J.M.; Day, N.U.; Melov, S.; Campisi, J. Mitochondrial oxidative stress caused by sod2 deficiency promotes cellular senescence and aging phenotypes in the skin. *Aging* **2012**, *4*, 3–12. [CrossRef] [PubMed]

89. Oh, S.H.; Swiderska-Syn, M.; Jewell, M.L.; Premont, R.T.; Diehl, A.M. Liver regeneration requires yap1-tgfbeta-dependent epithelial-mesenchymal transition in hepatocytes. *J. Hepatol.* **2018**, *69*, 359–367. [CrossRef]

90. Ezquer, M.; Ezquer, F.; Ricca, M.; Allers, C.; Conget, P. Intravenous administration of multipotent stromal cells prevents the onset of non-alcoholic steatohepatitis in obese mice with metabolic syndrome. *J. Hepatol.* **2011** *55*, 1112–1120. [CrossRef]

91. Watanabe, T.; Tsuchiya, A.; Takeuchi, S.; Nojiri, S.; Yoshida, T.; Ogawa, M.; Itoh, M.; Takamura, M.; Suganami, T.; Ogawa, Y.; et al. Development of a non-alcoholic steatohepatitis model with rapid accumulation of fibrosis, and its treatment using mesenchymal stem cells and their small extracellular vesicles. *Regen. Ther.* **2020**, *14*, 252–261. [CrossRef]

92. Chella Krishnan, K.; Kurt, Z.; Barrere-Cain, R.; Sabir, S.; Das, A.; Floyd, R.; Vergnes, L.; Zhao, Y.; Che, N.; Charugundla, S.; et al. Integration of multi-omics data from mouse diversity panel highlights mitochondrial dysfunction in non-alcoholic fatty liver disease. *Cell Syst.* **2018**, *6*, 103–115.e107. [CrossRef] [PubMed]

93. Sobaniec-Lotowska, M.E.; Lebensztejn, D.M. Ultrastructure of hepatocyte mitochondria in nonalcoholic steatohepatitis in pediatric patients: Usefulness of electron microscopy in the diagnosis of the disease. *Am. J. Gastroenterol.* **2003**, *98*, 1664–1665. [CrossRef] [PubMed]

94. Kimura, S.; Hase, K.; Ohno, H. The molecular basis of induction and formation of tunneling nanotubes. *Cell Tissue Res.* **2013**, *352*, 67–76. [CrossRef]

95. Rustom, A.; Saffrich, R.; Markovic, I.; Walther, P.; Gerdes, H.H. Nanotubular highways for intercellular organelle transport. *Science* **2004**, *303*, 1007–1010. [CrossRef]

96. Jash, E.; Prasad, P.; Kumar, N.; Sharma, T.; Goldman, A.; Sehrawat, S. Perspective on nanochannels as cellular mediators in different disease conditions. *Cell Commun. Signal. Ccs* **2018**, *16*, 76. [CrossRef]

97. Moravcova, A.; Cervinkova, Z.; Kucera, O.; Mezera, V.; Rychtrmoc, D.; Lotkova, H. The effect of oleic and palmitic acid on induction of steatosis and cytotoxicity on rat hepatocytes in primary culture. *Physiol. Res.* **2015**, *64*, S627–S636. [CrossRef] [PubMed]

98. Caballero, F.; Fernandez, A.; Matias, N.; Martinez, L.; Fucho, R.; Elena, M.; Caballeria, J.; Morales, A.; Fernandez-Checa, J.C.; Garcia-Ruiz, C. Specific contribution of methionine and choline in nutritional nonalcoholic steatohepatitis: Impact on mitochondrial s-adenosyl-l-methionine and glutathione. *J. Biol. Chem.* **2010**, *285*, 18528–18536. [CrossRef] [PubMed]

99. Alijani, N.; Johari, B.; Moradi, M.; Kadivar, M. A review on transcriptional regulation responses to hypoxia in mesenchymal stem cells. *Cell Biol. Int.* **2020**, *44*, 14–26. [CrossRef] [PubMed]

100. Newell, C.; Sabouny, R.; Hittel, D.S.; Shutt, T.E.; Khan, A.; Klein, M.S.; Shearer, J. Mesenchymal stem cells shift mitochondrial dynamics and enhance oxidative phosphorylation in recipient cells. *Front. Physiol.* **2018**, *9*, 1572. [CrossRef]

101. Marlein, C.R.; Piddock, R.E.; Mistry, J.J.; Zaitseva, L.; Hellmich, C.; Horton, R.H.; Zhou, Z.; Auger, M.J.; Bowles, K.M.; Rushworth, S.A. Cd38-driven mitochondrial trafficking promotes bioenergetic plasticity in multiple myeloma. *Cancer Res.* **2019**, *79*, 2285–2297. [CrossRef]

102. Jackson, M.V.; Morrison, T.J.; Doherty, D.F.; McAuley, D.F.; Matthay, M.A.; Kissenpfennig, A.; O'Kane, C.M.; Krasnodembskaya, A.D. Mitochondrial transfer via tunneling nanotubes is an important mechanism by which mesenchymal stem cells enhance macrophage phagocytosis in the in vitro and in vivo models of ards. *Stem Cells* **2016**, *34*, 2210–2223. [CrossRef]

103. Zhang, Y.; Yu, Z.; Jiang, D.; Liang, X.; Liao, S.; Zhang, Z.; Yue, W.; Li, X.; Chiu, S.M.; Chai, Y.H.; et al. Ipsc-mscs with high intrinsic miro1 and sensitivity to tnf-alpha yield efficacious mitochondrial transfer to rescue anthracycline-induced cardiomyopathy. *Stem Cell Rep.* **2016**, *7*, 749–763. [CrossRef]

104. Ahmad, T.; Mukherjee, S.; Pattnaik, B.; Kumar, M.; Singh, S.; Kumar, M.; Rehman, R.; Tiwari, B.K.; Jha, K.A.; Barhanpurkar, A.P.; et al. Miro1 regulates intercellular mitochondrial transport & enhances mesenchymal stem cell rescue efficacy. *EMBO J.* **2014**, *33*, 994–1010.

105. Han, D.; Zheng, X.; Wang, X.; Jin, T.; Cui, L.; Chen, Z. Mesenchymal stem/stromal cell-mediated mitochondrial transfer and the therapeutic potential in treatment of neurological diseases. *Stem Cells Int.* **2020**, *2020*, 8838046. [CrossRef]

106. Christ, B.; Dollinger, M.M. The generation of hepatocytes from mesenchymal stem cells and engraftment into the liver. *Curr. Opin. Organ Transplant.* **2011**, *16*, 69–75. [CrossRef]

107. Neumann, E. Kraftwerke unserer Zellen. *Top Life Aktuell* **2010**, *1005*. Available online: http://www.toplife.at/gesundheit/artikel172.html (accessed on 30 June 2020).

108. Kraft, E.; Stickl, H. Comparative measurement of the growth of rat liver by means of square grid and leitz' integration table on histological slices. *Virchows Archiv Fur Pathol. Anat. und Physiol. und fur Klin. Med.* **1954**, *324*, 650–661. [CrossRef] [PubMed]

4

Telomeres, NAFLD and Chronic Liver Disease

Benedetta Donati and Luca Valenti *

Department of Pathophysiology and Transplantation, Università degli Studi di Milano,
Fondazione IRCCS Ca' Granda Ospedale Policlinico Milano, 20122 Milano, Italy; benedetta.donati@unimi.it
* Correspondence: luca.valenti@unimi.it

Academic Editors: Amedeo Lonardo and Giovanni Targher

Abstract: Telomeres consist of repeat DNA sequences located at the terminal portion of chromosomes that shorten during mitosis, protecting the tips of chromosomes. During chronic degenerative conditions associated with high cell replication rate, progressive telomere attrition is accentuated, favoring senescence and genomic instability. Several lines of evidence suggest that this process is involved in liver disease progression: (a) telomere shortening and alterations in the expression of proteins protecting the telomere are associated with cirrhosis and hepatocellular carcinoma; (b) advanced liver damage is a feature of a spectrum of genetic diseases impairing telomere function, and inactivating germline mutations in the telomerase complex (including *human Telomerase Reverse Transcriptase (hTERT)* and *human Telomerase RNA Component (hTERC)*) are enriched in cirrhotic patients independently of the etiology; and (c) experimental models suggest that telomerase protects from liver fibrosis progression. Conversely, reactivation of telomerase occurs during hepatocarcinogenesis, allowing the immortalization of the neoplastic clone. The role of telomere attrition may be particularly relevant in the progression of nonalcoholic fatty liver, an emerging cause of advanced liver disease. Modulation of telomerase or shelterins may be exploited to prevent liver disease progression, and to define specific treatments for different stages of liver disease.

Keywords: telomere; telomerase; liver disease progression; nonalcoholic fatty liver disease; cirrhosis; hepatocellular carcinoma

1. Introduction

In humans, telomeres consist of thousands copies of six base repeats (TTAGGG) located at the extremities of the chromosomes that protect chromosomes tips from end-to-end fusion, rearrangement and translocation. Telomere length is progressively shortened at each mitosis, due to the inability of the DNA polymerase complex to replicate the very 5′ end of the lagging strand (attrition). For this reason, telomere shortening may function as a "mitotic clock" to sense somatic cells aging. When telomeres become critically short, a DNA-damage program is activated, leading to apoptosis or cell senescence. On the contrary, immortal cells (cancer, stem and germ cells) constitutionally express telomerase, a ribonuclear enzymatic complex associated with telomeres that is responsible for stabilizing telomere length by synthesizing new DNA sequences and adding them to the end of the chromosomes during DNA replication [1]. Telomerase comprises two essential components: Telomerase reverse transcriptase (hTERT) and its RNA template, the telomerase RNA component (hTERC). Dyskerin complex binds to hTERC, in order to protect it and to stabilize the telomerase complex. It includes four nucleolar proteins: Dyskerin (DKC1) and Nucleolar protein family A member 1, 2 and 3 (NOLA1-NOLA2-NOLA3) [2–4]. Besides telomerase, the Shelterin complex, which binds specifically to telomeres, plays a fundamental role in the protection of chromosome ends facilitating telomerase-based telomere elongation [5]. It is composed of six core proteins: the telomeric repeat binding factors 1 and 2 (TRF1-TRF2) that bind telomeric double strand DNA, the protection of telomeres

1 (POT1), which binds the 3′ telomeric region of single strand DNA avoiding the degradation by nuclease, and the TRF-1 interacting protein 2 (TIN2), the POT1-TIN2 organizing protein (TPP1) and the repressor/activator protein 1 (RAP1), that interact with the other proteins bound to telomere stabilizing the complex (Figure 1; [6,7]). Mutations of proteins involved in maintenance and repair of telomeres are responsible for telomeropathies [8,9]: a spectrum of progressive genetic diseases exemplified in the most severe cases by dyskeratosis congenita (DKC), whose common autosomal recessive form is caused by mutations in *DKC1*. They are degenerative and age-dependent diseases, characterized by premature senescence of the stem cell compartment, determining increased risk of organ failure and cancer, with possible involvement of the hematopoietic compartment, lungs, mucous membranes, skin, and also the liver. Consistently, loss-of-function mutations in *hTERT* and *hTERC* may cause a spectrum of familial liver diseases [10]. Telomere length is a strong hereditable tract and telomere shortening is accentuated in chronic degenerative condition associated with high cell replication rate. Thus, involvement of telomeres and telomerase mutations seems to be important in predisposition to liver disease progression towards hepatocellular carcinoma (HCC). Indeed, the incidence of HCC increases with age, and, in particular, in nonalcoholic fatty liver disease (NAFLD), where there is a strong aggregation of familial cases [11].

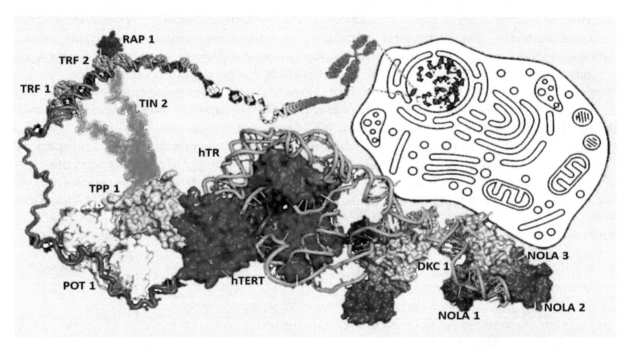

Figure 1. Model representing the telomeres associated proteins. Telomerase (including hTERT (**red**) and hTERC (**green**)) represents the principal catalytic subunit. The Shelterin complex is anchored by binding of the proteins TRF1 and TRF2 to double-stranded telomeric repeats. TRF1 and TRF2 are bridged to the single-stranded telomeric-repeat G-strand DNA-binding protein POT1 through TIN2 and TPP1. Additionally, shelterin RAP1 binds directly to TRF2. Dyskerin complex involving NOLA proteins, interacts and stabilizes the non-overlapping regions of hTERC.

2. Telomerase and Telomere Diseases

2.1. Telomere Shortening Related to Cellular Senescence Characterizes Human Cirrhosis

The role of ageing in liver fibrosis progression has been largely demonstrated, and older age and duration of liver disease remain the major and more validated risk factors for liver disease progression, together with male gender and alcohol abuse [12,13]. Cellular ageing is generally referred to as replicative senescence, a condition strictly linked to telomerase and telomere biology. Indeed, telomere shortening limited the replicative capacity of cells and the number of cells participating in tissue regeneration. Thus, the regenerative potential of an organ depends on the size of the population of cells with sufficient telomere reserves required for cell proliferation. Consistently, in chronic disease associated with tissue regeneration, such as cirrhosis, an elevated regenerative pressure is generated on the proliferating subpopulation of cells, which undergoes several rounds of cell division that, in turn, accelerate the rate of telomere shortening [14]. When telomeres become critically short, a DNA damage program is activated, leading to cell senescence or apoptosis (due to the Hayflick limit), further reducing the number of cell with regenerative capacity.

Several lines of evidence correlate shortened telomeres with liver fibrosis. Kitada *et al.* [15] first described a progressive reduction of telomere length during liver disease progression. Urabe *et al.* [16] confirmed these data and described telomerase re-activation in poorly differentiated HCC, consistently with an increase of telomere length compared to those well differentiated. In the normal liver, progressive telomere shortening has been correlated with age. Consistently, reduction of telomere length in cirrhotic tissue was more marked in patients who developed cirrhosis at younger age [17]. Additionally, reduction of telomere length is considered a hallmark of cirrhotic tissue independently of the etiology of liver disease (e.g., viral hepatitis, autoimmune hepatitis, alcohol abuse . . .) [18]. Thus, excessive telomere shortening, caused either by telomerase gene mutations or acquired factors, may impair the hepatocyte regenerative ability in response to chronic injury, facilitating fibrosis progression [19,20]. A causal role of telomere shortening in fibrosis progression has been experimentally demonstrated in telomerase deficient mice. After three generations, these mice developed shortened telomeres and displayed diminished capacity for liver regeneration, and with accelerated development of cirrhosis after liver injury. On the contrary, overexpression of TERT activity improved liver function and protected mice from development of hepatic steatosis and fibrosis [21].

Consistently, shortened telomere length in cirrhotic patients was correlated with the expression of known markers of cellular senescence, such as β-galactosidase, p16, p21 and p53 not only in hepatocytes but also in non-parenchymal cells, such as biliary cells [22,23]. The p53 protein represents the key regulator point for various signaling pathways of senescence: p53 phosphorylation and consequent activation inhibits cell division primarily inducing p21 expression, which, in turn, activates pRb through inhibition of a cyclin-dependent kinase (Cdk) complex. The activated pRb inhibits the transcription of E2F target genes that are required for cell cycle progression. pRB can alternatively be activated by p16, another Cdk inhibitor, that typically accumulates in senescent cells [23].

Cellular senescence may have a dual role in liver disease: in a first phase, it seems to contribute to liver impairment by reducing the hepatocytes and progenitor cell population, while, in a second phase, the subsequent senescence of HSC (epatic stellate cells) due to long-standing activation of fibrogenesis may protect from further fibrosis progression [24–26]. In particular, progression of human fibrosis is often characterized by a state of chronic inflammation that results in a condition of cell death and tissue regeneration, involving also a massive expansion of hepatic progenitor cells in order to restore the lost hepatocytes. Ductular reaction typical of this condition has been shown to produce chemotactic stimuli for induction of inflammatory cells and activation of pro-fibrotic hepatic stellate cells (HSC). Moreover, due to the epithelial to mesenchymal transition, progenitors and biliary epithelial cells may provide a portion of myofibroblasts, contributing to fibrosis progression [27]. When the wound is filled, the activated HSC undergo apoptosis or cellular senescence and consequently are eliminated by immune cells. In this way, HSC induce the recruitment of other immune cells at the site of tissue injury that, in turn, help in arresting liver fibrosis progression. However, it has recently been shown that later, senescent HSC may favor HCC development by secreting pro-carcinogenic mediators (the senescence associated secretory program: SASP) [28].

2.2. Telomerase Mutations Are Hallmarks of Liver Fibrosis

Genetic studies have proven that mutations in telomerase represent the underlying cause of accelerated telomere shortening and organ failure in some rare human diseases, including some forms of DKC [29], which may be characterized by liver injury and development of complications of portal hypertension. Moreover, evidence suggests that telomere attrition is also involved in liver disease progression in humans. Indeed, a spectrum of familial liver disease with autosomal dominant transmission and incomplete penetrance has been associated with inheritance of *hTERT* and *hTERC* mutations [10,30]. In these pedigrees, liver disease was characterized by development of steatosis, with possible progression to cirrhosis and HCC. Furthermore, a significant enrichment of missense mutations in the *hTERT* and *hTERC* genes was observed in 7% of patients and one patient, respectively, of a US cohort including 134 patients with cirrhosis of different etiologies (NAFLD, but also alcohol abuse and Hepatitis C virus infection), as compared to healthy controls. These mutations impaired hTERT enzymatic activity, as they were associated with reduced telomere length in the peripheral blood of patients and reduced telomerase activity *in vitro* [19]. These data were substantially confirmed in a larger series of 521 German patients with cirrhosis, of whom 3% carried functional *hTERT* mutations again independently from the etiology of the liver disease [31]. These observations indicate that, in at least a proportion of patients who developed cirrhosis, fibrosis progression may be favored by genetic risk variants facilitating telomere shortening and cell senescence in the presence of triggering factors.

2.3. Telomere Shortening Induces Genomic Instability in Hepatocellular Carcinoma (HCC)

Thus, telomere shortening is a hallmark of cirrhosis, the main risk factor for the development of liver cancer [32]. The state of chronic inflammation characteristic of injured liver, results *per se* in oxidative DNA damage leading to genomic and epigenomic alterations, pushing cells toward a malignant phenotype. Deregulation of key oncogenes and tumor-suppressor genes, such as *TP53*, *β-catenin, ErbB receptor family members* and *p16(INK4a)* have been observed both in early and advance HCC. Impaired function of p53 most likely induces alterations in DNA damage response machinery, resulting in loss of DNA repairing and avoiding cellular apoptosis, thus contributing to an increased mutation rate. Moreover, aberrant DNA methylation patterns have been reported in the earliest stages of hepatocarcinogenesis, and to a greater extent in tumor progression. Finally, karyotypic analysis of HCCs revealed that recurrent regions of copy number change and allelic imbalances are present in 90% of cases, thus highlighting the possibility for new cancer gene targets reside in these loci [33,34]. In this context, telomere shortening may favor carcinogenesis by directly facilitating genomic instability. Telomere shortening plays a pivotal role in inducing genomic alteration first favoring chromosomes segregation defect. Indeed, shortened telomeres have been associated with the typical karyotipic alterations in HCC (chromosome 8 alterations), especially in the presence of *TP53* mutations [33,35].

Moreover, loss of *hTERT* has been shown to affect the overall configuration of chromatin and to diminish the capacity for DNA repair of double strand breaks (DSB) [36]. Therefore, current data suggest a model whereby telomere shortening drives chromosomal instability during early stages of hepatic carcinogenesis, while telomerase re-activation is involved in malignant progression, as it restores chromosomal stability necessary for cellular immortalization.

2.4. Elongation of Telomeres and Telomerase Complex Reactivation during Advance Hepatocarcinogenesis

While the majority of tumors display shortened telomeres compared to non-neoplastic tissues, nevertheless telomere lengthening has been observed in various tumors at advanced stage, including colorectal, and head and neck cancers [37]. In HCC tissues, long telomeres and increased telomerase activity were also shown to be a significant reflection of poor prognostic factors, associated with clinicopathological features of aggressive behavior [38]. Indeed, HCC tumor progression is associated with the reactivation of telomerase, which is necessary for the immortalization of the neoplastic clone [39,40]. Accordingly, *hTERT* was found upregulated in dysplastic liver nodules and to be more than 10-fold induced in overt HCC tissue compared to the surrounding non-neoplastic tissue [41] independently from the etiology of liver disease [42].

On the contrary, a specific gene signature of the Shelterin complex has been identified for each cause of liver disease. Indeed, Shelterin overexpressed in HCC developed upon HCV infection or in the presence of alcohol abuse, and displayed a diminished expression in HCC developed upon

HBV infection [5]. In particular, longer telomeres have been observed in HCCs expressing markers of stemness, such as CK19, EpCAM and CD133, generally considered more aggressive than the conventional, negative for these markers [43,44]. It is known that there is heterogeneity in the expression patterns of stemness-related markers within the same tumors. Interestingly, the analysis of telomere length among different cells according to EpCAM expression status has shown that longer telomeres were present in HCC tumor cells that expressed EpCAM, compared to tumor cells that were EpCAM-negative [45]. Additionally, stemness–related markers were correlated with the expression of the Shelterin proteins. Increased TPP1, TRF2, RAP1, and POT1 expression were observed in HCC tissues expressing "stemness"-related markers compared to conventional HCCs, and their expression was correlated with poorer prognosis and reduced disease-free survival [45]. On the other hand, shortened telomeres and low POT1 expression have been observed in HCCs expressing HepPar1, a marker of hepatocytes differentiation. Additionally, Kim *et al.* [46] demonstrated that TPP1 expression was correlated with hTERT expression, supporting previous findings indicating TPP1 as a positive regulator of telomere maintenance that may represent a good target for cancer therapy as it plays a dominant role in the recruitment of hTERT to telomeres.

Elongation of telomere may also be due to higher expression of DKC1 in HCC compared to noncancerous liver tissue where the level of the protein was absent or very low. DKC1 expression has been validated as an independent risk factor for adverse overall mortality, and it was correlated with advanced HCC clinical stage (grade III–IV) and recurrence independently of hTERT expression [47]. Considering that *DKC1* is the direct and conserved transcriptional target of c-myc responsible for proliferative activity of cancer cells [48], this suggests that the role of DKC1 on cancer progression may be independent of its involvement in telomerase complex function.

Additionally, elongation of telomeres in 7% of HCC cases is associated with alternative lengthening of telomeres (ALT), the telomerase-independent telomere maintenance mechanism, which is thought to be dependent on homologous recombination. The ALT-positive cells are characterized by telomere length heterogeneity, as well as increased chromosomal instability [49].

2.5. Mechanisms of Reactivation of Telomerase in HCC Tissue

Several mechanisms have been shown to lead to telomerase activation during hepatic carcinogenesis. *hTERT* promoter mutations have been described as the most frequent somatic genetic alteration in HCC, with an overall frequency of 60% in Western countries, in particular in patients with chronic HCV infection [50,51]. Interestingly, these somatic mutations occur not only in cancer tissue but in 6%–19% of the cases have been observed also in the early cirrhotic tissue, while usually somatic mutations in oncogene or oncosuppressor genes occur in a more advanced stage of tumorigenesis [51,52]. These promoter mutations represent the most important mechanism of reactivation of telomerase during hepatocarcinogenesis. Indeed, they create new binding sites for specific transcription factors, which consequently induce hTERT overexpression [53,54]. No promoter mutations have been individuated in studies involving cholangiocarcinoma [52] and hepatoblastoma [55], while a minority of patients affected by hepatocholangiocarcinoma presented these kinds of mutations. This evidence suggests that telomerase involvement is dependent on the origin of the cancer cells [56]. In HCC, due to HBV infection, the reactivation of telomerase is generally due to the insertion of the HBV virus in *hTERT* gene, more frequently in the promoter [57,58]. Integration of HBV was detected in 22% of the HBV positive samples, whereas *hTERT* focal amplification, another mechanism likely inducing increased telomerase activity, in 6.7% of the cases. In the same study, *hTERT* promoter mutations were mutually exclusive with HBV genome integration in the *hTERT* locus and were almost mutually exclusive with *hTERT* focal amplifications [59].

2.6. Telomerase Promotes Hepatic Carcinogenesis by Multiple Pathways

Besides telomere protection and maintenance, several *in vitro* and *in vivo* studies in which *hTERT* has been exogenously expressed revealed novel telomerase functions in tumorigenesis independently of *hTERC* [60]. First, hTERT can act as a transcription factor in the Wnt-β-catenin signaling pathway, regulating the expression of Wnt target genes, which play a role in tumorigenesis. Indeed, hTERT interacts with BRG1, a chromatin remodeler binding to β-catenin and involved in the Wnt signaling [61], and promotes the expression of several β-catenin target genes in a BRG1-dependent way. Consistently, *hTERT* was found to interact with the same promoter elements recognized by BRG1 and β-catenin [62]. Actually, the relationship between hTERT and the Wnt-β-catenin pathway is bidirectional: indeed, *β-catenin* deficient human cell lines showed shorter telomere and reduced telomerase activity, and *hTERT* appears as a direct target of β-catenin through the binding to TCF4 transcription factor [63]. Furthermore, hTERT and BRG1 interact with nucleostemin, a GTP-binding protein overexpressed in stem cells and cancers [64], which is essential to drive transcriptional programs relevant for the maintenance of the cancer stem cells phenotype [65]. In this case, hTERT contributes to tumorigenesis increasing the proportion of stem cells within a tumor.

Further functions of hTERT in tumorigenesis are related to its localization in mitochondria. Here, telomerase plays a role as an RNA-dependent RNA polymerase (RdRP) paired to a mitochondrial non-coding RNA, the mitochondrial RNA processing endoribonuclease (RMRP) [66]. hTERT represents the only RdRP identified in mammals and hTERT-RMRP complex leads to the production of double-stranded RMRP RNA molecules, subsequently processed into 22-nucleotide siRNAs by RNA-induced silencing complex (RISC) [66]. Since RMRP has several cellular functions, including mRNA cleavage of cell cycle genes [67], hTERT may influence cellular proliferation, both increasing cell division and reducing apoptosis, independently of activation of Wnt signaling.

Finally, hTERT can increase cancer cell fitness, improving mitochondrial activity and resistance to apoptosis. Indeed, mt-TERT, through its reverse transcriptase domain, can provide mt-DNA replication and repair using mt-tRNAs as the template [68]. Additionally, Sahin *et al.* [60,69] noticed that *Tert* and *Terc* late generation knockout mice showed a p53-mediated repression of peroxisome proliferator-activated receptor gγ coactivator-1 α and β (Pgc-1α and Pgc-1β), the master regulators of mitochondrial physiology and metabolism, resulting in altered mitochondrial biogenesis and function and increased reactive oxygen species.

2.7. Telomeres and Nonalcoholic Fatty Liver Disease (NAFLD)

Following the epidemic of obesity and type 2 diabetes, NAFLD is becoming the most frequent liver disease in Western countries. Established risk factors for disease progression in NAFLD include older age and presence of features of the metabolic syndrome, such as obesity, insulin resistance, and hypertension. However, progression of liver disease to cirrhosis and HCC is generally limited to the subgroup of patients who developed non-alcoholic steatohepatitis (NASH), a condition characterized by active inflammation and fibrosis [70]. Genetic factors have also been shown to influence disease progression in NAFLD. Besides the most validated factors influencing lipid metabolism, such as the I148M variant of *PNPLA3*, the influence of variants involved in fibrogenesis has recently been described.

Genetic data indicate that NAFLD is commonly observed in patients with telomeropathies, suggesting that steatosis may either be a consequence of hepatocellular senescence, as also observed in animal models, or a trigger for liver disease progression [10,21]. Fibrosis stage and liver disease progression are also strictly linked to cell senescence. Consistently, hepatocyte expression of p21, playing a pivotal role in the induction and maintenance of cellular senescence, was associated with fibrosis stage in NAFLD and increase liver related morbidity and mortality [71]. Additionally, the rs762623 variant in the promoter region of *Cyclin-dependent Kinase 1A (CDKN1A)* gene, encoding for p21 protein, was associated with the development but not the progression of fibrosis in NAFLD independently from well-recognized *PNPLA3* I148M status [72]. This polymorphism has been associated with reduced p21 expression by abolishing an E2F transcription factor binding site. Thereby these data suggest that *CDKN1A* rs762623 G > A polymorphism favors HSC proliferation by limiting p21 induction, due to DNA damage and telomere shortening, but it may not predispose to severe fibrosis because it antagonizes cellular senescence [73]. Interestingly, *CDKN1A* variants have previously been described in association with rapid progression of idiopathic pulmonary fibrosis, another degenerative condition characterized by cellular senescence and impairment of telomeres [74].

Telomere attrition may also be involved in mediating cancer susceptibility in NAFLD. We reported the occurrence of HCC in NAFLD in a family where a novel missense *hTERT* mutation was segregated with idiopathic familial pulmonary fibrosis and NAFLD. This rare Glu668Asp variant located in the motif 3c of the reverse transcriptase domain of the protein likely led to reduced telomeres length by directly interfering with hTERT enzymatic activity [75]. This finding suggested us to investigate the presence of *hTERT* germline coding mutations in a cohort of patients who developed HCC without recognized risk factors (cryptogenic) or were affected only by NAFLD, which, in the absence of other predisposing conditions, is *per se* a relatively weak risk factor for progressive liver disease. We observed a highly significant enrichment of germline coding mutations in NAFLD HCC. In fact, 10% of NASH HCC were carriers of mutations, while no mutations were identified in 30 NASH cirrhosis and in healthy controls. The rare mutations modifying the sequence of the protein identified (three missense and one frameshift) were located in the N-terminal domain of interaction with hTERC or in the catalytic domain, likely impairing the activity of the telomerase complex. However, the relatively small number of patients analyzed did not allow for correlation of the presence of *hTERT* mutations with HCC prognosis. Additionally, in the same study, we found that telomeres are progressively shortened in peripheral blood leukocytes of NAFLD HCC patients compared to cirrhosis and controls [76]. These data point out a possible causal role for telomere attrition and telomerase mutations in influencing susceptibility towards HCC in NAFLD patients. As telomere shortening was not always correlated with the presence of *hTERT* mutations, this suggests that mutations in other genes contributing to the maintenance of telomeres or epigenetic mechanisms may result in a similar phenotype (genetic heterogeneity) and contribute to the phenotypic expression of heterozygous *hTERT* mutations.

3. Conclusions

Telomeres and telomerase play an important role in the onset and progression of liver disease independently of the underlying etiology. However, the role of telomere attrition and cell senescence is most likely magnified in NAFLD, where genetic risk factors and ageing have a large impact on the predisposition to advanced liver damage in combination with acquired risk factors. The role of telomeres in the pathogenesis of liver disease may be explained by the following hypothesis. Triggering factors, such as obesity and insulin resistance in the case of NAFLD, induce a condition of chronic hepatic damage and regeneration characterized by progressive hepatocytes telomere shortening and senescence. When hepatocytes reach senescence, liver regeneration decreases, but chronic damage remains. Concomitantly, other cell types, such as HSCs, become activated and form fibrotic tissue in area of hepatocyte loss. In this context, germline *hTERT* loss-of-function mutations accelerate telomere shortening, favoring fibrosis development and thus creating a favorable microenvironment for cancer onset. Moreover, telomere attrition and germline *hTERT* loss-of-function mutations may exert a direct pro-carcinogenic effect by promoting genomic instability, both inducing telomere shortening and impairing telomerase activity in DNA repair and chromatin organization [36]. Within this context, the presence of heterozygous mutations does not prevent the reactivation of the telomerase wild type allele at later stages of carcinogenesis, which is necessary for the indefinite replication of the neoplastic clone (Figure 2).

Several studies suggest the use of telomerase inhibitors for HCC treatment. These molecules will hopefully be able to arrest early tumor growth by blocking telomerase, having an almost immediate effect since they likely act on a phenotype of still short telomeres [77]. Moreover, they could arrest inflammatory and HSC telomerase activity, and, consequently, telomere elongation, which has been described as a feature of cirrhotic tissue surrounding tumors [18], thus having a beneficial effect both on the cirrhotic and the cancer tissue. Additionally, inhibition of telomerase may enhance chemosensitivity of cancer cells to chemotherapeutic agents [78]. *Vice versa*, treatment based on molecules that activate telomerase may be useful at the first stage of liver disease and in patients carrying telomerase complex mutations, in order to permit tissue regeneration by avoiding hepatocyte telomere shortening and senescence. This could be exploited by transplantation of liver cells engineered for *hTERT* gene expression, by directly delivering hTERT to the organ, or by small molecules enhancing telomerase activity. However, to date, it is not known how to manage both the carcinogenic potential of *hTERT*-immortalized hepatocytes, and the hepatotoxicity linked to gene delivery [77].

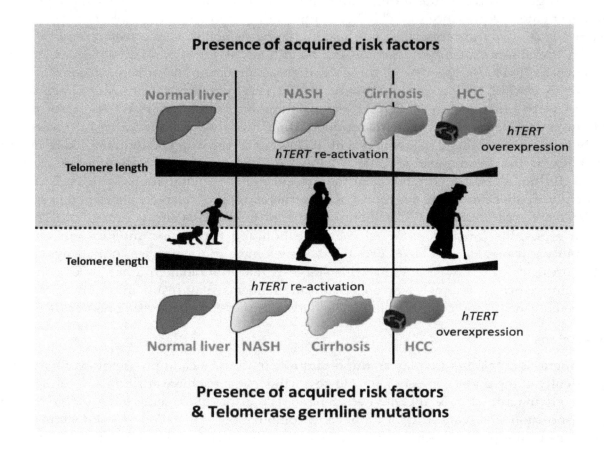

Figure 2. Hypothesis for telomeres' role in pathogenesis of nonalcoholic fatty liver disease (NAFLD) progression toward cirrhosis and hepatocellular carcinoma (HCC). The model shows that, in the presence of triggering acquired risk factors such as obesity and insulin resistance, the liver undergoes cycle of damage and regeneration that requires telomerase re-activation. However, degenerative chronic conditions lead to telomere shortening and fibrosis progression towards cirrhosis, the main risk factor for HCC. In carriers of telomerase germline loss-of-function mutations, this process is accelerated due to telomerase inability to elongate telomeres, thus impairing tissue regeneration. Moreover, telomerase mutations may have a direct pro-carcinogenic effect by inducing genomic instability. Finally, telomere re-elongation in cancer tissue was triggered by different mechanisms, among which, overexpression of *hTERT* is necessary for the immortalization of the neoplastic clone.

Interestingly, both the inhibition and the activation of telomerase may be useful in different stages of liver disease, and, at the same time, may have important side effects due also to the impairment of the physiological expression of this gene in other organs and tissues. Thus, how to act in order to modulate telomerase activity remains controversial. Further studies are necessary in order to better understand the impact of telomeres and telomerase on the different levels of liver disease progression, and consequently how to act to prevent telomerase related damage.

Abbreviations

The following abbreviations are used in this manuscript:

NAFLD	Non-alcoholic fatty liver disease
HCC	Hepatocellular carcinoma
hTERT	Human telomerase Reverse Transcriptase
hTERC	Human telomerase RNA Component
DKC1	Dyskerin
NOLA1-NOLA2- NOLA3	Nucleolar protein family A member 1, 2 and 3
TRF1-TRF2	Telomeric repeat- binding factors 1 and 2
POT1	Protection of telomeres 1
TIN2	TRF-1 interacting protein 2
TPP1	POT1-TIN2 organizing protein
RAP1	repressor/activator protein 1
pRb	Retinoblastoma 1
Cdk	Cyclin-dependent kinase
E2F	Transcription factor E2F
ErbB	Epidermal Growth Factor Receptor family members
INK4a	Cyclin-dependent kinase inhibitor 2A
K19	Keratin 19
EpCAM	Epithelial Cell Adhesion Molecule
ALT	Alternative Lengthening of Telomeres
BRG1	SWI/SNF related, matrix associated, actin dependent regulator of chromatin, subfamily a, member 4
TCF4	Transcription factor 4
RdRP	RNA-dependent RNA polymerase
RMRP	RNA component of mitochondrial RNA processing endoribonuclease
siRNA	Silencing RNA
RISC	RNA-induced silencing complex
Pgc-1α/β	Peroxisome proliferator-activated receptor γ coactivator-1 α/β
NASH	Non-alcoholic steatohepatitis
CDKN1A	Cyclin-dependent kinase inhibitor 1A

References

1. Blackburn, E.H. Structure and function of telomeres. *Nature* **1991**, *350*, 569–573. [CrossRef] [PubMed]
2. Egan, E.D.; Collins, K. Specificity and stoichiometry of subunit interactions in the human telomerase holoenzyme assembled *in vivo*. *Mol. Cell. Biol.* **2010**, *30*, 2775–2786. [CrossRef] [PubMed]
3. Reichow, S.L.; Hamma, T.; Ferre-D'Amare, A.R.; Varani, G. The structure and function of small nucleolar ribonucleoproteins. *Nucleic Acids Res.* **2007**, *35*, 1452–1464. [CrossRef] [PubMed]
4. Wang, C.; Meier, U.T. Architecture and assembly of mammalian H/ACA small nucleolar and telomerase ribonucleoproteins. *EMBO J.* **2004**, *23*, 1857–1867. [CrossRef] [PubMed]
5. El Idrissi, M.; Hervieu, V.; Merle, P.; Mortreux, F.; Wattel, E. Cause-specific telomere factors deregulation in hepatocellular carcinoma. *J. Exp. Clin. Cancer Res.* **2013**, *32*, 64. [CrossRef] [PubMed]
6. De Lange, T. Shelterin: The protein complex that shapes and safeguards human telomeres. *Genes Dev.* **2005**, *19*, 2100–2110. [CrossRef] [PubMed]
7. Xin, H.; Liu, D.; Wan, M.; Safari, A.; Kim, H.; Sun, W.; O'Connor, M.S.; Songyang, Z. TPP1 is a homologue of ciliate TEBP-β and interacts with POT1 to recruit telomerase. *Nature* **2007**, *445*, 559–562. [CrossRef] [PubMed]
8. Dokal, I. Dyskeratosis congenita. A disease of premature ageing. *Lancet* **2001**, *358*, S27. [CrossRef]
9. Calado, R.T.; Young, N.S. Telomere diseases. *N. Eng. J. Med.* **2009**, *361*, 2353–2365. [CrossRef] [PubMed]
10. Calado, R.T.; Regal, J.A.; Kleiner, D.E.; Schrump, D.S.; Peterson, N.R.; Pons, V.; Chanock, S.J.; Lansdorp, P.M.; Young, N.S. A spectrum of severe familial liver disorders associate with telomerase mutations. *PLoS ONE* **2009**, *4*, e7926. [CrossRef] [PubMed]

11.   Dongiovanni, P.; Romeo, S.; Valenti, L. Hepatocellular carcinoma in nonalcoholic fatty liver: Role of environmental and genetic factors. *World J. Gastroenterol.* **2014**, *20*, 12945–12955. [CrossRef] [PubMed]

12.   Pinzani, M. Pathophysiology of liver fibrosis. *Dig. Dis.* **2015**, *33*, 492–497. [CrossRef] [PubMed]

13.   Poynard, T.; Mathurin, P.; Lai, C.L.; Guyader, D.; Poupon, R.; Tainturier, M.H.; Myers, R.P.; Muntenau, M.; Ratziu, V.; Manns, M.; *et al.* A comparison of fibrosis progression in chronic liver diseases. *J. Hepatol.* **2003**, *38*, 257–265.

14.   Satyanarayana, A.; Wiemann, S.U.; Buer, J.; Lauber, J.; Dittmar, K.E.; Wustefeld, T.; Blasco, M.A.; Manns, M.P.; Rudolph, K.L. Telomere shortening impairs organ regeneration by inhibiting cell cycle re-entry of a subpopulation of cells. *EMBO J.* **2003**, *22*, 4003–4013. [CrossRef] [PubMed]

15.   Kitada, T.; Seki, S.; Kawakita, N.; Kuroki, T.; Monna, T. Telomere shortening in chronic liver diseases. *Biochem. Biophys. Res. Commun.* **1995**, *211*, 33–39. [CrossRef] [PubMed]

16.   Urabe, Y.; Nouso, K.; Higashi, T.; Nakatsukasa, H.; Hino, N.; Ashida, K.; Kinugasa, N.; Yoshida, K.; Uematsu, S.; Tsuji, T. Telomere length in human liver diseases. *Liver* **1996**, *16*, 293–297. [CrossRef] [PubMed]

17.   Aikata, H.; Takaishi, H.; Kawakami, Y.; Takahashi, S.; Kitamoto, M.; Nakanishi, T.; Nakamura, Y.; Shimamoto, F.; Kajiyama, G.; Ide, T. Telomere reduction in human liver tissues with age and chronic inflammation. *Exp. Cell Res.* **2000**, *256*, 578–582. [CrossRef] [PubMed]

18.   Wiemann, S.U.; Satyanarayana, A.; Tsahuridu, M.; Tillmann, H.L.; Zender, L.; Klempnauer, J.; Flemming, P.; Franco, S.; Blasco, M.A.; Manns, M.P.; *et al.* Hepatocyte telomere shortening and senescence are general markers of human liver cirrhosis. *FASEB J.* **2002**, *16*, 935–942. [CrossRef] [PubMed]

19.   Calado, R.T.; Brudno, J.; Mehta, P.; Kovacs, J.J.; Wu, C.; Zago, M.A.; Chanock, S.J.; Boyer, T.D.; Young, N.S. Constitutional telomerase mutations are genetic risk factors for cirrhosis. *Hepatology* **2011**, *53*, 1600–1607. [CrossRef] [PubMed]

20.   Chaiteerakij, R.; Roberts, L.R. Telomerase mutation: A genetic risk factor for cirrhosis. *Hepatology* **2011**, *53*, 1430–1432. [CrossRef] [PubMed]

21.   Rudolph, K.L.; Chang, S.; Millard, M.; Schreiber-Agus, N.; Depinho, R.A. Inhibition of experimental liver cirrhosis in mice by telomerase gene delivery. *Science* **2000**, *287*, 1253–1258. [CrossRef] [PubMed]

22.   Sasaki, M.; Ikeda, H.; Yamaguchi, J.; Nakada, S.; Nakanuma, Y. Telomere shortening in the damaged small bile ducts in primary biliary cirrhosis reflects ongoing cellular senescence. *Hepatology* **2008**, *48*, 186–195. [CrossRef] [PubMed]

23.   Gutierrez-Reyes, G.; del Carmen Garcia de Leon, M.; Varela-Fascinetto, G.; Valencia, P.; Perez Tamayo, R.; Rosado, C.G.; Labonne, B.F.; Rochilin, N.M.; Garcia, R.M.; Valadez, J.A.; *et al.* Cellular senescence in livers from children with end stage liver disease. *PLoS ONE* **2010**, *5*, e10231. [CrossRef]

24.   Krizhanovsky, V.; Yon, M.; Dickins, R.A.; Hearn, S.; Simon, J.; Miething, C.; Yee, H.; Zender, L.; Lowe, S.W. Senescence of activated stellate cells limits liver fibrosis. *Cell* **2008**, *134*, 657–667. [CrossRef] [PubMed]

25.   Schnabl, B.; Purbeck, C.A.; Choi, Y.H.; Hagedorn, C.H.; Brenner, D. Replicative senescence of activated human hepatic stellate cells is accompanied by a pronounced inflammatory but less fibrogenic phenotype. *Hepatology* **2003**, *37*, 653–664. [CrossRef] [PubMed]

26.   Ramakrishna, G.; Rastogi, A.; Trehanpati, N.; Sen, B.; Khosla, R.; Sarin, S.K. From cirrhosis to hepatocellular carcinoma: New molecular insights on inflammation and cellular senescence. *Liver Cancer* **2013**, *2*, 367–383. [CrossRef] [PubMed]

27.   Richardson, M.M.; Jonsson, J.R.; Powell, E.E.; Brunt, E.M.; Neuschwander-Tetri, B.A.; Bhathal, P.S.; Dixon, J.B.; Weltman, M.D.; Tilg, H.; Moschen, A.R.; *et al.* Progressive fibrosis in nonalcoholic steatohepatitis: Association with altered regeneration and a ductular reaction. *Gastroenterology* **2007**, *133*, 80–90. [CrossRef] [PubMed]

28.   Yoshimoto, S.; Loo, T.M.; Atarashi, K.; Kanda, H.; Sato, S.; Oyadomari, S.; Iwakura, Y.; Oshima, K.; Morita, H.; Hattori, M.; *et al.* Obesity-induced gut microbial metabolite promotes liver cancer through senescence secretome. *Nature* **2013**, *499*, 97–101. [CrossRef] [PubMed]

29.   Vulliamy, T.; Marrone, A.; Goldman, F.; Dearlove, A.; Bessler, M.; Mason, P.J.; Dokal, I. The RNA component of telomerase is mutated in autosomal dominant dyskeratosis congenita. *Nature* **2001**, *413*, 432–435. [CrossRef] [PubMed]

30.   Armanios, M.Y.; Chen, J.J.-L.; Cogan, J.D.; Alder, J.K.; Ingersoll, R.G.; Markin, C.; Lawson, W.E.; Xie, M.; Vulto, I.; Phillips, J.A.; *et al.* Telomerase Mutations in Families with Idiopathic Pulmonary Fibrosis. *N. Eng. J. Med.* **2007**, *356*, 1317–1326. [CrossRef] [PubMed]

31. Hartmann, D.; Srivastava, U.; Thaler, M.; Kleinhans, K.N.; N'Kontchou, G.; Scheffold, A.; Bauer, K.; Kratzer, R.F.; Kloos, N.; Katz, S.F.; *et al.* Telomerase gene mutations are associated with cirrhosis formation. *Hepatology* **2011**, *53*, 1608–1617. [CrossRef] [PubMed]

32. El-Serag, H.B.; Rudolph, K.L. Hepatocellular carcinoma: Epidemiology and molecular carcinogenesis. *Gastroenterology* **2007**, *132*, 2557–2576. [CrossRef] [PubMed]

33. Plentz, R.R.; Schlegelberger, B.; Flemming, P.; Gebel, M.; Kreipe, H.; Manns, M.P.; Rudolph, K.L.; Wilkens, L. Telomere shortening correlates with increasing aneuploidy of chromosome 8 in human hepatocellular carcinoma. *Hepatology* **2005**, *42*, 522–526. [CrossRef] [PubMed]

34. Farazi, P.A.; DePinho, R.A. Hepatocellular carcinoma pathogenesis: From genes to environment. *Nat. Rev. Cancer* **2006**, *6*, 674–687. [CrossRef] [PubMed]

35. Farazi, P.A.; Glickman, J.; Jiang, S.; Yu, A.; Rudolph, K.L.; DePinho, R.A. Differential impact of telomere dysfunction on initiation and progression of hepatocellular carcinoma. *Cancer Res.* **2003**, *63*, 5021–5027. [PubMed]

36. Masutomi, K.; Possemato, R.; Wong, J.M.; Currier, J.L.; Tothova, Z.; Manola, J.B.; Ganesan, S.; Lansdorp, P.M.; Collins, K.; Hahn, W.C. The telomerase reverse transcriptase regulates chromatin state and DNA damage responses. *Proc. Nat. Acad. Sci. USA* **2005**, *102*, 8222–8227. [CrossRef] [PubMed]

37. Plentz, R.R.; Wiemann, S.U.; Flemming, P.; Meier, P.N.; Kubicka, S.; Kreipe, H.; Manns, M.P.; Rudolph, K.L. Telomere shortening of epithelial cells characterises the adenoma-carcinoma transition of human colorectal cancer. *Gut* **2003**, *52*, 1304–1307.

38. Oh, B.K.; Kim, H.; Park, Y.N.; Yoo, J.E.; Choi, J.; Kim, K.S.; Lee, J.J.; Park, C. High telomerase activity and long telomeres in advanced hepatocellular carcinomas with poor prognosis. *Lab. Invest.* **2008**, *88*, 144–152.

39. Oh, B.K.; Jo Chae, K.; Park, C.; Kim, K.; Lee, W.J.; Han, K.H.; Park, Y.N. Telomere shortening and telomerase reactivation in dysplastic nodules of human hepatocarcinogenesis. *J. Hepatol.* **2003**, *39*, 786–792. [CrossRef]

40. Ju, Z.; Rudolph, K.L. Telomeres and telomerase in cancer stem cells. *Eur. J. Cancer* **2006**, *42*, 1197–1203. [CrossRef] [PubMed]

41. Llovet, J.M.; Chen, Y.; Wurmbach, E.; Roayaie, S.; Fiel, M.I.; Schwartz, M.; Thung, S.N.; Khitrov, G.; Zhang, W.; Villanueva, A.; *et al.* A molecular signature to discriminate dysplastic nodules from early hepatocellular carcinoma in HCV cirrhosis. *Gastroenterology* **2006**, *131*, 1758–1767. [CrossRef] [PubMed]

42. Saini, N.; Srinivasan, R.; Chawla, Y.; Sharma, S.; Chakraborti, A.; Rajwanshi, A. Telomerase activity, telomere length and human telomerase reverse transcriptase expression in hepatocellular carcinoma is independent of hepatitis virus status. *Liver Int.* **2009**, *29*, 1162–1170. [CrossRef] [PubMed]

43. Yamashita, T.; Forgues, M.; Wang, W.; Kim, J.W.; Ye, Q.; Jia, H.; Budhu, A.; Zanetti, K.A.; Chen, Y.; Qin, L.X.; *et al.* EpCAM and alpha-fetoprotein expression defines novel prognostic subtypes of hepatocellular carcinoma. *Cancer Res.* **2008**, *68*, 1451–1461. [CrossRef] [PubMed]

44. Kim, H.; Choi, G.H.; Na, D.C.; Ahn, E.Y.; Kim, G.I.; Lee, J.E.; Cho, J.Y.; Yoo, J.E.; Choi, J.S.; Park, Y.N. Human hepatocellular carcinomas with "Stemness"-related marker expression: Keratin 19 expression and a poor prognosis. *Hepatology* **2011**, *54*, 1707–1717. [CrossRef] [PubMed]

45. Kim, H.; Yoo, J.E.; Cho, J.Y.; Oh, B.K.; Yoon, Y.S.; Han, H.S.; Lee, H.S.; Jang, J.J.; Jeong, S.H.; Kim, J.W.; *et al.* Telomere length, TERT and shelterin complex proteins in hepatocellular carcinomas expressing "stemness"-related markers. *J. Hepatol.* **2013**, *59*, 746–752. [CrossRef] [PubMed]

46. Tejera, A.M.; Stagno d'Alcontres, M.; Thanasoula, M.; Marion, R.M.; Martinez, P.; Liao, C.; Flores, J.M.; Tarsounas, M.; Blasco, M.A. TPP1 is required for TERT recruitment, telomere elongation during nuclear reprogramming, and normal skin development in mice. *Dev. Cell* **2010**, *18*, 775–789. [CrossRef] [PubMed]

47. Liu, B.; Zhang, J.; Huang, C.; Liu, H. Dyskerin overexpression in human hepatocellular carcinoma is associated with advanced clinical stage and poor patient prognosis. *PLoS ONE* **2012**, *7*, e43147. [CrossRef] [PubMed]

48. Alawi, F.; Lee, M.N. DKC1 is a direct and conserved transcriptional target of c-MYC. *Biochem. Biophys. Res. Commun.* **2007**, *362*, 893–898. [CrossRef] [PubMed]

49. Heaphy, C.M.; Subhawong, A.P.; Hong, S.M.; Goggins, M.G.; Montgomery, E.A.; Gabrielson, E.; Netto, G.J.; Epstein, J.I.; Lotan, T.L.; Westra, W.H.; *et al.* Prevalence of the alternative lengthening of telomeres telomere maintenance mechanism in human cancer subtypes. *Am. J. Pathol.* **2011**, *179*, 1608–1615. [PubMed]

50. Cevik, D.; Yildiz, G.; Ozturk, M. Common telomerase reverse transcriptase promoter mutations in hepatocellular carcinomas from different geographical locations. *World J. Gastroenterol.* **2015**, *21*, 311–317. [CrossRef] [PubMed]

51. Nault, J.C.; Mallet, M.; Pilati, C.; Calderaro, J.; Bioulac-Sage, P.; Laurent, C.; Laurent, A.; Cherqui, D.; Balabaud, C.; Zucman-Rossi, J. High frequency of telomerase reverse-transcriptase promoter somatic mutations in hepatocellular carcinoma and preneoplastic lesions. *Nat. Commun.* **2013**, *4*, 2218. [CrossRef] [PubMed]

52. Quaas, A.; Oldopp, T.; Tharun, L.; Klingenfeld, C.; Krech, T.; Sauter, G.; Grob, T.J. Frequency of TERT promoter mutations in primary tumors of the liver. *Virchows Arch.* **2014**, *465*, 673–677. [CrossRef] [PubMed]

53. Horn, S.; Figl, A.; Rachakonda, P.S.; Fischer, C.; Sucker, A.; Gast, A.; Kadel, S.; Moll, I.; Nagore, E.; Hemminki, K.; *et al.* TERT promoter mutations in familial and sporadic melanoma. *Science* **2013**, *339*, 959–961. [CrossRef] [PubMed]

54. Huang, F.W.; Hodis, E.; Xu, M.J.; Kryukov, G.V.; Chin, L.; Garraway, L.A. Highly recurrent TERT promoter mutations in human melanoma. *Science* **2013**, *339*, 957–959. [CrossRef] [PubMed]

55. Eichenmuller, M.; Trippel, F.; Kreuder, M.; Beck, A.; Schwarzmayr, T.; Haberle, B.; Cairo, S.; Leuschner, I.; von Schweinitz, D.; Strom, T.M.; *et al.* The genomic landscape of hepatoblastoma and their progenies with HCC-like features. *J. Hepatol.* **2014**, *61*, 1312–1320. [CrossRef] [PubMed]

56. Nault, J.C.; Zucman-Rossi, J. TERT promoter mutations in primary liver tumors. *Clin. Res. Hepatol. Gastroenterol.* **2016**, *40*, 9–14. [CrossRef] [PubMed]

57. Paterlini-Brechot, P.; Saigo, K.; Murakami, Y.; Chami, M.; Gozuacik, D.; Mugnier, C.; Lagorce, D.; Brechot, C. Hepatitis B virus-related insertional mutagenesis occurs frequently in human liver cancers and recurrently targets human telomerase gene. *Oncogene* **2003**, *22*, 3911–3916. [CrossRef] [PubMed]

58. Sung, W.K.; Zheng, H.; Li, S.; Chen, R.; Liu, X.; Li, Y.; Lee, N.P.; Lee, W.H.; Ariyaratne, P.N.; Tennakoon, C.; *et al.* Genome-wide survey of recurrent HBV integration in hepatocellular carcinoma. *Nat. Genet.* **2012**, *44*, 765–769. [CrossRef] [PubMed]

59. Totoki, Y.; Tatsuno, K.; Covington, K.R.; Ueda, H.; Creighton, C.J.; Kato, M.; Tsuji, S.; Donehower, L.A.; Slagle, B.L.; Nakamura, H.; *et al.* Trans-ancestry mutational landscape of hepatocellular carcinoma genomes. *Nat. Gene.* **2014**, *46*, 1267–1273. [CrossRef] [PubMed]

60. Chiodi, I.; Mondello, C. Telomere-independent functions of telomerase in nuclei, cytoplasm, and mitochondria. *Front. Oncol.* **2012**, *2*, 133. [CrossRef] [PubMed]

61. Barker, N.; Hurlstone, A.; Musisi, H.; Miles, A.; Bienz, M.; Clevers, H. The chromatin remodelling factor BRG-1 interacts with β-catenin to promote target gene activation. *EMBO J.* **2001**, *20*, 4935–4943. [CrossRef] [PubMed]

62. Park, J.I.; Venteicher, A.S.; Hong, J.Y.; Choi, J.; Jun, S.; Shkreli, M.; Chang, W.; Meng, Z.; Cheung, P.; Ji, H.; *et al.* Telomerase modulates Wnt signalling by association with target gene chromatin. *Nature* **2009**, *460*, 66–72. [CrossRef] [PubMed]

63. Zhang, Y.; Toh, L.; Lau, P.; Wang, X. Human telomerase reverse transcriptase (hTERT) is a novel target of the Wnt/β-catenin pathway in human cancer. *J. Biol. Chem.* **2012**, *287*, 32494–32511. [CrossRef] [PubMed]

64. Tsai, R.Y.; McKay, R.D. A nucleolar mechanism controlling cell proliferation in stem cells and cancer cells. *Genes Dev.* **2002**, *16*, 2991–3003. [PubMed]

65. Okamoto, N.; Yasukawa, M.; Nguyen, C.; Kasim, V.; Maida, Y.; Possemato, R.; Shibata, T.; Ligon, K.L.; Fukami, K.; Hahn, W.C.; *et al.* Maintenance of tumor initiating cells of defined genetic composition by nucleostemin. *Proc. Nat. Acad. Sci. USA* **2011**, *108*, 20388–20393.

66. Maida, Y.; Yasukawa, M.; Furuuchi, M.; Lassmann, T.; Possemato, R.; Okamoto, N.; Kasim, V.; Hayashizaki, Y.; Hahn, W.C.; Masutomi, K. An RNA-dependent RNA polymerase formed by TERT and the RMRP RNA. *Nature* **2009**, *461*, 230–235. [CrossRef] [PubMed]

67. Esakova, O.; Krasilnikov, A.S. Of proteins and RNA: The RNase P/MRP family. *Rna* **2010**, *16*, 1725–1747. [CrossRef] [PubMed]

68. Sharma, N.K.; Reyes, A.; Green, P.; Caron, M.J.; Bonini, M.G.; Gordon, D.M.; Holt, I.J.; Santos, J.H. Human telomerase acts as a hTR-independent reverse transcriptase in mitochondria. *Nucleic Acids Res.* **2012**, *40*, 712–725. [CrossRef] [PubMed]

69. Sahin, E.; DePinho, R.A. Axis of ageing: Telomeres, p53 and mitochondria. *Nat. Rev. Mol. Cell Biol.* **2012**, *13*, 397–404. [CrossRef] [PubMed]

70.   Dongiovanni, P.; Valenti, L. Genetics of nonalcoholic fatty liver disease. *Metabolism* **2015**. (in press). [CrossRef] [PubMed]

71.   Aravinthan, A.; Scarpini, C.; Tachtatzis, P.; Verma, S.; Penrhyn-Lowe, S.; Harvey, R.; Davies, S.E.; Allison, M.; Coleman, N.; Alexander, G. Hepatocyte senescence predicts progression in non-alcohol-related fatty liver disease. *J. Hepatol.* **2013**, *58*, 549–556. [CrossRef] [PubMed]

72.   Aravinthan, A.; Mells, G.; Allison, M.; Leathart, J.; Kotronen, A.; Yki-Jarvinen, H.; Daly, A.K.; Day, C.P.; Anstee, Q.M.; Alexander, G. Gene polymorphisms of cellular senescence marker p21 and disease progression in non-alcohol-related fatty liver disease. *Cell Cycle* **2014**, *13*, 1489–1494.

73.   Valenti, L.; Dongiovanni, P. CDKN1A: A double-edged sword in fatty liver? *Cell Cycle* **2014**, *13*, 1371–1372. [CrossRef] [PubMed]

74.   Korthagen, N.M.; van Moorsel, C.H.; Barlo, N.P.; Kazemier, K.M.; Ruven, H.J.; Grutters, J.C. Association between variations in cell cycle genes and idiopathic pulmonary fibrosis. *PLoS ONE* **2012**, *7*, e30442. [CrossRef] [PubMed]

75.   Valenti, L.; Dongiovanni, P.; Maggioni, M.; Motta, B.M.; Rametta, R.; Milano, M.; Fargion, S.; Reggiani, P.; Fracanzani, A.L. Liver transplantation for hepatocellular carcinoma in a patient with a novel telomerase mutation and steatosis. *J. Hepatol.* **2013**, *58*, 399–401. [CrossRef] [PubMed]

76.   Donati, B.; Vanni, E.; Dongiovanni, P.; Iavarone, M.; Rametta, R.; Rosso, C.; Carnelutti, A.; Petta, S.; Fracanzani, A.L.; Reeves, H.L.; *et al.* O071: Telomerase reverse transcriptase mutations are associated with hepatocellular carcinoma in nash. *J. Hepatol.* **2015**, *62*, S226. [CrossRef]

77.   Lechel, A.; Manns, M.P.; Rudolph, K.L. Telomeres and telomerase: New targets for the treatment of liver cirrhosis and hepatocellular carcinoma. *J. Hepatol.* **2004**, *41*, 491–497. [CrossRef] [PubMed]

78.   Lee, K.H.; Rudolph, K.L.; Ju, Y.J.; Greenberg, R.A.; Cannizzaro, L.; Chin, L.; Weiler, S.R.; DePinho, R.A. Telomere dysfunction alters the chemotherapeutic profile of transformed cells. *Proc. Nat. Acad. Sci. USA* **2001**, *98*, 3381–3386. [CrossRef] [PubMed]

5

Different Serum Free Fatty Acid Profiles in NAFLD Subjects and Healthy Controls after Oral Fat Load

Roberto Gambino *, Elisabetta Bugianesi, Chiara Rosso, Lavinia Mezzabotta, Silvia Pinach, Natalina Alemanno, Francesca Saba and Maurizio Cassader

Department of Medical Sciences, University of Turin, C.so Dogliotti 14, 10126 Torino, Italy; elisabetta.bugianesi@unito.it (E.B.); crosso3@cittadellasalute.to.it (C.R.); lavinia.mezzabotta@unito.it (L.M.); silvia.pinach@unito.it (S.P.); natalina.alemanno@unito.it (N.A.); francescasaba85@yahoo.it (F.S.); maurizio.cassader@unito.it (M.C.)
* Correspondence: roberto.gambino@unito.it

Academic Editors: Amedeo Lonardo and Giovanni Targher

Abstract: Background: Free fatty acid (FFA) metabolism can impact on metabolic conditions, such as obesity and nonalcoholic fatty liver disease (NAFLD). This work studied the increase in total FFA shown in NAFLD subjects to possibly characterize which fatty acids significantly accounted for the whole increase. Methods: 21 patients with NAFLD were selected according to specified criteria. The control group consisted of nine healthy subjects. All subjects underwent an oral standard fat load. Triglycerides; cholesterol; FFA; glucose and insulin were measured every 2 h with the determination of fatty acid composition of FFA. Results: higher serum FFA levels in NAFLD subjects are mainly due to levels of oleic, palmitic and linoleic acids at different times. Significant increases were shown for docosahexaenoic acid, linolenic acid, eicosatrienoic acid, and arachidonic acid, although this was just on one occasion. In the postprandial phase, homeostatic model assessment HOMA index positively correlated with the ω3/ω6 ratio in NAFLD patients. Conclusions: the higher serum levels of FFA in NAFLD subjects are mainly due to levels of oleic and palmitic acids which are the most abundant circulating free fatty acids. This is almost exactly corresponded with significant increases in linoleic acid. An imbalance in the n-3/n-6 fatty acids ratio could modulate postprandial responses with more pronounced effects in insulin-resistant subjects, such as NAFLD patients.

Keywords: nonalcoholic fatty liver disease; free fatty acids; insulin resistance

---

1. Introduction

Free fatty acid (FFA) metabolism can widely impact on metabolic health. Several metabolic conditions, such as obesity, insulin resistance, type 2 diabetes, and non-alcoholic steatohepatitis, are associated with increased total concentrations of serum free fatty acids [1,2]. Nonalcoholic fatty liver disease (NAFLD) encompasses a spectrum of conditions characterized histologically by hepatic steatosis in individuals without significant alcohol consumption and negative viral, congenital and autoimmune liver disease markers. Hepatic lipid accumulation results from an imbalance between lipid availability and lipid disposal [3,4]. In this context, the composition of serum FFA has been poorly studied so far, especially in the postprandial state [5]. High levels of saturated fatty acids (SFA) were reported to increase coronary risk [6,7].

The liver is the main organ regulating fatty acid metabolism. Several sources supply the liver with a continuous flux of fatty acids [8]. In particular, in the fasting state free fatty acids coming from the lipolysis in adipose tissue fuel the liver. In the fed state, there are two major forms of dietary fatty acids which are available to the liver. In esterified forms, fatty acids are carried to the liver by triacylglycerol–rich chylomicron remnant particles and, as FFA, they stem from the so called spillover mechanism: in the spillover mechanism, FFA are released from chylomicron triacylglycerol by the activity of lipoprotein lipase (LPL, n. EC 3.1.1.34) in peripheral tissues, mainly adipose tissue [9]. Moreover, hepatic "*de novo*" lipogenesis (DNL) from non-lipid precursor increases the content of fatty acid in the liver.

After SFA exposure, *in vitro* experiments had shown that different cell types were induced to synthetize proinflammatory cytokines; they were more prone to apoptosis and had impaired insulin signaling [10,11]. By contrast, the exposure of monounsaturated fatty acids does not seem to trigger apoptosis [12]. Different signaling mechanisms were suggested in order to explain how SFA triggers apoptosis in hepatic cells. Endoplasmic reticulum (ER) stress, mitochondrial dysfunction, Jun N-terminal kinase (JNK) signaling and lipotoxicity are the main molecular mechanisms through which fatty acids exert their deleterious effects on the human metabolism. Wistar rats fed with a diet high in saturated fats showed liver damage and hepatic ER stress [13]. ER stress was due to a decreased fluidity of the lipid bilayer for abnormal incorporation of saturated phospholipids [14]. Excess of unesterified SFA is assembled into saturated phospholipid species leading to stiffening of cellular membranes [15]. Dysregulation of mitochondrial metabolism is due to an imbalance between the glycolytic fluxes and tricarboxylic acid (TCA) cycle since palmitate inhibits glycolytic flux and up regulates TCA cycle and anaplerotic fluxes [16]. The altered mitochondrial metabolism generates an elevated level of reacting oxygen species (ROS) stimulating apoptosis. An accelerated mitochondrial metabolism was observed in NAFLD patients [17]. Additionally, under either ER stress or oxidative stress, molecular signaling arises from JNK activation. Palmitate-induced JNK phosphorylation can be reversed in hepatic cells with administration of antioxidants [18]. SFA shows also a high degree of lipotoxicity. For instance, ceramide synthesis was associated with apoptosis in a hemopoietic precursor cell line [19] and with insulin resistance [20]. In this context, circulating FFAs, which should provide the substrate for triacylglycerol formation, may turn out to be cytotoxic in certain circumstances, such as under insulin resistance. NAFLD is characterized by elevated serum concentration of FFAs, hepatocyte apoptosis, progressive inflammation and fibrosis. In this work, we investigated the composition of circulating FFA in normal and NAFLD subjects during fasting and after a standard oral lipid load. Cultured hepatocytes incubated with FFA of various lengths demonstrated an inverse correlation between FA chain lengths and NAFLD induction [21].

The aim of our work was to study in depth the well-known significant increase in total free fatty acids shown in NAFLD subjects, and to possibly characterize which fatty acids significantly accounted for the whole increase, with specific regard to their classification (saturated, n-3, n-6 polyunsaturated fatty acids).

2. Results

Main basal features of the patients and control subjects are reported in Table 1. After oral fat load in NAFLD patients, triglycerides reached their maximum peak after around 4 h and they circulated at higher levels than in control subjects. The differences were significant at all times (Figure 1a). The trend of FFA over a 4 h period after the oral fat load is different between NAFLD patients and control subjects (Figure 1b). NAFLD patients showed higher FFA levels than control subjects from baseline through the end of the oral fat load with significant differences at times 60, 150, 180 and 210 min.

Table 1. Subjects baseline physical characteristics and fasting blood measurements.

Parameters	Control Group ($n = 9$)	NAFLD Group ($n = 21$)	p
Age (year)	27 ± 2	40 ± 9	0.001
BMI (kg/m^2)	21 ± 2	28 ± 4	0.002
Systolic blood pressure (mmHg)	119 ± 4	125 ± 8	0.049
Waist (cm)	73 ± 6	94 ± 8	0.000001
Diastolic blood pressure (mmHg)	80 ± 0	82 ± 9	0.615
Glucose (mg/dL)	91 ± 5	98 ± 11	0.097
Triglycerides (mg/dL)	59 ± 19	100 ± 49	0.021

Table 1. *Cont.*

Parameters	Control Group ($n = 9$)	NAFLD Group ($n = 21$)	p
Cholesterol (mg/dL)	168 ± 27	182 ± 34	0.306
HDL-Chol (mg/dL)	54 ± 13	42 ± 8	0.007
HDL$_2$-Chol (mg/dL)	20 ± 8	12 ± 4	0.003
HDL$_3$-Chol (mg/dL)	34.22 ± 5	30 ± 5	0.072
LDL-Chol (mg/dL)	107 ± 27	125 ± 29	0.139
FFA (mmol/L)	0.73 ± 0.41	1.07 ± 0.59	0.131
sdLDL (mg/dL)	21 ± 11	31 ± 18	0.127
c-Peptide (pM/mL)	0.54 ± 0.13	0.92 ± 0.35	0.004
Insulin (µU/mL)	6.28 ± 1.99	12.7 ± 7.68	0.021
AST (U/L)	20 ± 4	33 ± 10	0.002
ALT (U/L)	16 ± 4	64 ± 30	0.001
GGT (U/L)	14 ± 12	80 ± 74	0.021
ALP (U/L)	51 ± 21	75 ± 23	0.016
HOMA-IR	1.42 ± 0.49	3.16 ± 2.13	0.024
QUICKI index	0.367 ± 0.02	0.333 ± 0.03	0.008

Abbreviations: HDL-Chol, High density lipoprotein-Cholesterol; HDL$_2$-Chol, High density lipoprotein 2-Cholesterol; HDL$_3$-Chol, High density lipoprotein 3-Cholesterol; LDL-Chol, Low density lipoprotein-Cholesterol; FFA, free fatty acids; sdLDL, small dense low-density lipoproteins; AST, aspartate aminotransferase; ALT, alanine aminotransferase; GGT, gamma-glutamyltransferase; ALP, alkaline phosphatase; HOMA-IR, homeostatic model assessment-insulin resistance; QUICKI index, quantitative insulin sensitivity check index.

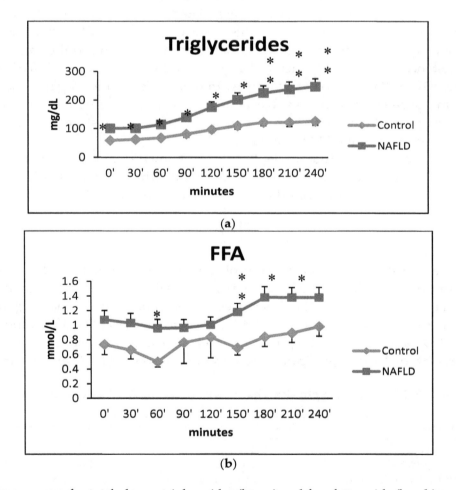

(a)

(b)

Figure 1. Time courses for total plasma triglycerides (box **a**) and free fatty acids (box **b**) concentrations during the oral fat meal in control (filled diamonds) and nonalcoholic fatty liver disease (NAFLD) (filled squares) subjects. Values are expressed as mean ±SEM. * $p < 0.05$, ** $p < 0.01$.

The trend of glycemia is dotted in Figure 2a and it shows a slight decrease from baseline to 90 min both in NAFLD and control group and then a constant course up to 240 min with a statistically significant difference at 210 min. Insulin curve showed in NAFLD patients a major peak at 30 min and higher levels than in control subjects. At all times, except at 180 min, there were statistically significant differences (Figure 2b).

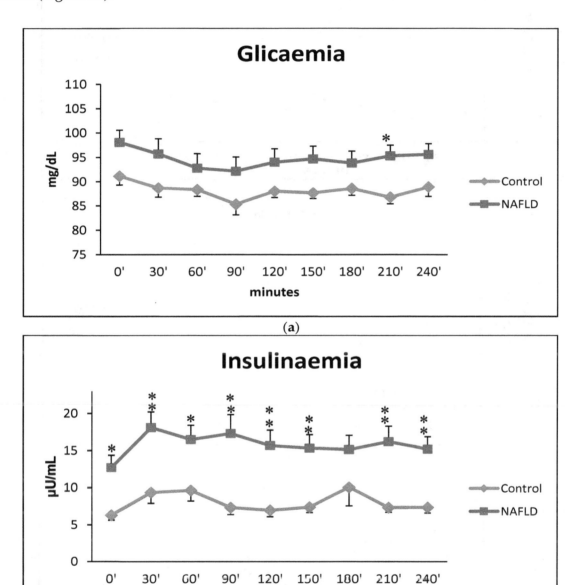

(a)

(b)

Figure 2. Time courses for glucose (box **a**) and insulin (box **b**) concentrations during the oral fat meal in control (filled diamonds) and NAFLD (filled squares) subjects. Values are expressed as mean ± SEM. * $p < 0.05$, ** $p < 0.01$.

Fatty acid values are given as percentage contents (mmol/100 mmol total fatty acids) since the between-individual variations in the molar concentration of total serum FFA is very high [22]. Figure 3 shows the trends of saturated fatty acids lauric (12:0) (a), myristic (14:0) (b) and stearic (18:0) (STA) (c) which did not present significant statistical differences between the two groups.

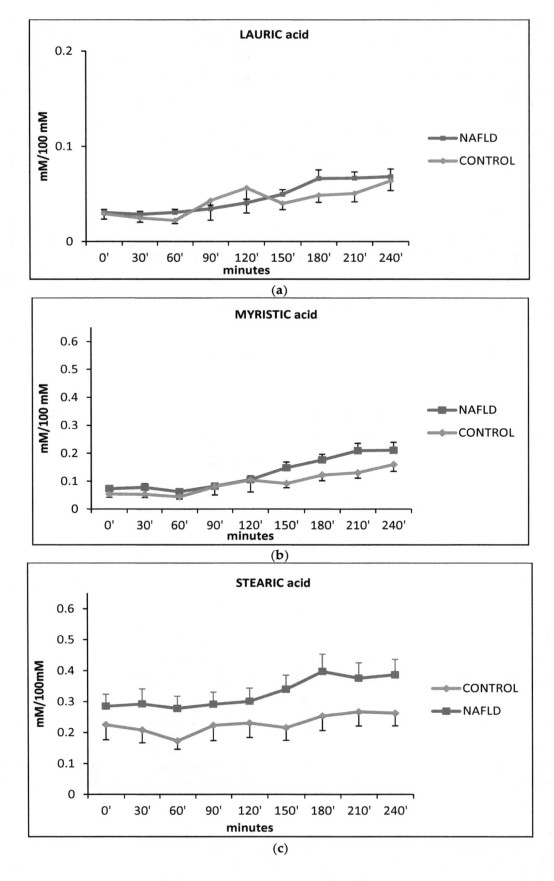

Figure 3. Change in plasma levels of saturated lauric (box **a**), myristic (box **b**) and stearic (box **c**) acid during the oral fat meal in control (filled diamonds) and NAFLD (filled squares) subjects. Values are expressed as mean ± SEM.

Figure 4 shows the trends of oleic acid (18:1*n*-9) (OLA) eluted with palmitic acid (16:0) (PAL), a saturated fatty acid. Oleic and palmitic acids amounts reached their peak at 180 min in NAFLD patients and were statistically higher in NAFLD patients than in control subjects at times 60, 150, and 210 min.

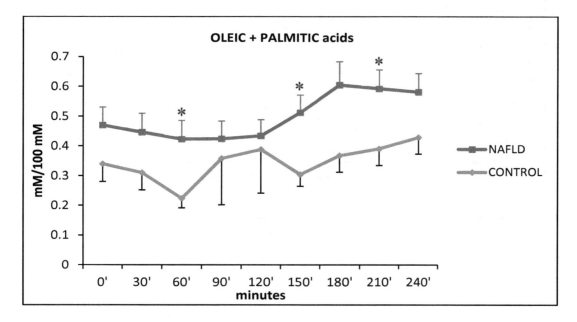

Figure 4. Change in plasma levels of oleic + palmitic acid during the oral fat meal in control (filled diamonds) and NAFLD (filled squares) subjects. Values are expressed as mean ± SEM. * $p < 0.05$.

The monounsaturated palmitoleic acid (16:1*n*-7) fell from baseline to 90 min in NAFLD subjects and from baseline to 150 min in control subjects. Then, in both group palmitoleic acids rose progressively up until the end of the test. No significant differences were observed between NAFLD and control subjects (Figure 5a).

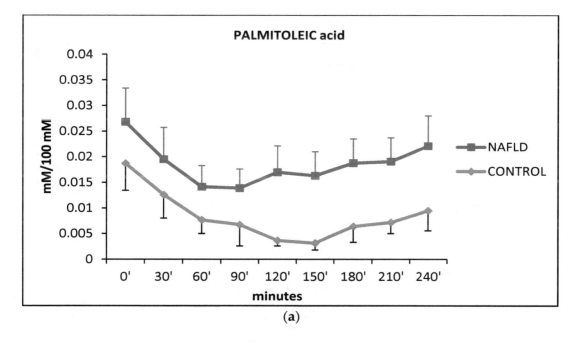

(a)

Figure 5. *Cont.*

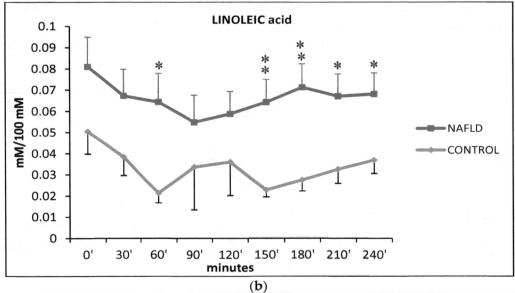

(b)

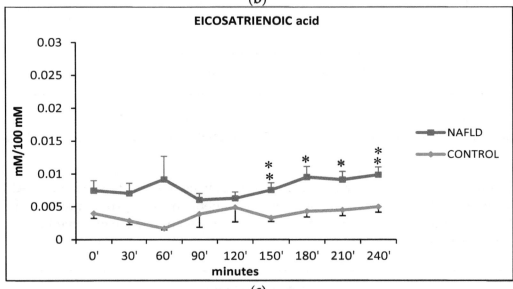

(c)

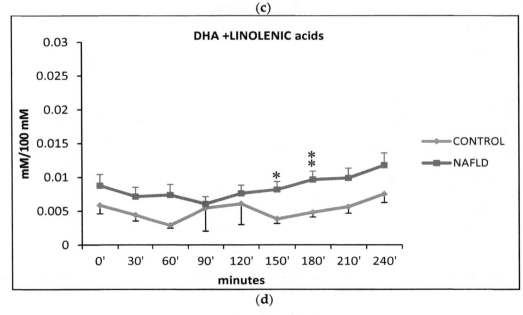

(d)

Figure 5. *Cont.*

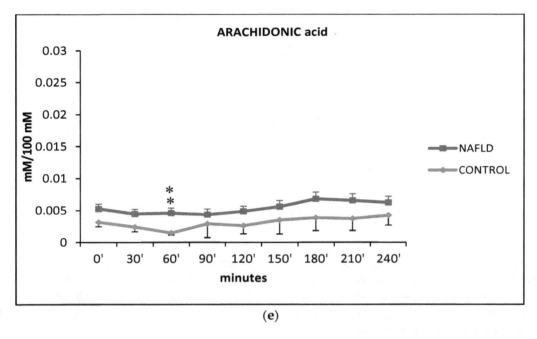

(e)

Figure 5. Change in plasma levels of palmitoleic (box **a**), linoleic (box **b**) eicosatrienoic (box **c**), DHA + linolenic (**d**) and arachidonic (**e**) acids during the oral fat meal in control (filled diamonds) and NAFLD (filled squares) subjects. Values are expressed as mean $\pm$ SEM. * $p < 0.05$, ** $p < 0.01$.

Linoleic acid (18:2n-6) (LNA) throughout the fat load showed significant differences at times 60, 150, 180, 210, and 240 min between NAFLD and control subjects (Figure 5b).

Eicosatrienoic acid (20:3n-9) in NAFLD patients had higher levels than in control subjects with significant differences from 150 min to the end of the fat oral test (Figure 5c).

Docosahexaenoic (22:6n-3) (DHA) and linolenic acids (18:3n-3) (ALA), two polyunsaturated fatty acids, are significantly increased in NAFLD patients at 150 and 180 min, compared to control subjects (Figure 5d).

Arachidonic acid (20:4n-6) (ARA) showed an almost flat trend in both NAFLD and control group with a significant difference at 60 min (Figure 5e).

The n-3/n-6 ratio measured at every time is not statistically different between control and NAFLD groups. HOMA-IR was higher in NAFLD subjects compared to the control subjects (3.16 ± 2.13 vs. 1.42 ± 0.49, $p = 0.024$). HOMA index positively correlated with the n-3/n-6 ratio at time 210 and 240 min in NAFLD patients ($r = 0.55$, $p = 0.0122$ and $r = 0.47$, $p = 0.035$, respectively) (Figure 6a,b).

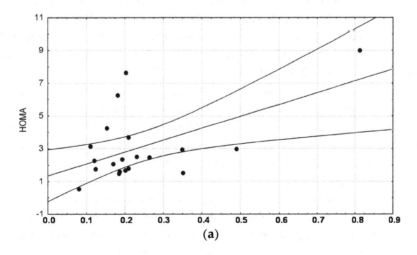

(a)

Figure 6. *Cont.*

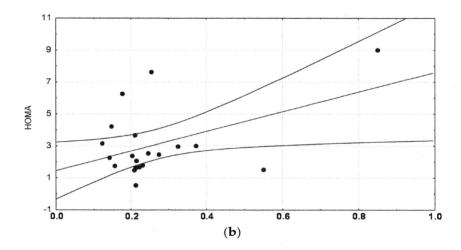

Figure 6. Correlation between homeostatic model assessment HOMA index and n-3/n-6 ratio at time 210 min in NAFLD patients (box **6a**); correlation between HOMA index and n-3/n-6 ratio at time 240 min in NAFLD patients (box **6b**); Figure 6a: PUFA n-3/n-6 at 210 min *vs.* HOMA in NAFLD; *r* = 0.54883, PUFA n-3/n-6 at 210 min; Figure 6b: PUFA n-3/n-6 at 240 min *vs.* HOMA in NAFLD; *r* = 0.47351, PUFA n-3/n-6 at 240 min.

3. Discussion

Free fatty acids derived from the diet can directly enter the circulation through spillover into the plasma FFA pool [23]. Other potential sources of fats causing fatty liver include adipose tissue from where non-esterified fatty acids flow to the liver, *de novo* lipogenesis and through the uptake of intestinally derived chylomicron remnants [24]. After a fatty meal, the FFA profile mirrors that of the meal [25]. We performed an abbreviated 4-hour postprandial fat load which was a valid surrogate for longer oral fat loads [26].

In the postprandial phase, the high insulinaemia and triglyceridemia observed in NAFLD patients confirms the insulin resistance state in these subjects [27]. Insulin does not suppress hormone-sensitive lipase in adipose tissue as in healthy subjects; therefore, in the postprandial phase, adipocyte-derived FFA mix with fatty acids coming from the diet and they can reach the liver.

The peak of triglycerides starts at around 4 h after the fatty meal in NAFLD subjects whilst in control subjects the peak is reached earlier. That means a delayed clearance of triglyceride-rich lipoproteins in NAFLD patients [28].

FFA levels are high in NAFLD patients compared to normal subjects with a trend similar to that of oleic and palmitic acid levels (Figures 1b and 4). This study shows that the higher serum levels of free fatty acids in NAFLD subjects are mainly due to levels of oleic (n9) and palmitic acids (reported as unique value in the data presented) which are the most abundant circulating free fatty acids (60, 150, and 210 min after the oral fat load) (Figures 1b and 4). Almost at the same time, linoleic acid (n6) levels increase significantly (60, 150, 180, 210, 240 min) (Figure 5b). Significant increases were also shown for docosahexaenoic acid (n3), linolenic acid (n-3) (Figure 5d), eicosatrienoic acid (n-9) (Figure 5c), and arachidonic acid (n6) (Figure 5e), although just on one occasion.

High levels of oleic and palmitic acids have molecular implications: oleic acid is the preferred substrate for the synthesis of triglycerides, and cholesteryl esters [29]. Palmitic acid is the substrate for isoforms 1 and 6 of fatty acid elongase (Elov-1 and Elov-6) which are converted into stearic acid [30]. Stearic acid is rapidly converted to oleic acid by the enzyme stearoyl-CoA 9-desaturase (SCD, No. EC 1.14.19.1) in mammalian cells [31]. A single double bond between carbon 9 and 10 is introduced in the chain of palmitic and stearic acids to be converted to palmitoleate and oleate, respectively [24]. The cellular ratio of oleic and stearic acids can affect membrane fluidity and signal transduction leading to an altered composition of membrane phospholipids, triglycerides and cholesterol esters [32]. Subjects exhibiting a hypertriglyceridemic response to a low-fat, high-carbohydrate diet show an increase in the oleic to stearic acids ratio [33].

Eicosatrienoic acid is significantly increased towards the end of the test in NAFLD subjects (Figure 5c). This increase is unlikely to be due to the meal composition since eicosatrienoic acid is of a negligible amount in dairy cream. Rather, eicosatrienoic acid might be derived from oleic acid metabolism [34].

Linolenic and DHA acids are two PUFA n-3 that coelute in our HPLC method. They significantly increase in NAFLD subjects at time 150 and 180 min. Humans have the ability to metabolize linolenic acids to their longer chain DHA even if this conversion is less than 1% in adults [35]. Further studies are needed to verify its physiological functions. The competition between n-3 and n6 fatty acids for the same enzymes and transport systems might explain why linoleic acid showed a flat trend throughout the test, even though they were found at higher concentrations in NAFLD patients than in control subjects.

The n-3/n-6 ratio measured every 30 min is not statistically different even if the ratio is slightly higher in control subjects than in NAFLD patients. When the n-3/n-6 ratio was correlated with HOMA-IR, it was found that HOMA index positively correlated with the n-3/n-6 ratio at times 210 and 240 min only in NAFLD patients (Figure 6a,b). Therefore, subjects who have a basal insulin resistance have higher n-3/n-6 ratio towards the end of the test as if higher n-3 fatty acids could worsen the clearance of triglycerides in NAFLD subjects. On the contrary, in healthy subjects with optimal insulin sensitivity, n-3 fatty acids could have beneficial influence on the lipid clearance. Our data seem to be in contrast with previous studies suggesting that increasing consumption of n-3 PUFA could improve lipid metabolism both in the fasting and postprandial states [36] even if modifying the n-3/n-6 polyunsaturated fatty acid ratio of a high-saturated fat challenge did not acutely change postprandial triglyceride response in men with metabolic syndrome [37]. It is likely for n-3 PUFA to need more than 8 h to exert beneficial effects in subjects with an impaired lipid metabolism [35]. Amount and type of dietary fatty acids can influence postprandial response [38]. Therefore, an imbalance in the n-3/n-6 fatty acids ratio could modulate postprandial response with more pronounced effects in insulin resistant subjects, such as NAFLD patients.

This preliminary study has some limitations due to the reduced number of control subjects available for the study which prevents us from matching by age, sex, BMI and also by physical activity on daily bases. The patients enrolled should be matched for a *de novo* clinical investigation to expand these preliminary results.

4. Experimental Section

4.1. Subjects

Twenty-one patients (ethics committee of University Hospital San Giovanni Battista of Torino, 00096648, 30 December 2009) with NAFLD (mean age $\pm$ SD, 40 ± 9 years, BMI 27.5 ± 3.9 kg/m^2) attending our Liver Unit were selected according to the following criteria: persistently (at least 12 months) elevated aspartate aminotransferases (AST) and alanine aminotransferases (ALT) in the absence of significant alcohol consumption (defined as <20 in men and <10 g/day in women); ultrasonographic presence of bright liver without any other liver or biliary tract disease. At ultrasounds, the diagnosis of NAFLD was based on four parameters: diffuse hyperechoic echotexture ("bright liver"), increased liver echotexture compared with the kidneys, vascular blurring and deep attenuation. Control subjects had a normal ultrasound liver scan.

Conditions known to be associated with fatty liver were ruled out by the following exclusion criteria: a Body Mass Index (BMI) $\geqslant 35$ kg/m^2; positive serum markers of viral, autoimmune or celiac disease; abnormal copper metabolism or thyroid function indices; a diagnosis of diabetes mellitus based on plasma glucose $\geqslant 126$ mg/dL in fasting conditions or $\geqslant 200$ mg/dL at +2 h on a standard oral glucose tolerance test, serum total cholesterol $\geqslant 220$ mg/dL, serum triglycerides

$\geqslant$160 mg/dL. The patients did not take drugs known to be steatogenic or to affect glucose metabolism and were not exposed to occupational hepatotoxins. The control group consisted of 9 healthy subjects (mean age $\pm$ SD, 27 $\pm$ 2 years, BMI 21.2 $\pm$ 1.6 kg/m^2) with normal liver enzymes and abdomen ultrasound scan (see Table 1).

4.2. Oral Fat Load

NAFLD patients and controls underwent a standard oral fat load to investigate the metabolism of triglyceride-rich lipoproteins and FFAs. The standard fat load consisted of a mixture of dairy cream (38% fat) and egg yolk for a total energy content of 745.22 Kcal. The fat meal was composed of 79.96 g fats, whose 54.32 g was of saturated fatty acids, 21.80 g of monounsaturated fatty acids, 2.82 g of polyunsaturated fatty acids, and 0.45 g of cholesterol. The Table 2 shows the amounts of the most represented fatty acids in the fat meal given to every participant.

Table 2. Fatty acid composition of lipid mixture prepared for the oral fat load.

Fatty Acids	200 g Dairy Cream (38% fat)	NO. 1 Egg Yolk	Total Fat Load
C12:0 (g)	3.02		
C14:0 (g)	9.18	0.013	
C16:0 (g)	21.40	1.020	
C18:0 (g)	7.54	0.630	
Total SFA (g)	52.75	1.67	54.32
C18:1 (g)	18.00	1.30	
Total MUFA (g)	20.48	1.33	21.81
C18:2 (g)	1.52	0.650	
C18:3 (g)	0.20	0.019	
C20:4 (g)		0.120	
Total PUFA (g)	2.07	0.74	2.82
Total fat (g)	75.30	4.66	79.96
Cholesterol (mg)	228.00	213.92	441.92
Proteins (g)	1.60	2.53	4.12
Carbohydrates (g)	2.28		2.28
Kcal	693.20	52.02	745.22

The fat load was consumed during a period of 5 min; subjects kept fasting and strenuous activity was forbidden during the test, since exercise can reduce postprandial lipemia. A catheter (Venflon Viggo AB, Helsingborg, Sweden) inserted in the antecubital vein and kept patent during the test was used to draw blood samples at baseline and every 30 min for 4 h for biochemical determinations. Blood samples were collected in tubes containing EDTA as anticoagulant and plasma was immediately frozen. All subjects provided their informed consent for the study, which was conducted in conformance with the Helsinki Declaration.

4.3. Biochemical Analyses

Serum glucose was measured by the glucose oxidase method (Sentinel, Milan, Italy) with an intra-assay variation coefficient of 1.07% and an inter-assay variation coefficient of 2.33%.

Triglycerides (Tg) and cholesterol (Chol) were assayed by enzymatic colorimetric assays (Sentinel, Milan, Italy) with an intra-assay variation coefficient of 2.99% and an inter-assay variation coefficient of 3.46% for triglycerides and with an intra-assay variation coefficient of 2.2% and an inter-assay variation coefficient of 3.38% for cholesterol.

HDL-Chol was determined by enzymatic colorimetric assay after precipitation of LDL and VLDL fractions using heparin-MnCl$_2$ solution and centrifugation at 4 °C [39], and it had an intra-assay variation coefficient of 2.5% and an inter-assay variation coefficient of 4.1%.

HDL$_2$- and HDL$_3$-Chol levels were determined according to Gidez *et al.* [40]: HDL$_2$ and HDL$_3$ lipoproteins were separated after precipitation of Apo B-containing lipoproteins with heparin-MnCl$_2$, and HDL_2 particles were further precipitated with dextran sulphate. HDL_3-Chol was determined in the supernatant. HDL_2-Chol was obtained by subtracting HDL_3-Chol from total HDL-Chol.

LDL-Chol was measured with a standardized homogeneous enzymatic colorimetric method in order to avoid triglycerides effects on LDL-Chol determination (Sentinel, Milan, Italy).

QUICKI was calculated from fasting glucose and insulin values as previously reported [41].

HOMA was calculated using units of millimoles per liter for glucose and microunits per milliliter for insulin [42].

The determination of fatty acid composition of free fatty acids was performed by high performance liquid chromatography (HPLC) coupled with a fluorescence detector [43]. This procedure enables the analyses of the content and profile of free fatty acids in total lipids extract. For free fatty acids' analyses, we prepared an acidified sample mixture containing a small volume of serum and 10% acetic acid. The mixture was applied onto C_{18} minicolumn and the column was washed with 10% acetic acid. The fatty acids were eluted with ethyl ether. The ether phase was evaporated and dried under vacuum at room temperature; the residue was dissolved into the derivatization solution containing the labeling fluorescent compound. A very small volume was injected in a HPLC reverse phase column and the free fatty acids profile was obtained within 45 min. Concentrations of each free fatty acid were obtained from a calibration curve made of 10 fatty acids run at 5 levels.

4.4. Statistical Analysis

Data were expressed as means ± SD. Between-group comparisons (NAFLD *vs.* control groups) were performed by using independent "*t*-test". To assess correlations between data, the Pearson correlation coefficient was calculated. Differences were considered statistically significant at $p < 0.05$.

5. Conclusions

The postprandial lipid metabolism in NAFLD subjects is very complex and partially understood. Although the excessive flow of FFA from adipose tissue, especially from abdominal obesity (Table 1), to the liver is considered to be the most important trigger of the NAFLD, little is known about the type of free fatty acids reaching the liver. In literature, there are few data dealing with levels of different circulating free fatty acids, but these data were usually measured only at baseline and come from small groups of subjects [5]; however, they confirmed a significant increase of oleic, palmitoleic and palmitic acids at baseline.

Taking into account the results coming out of this study, it would seem advisable for NAFLD subjects to not only follow a saturated fatty acid-free diet, but also be careful not to consume large amounts of n-3/n-6 PUFA. Obviously, these preliminary data should be further confirmed with larger clinical trials which could help to develop tailored nutritional interventions aimed to improving lipid metabolism in NAFLD subjects with the use of dynamic tests.

Acknowledgments: Funded by FP7/2007-2013 under grant agreement No. HEALTH-F2-2009-241762 for the project FLIP and by PRIN 2009ARYX4T.

Author Contributions: Roberto Gambino conceived of the study, performed HPLC analyses and participated in its design and coordination and helped to draft the manuscript; Elisabetta Bugianesi was involved in the planning of the study and commented on the draft manuscript; Chiara Rosso was involved in the planning of the study and selection of subjects; Lavinia Mezzabotta was involved in the planning of the study and selection of subjects; Silvia Pinach carried out biochemical analyses and commented on the draft manuscript; Natalina Alemanno carried out biochemical analyses; Francesca Saba performed HPLC analyses; Maurizio Cassader was involved in the planning of the study and commented on the draft manuscript; All authors read and approved the final manuscript.

References

1. Kooner, J.S.; Baliga, R.R.; Wilding, J.; Crook, D.; Packard, C.J.; Banks, L.M.; Peart, S.; Aitman, T.J.; Scott, J. Abdominal obesity, impaired nonesterified fatty acid suppression, and insulin-mediated glucose disposal are early metabolic abnormalities in families with premature myocardial infarction. *Arterioscler. Thromb. Vasc. Biol.* **1998**, *18*, 1021–1026. [CrossRef] [PubMed]

2. Zoratti, R.; Godsland, I.F.; Chaturvedi, N.; Crook, D.; Crook, D.; Stevenson, J.C.; McKeigue, P.M. Relation of plasma lipids to insulin resistance, nonesterified fatty acid levels, and body fat in men from three ethnic groups: Relevance to variation in risk of diabetes and coronary disease. *Metabolism* **2000**, *49*, 245–252. [CrossRef]

3. Musso, G.; Gambino, R.; Cassader, M. Recent insights into hepatic lipid metabolism in non-alcoholic fatty liver disease (NAFLD). *Prog. Lipid Res.* **2009**, *48*, 1–26. [CrossRef] [PubMed]

4. Musso, G.; Gambino, R.; de Michieli, F.; Biroli, G.; Fagà, E.; Pagano, G.; Cassader, M. Association of liver disease with postprandial large intestinal triglyceride-rich lipoprotein accumulation and pro/antioxidant imbalance in normolipidemic non-alcoholic steatohepatitis. *Ann. Med.* **2008**, *40*, 383–394. [CrossRef] [PubMed]

5. De Almeida, I.T.; Cortez-Pinto, H.; Fidalgo, G.; Rodrigues, D.; Camilo, M.E. Plasma total and free fatty acids composition in human non-alcoholic steatohepatitis. *Clin. Nutr.* **2002**, *21*, 219–223. [CrossRef] [PubMed]

6. Seidelin, K.N.; Myrup, B.; Fischer-Hansen, B. *n*-3 fatty acids in adipose tissue and coronary artery disease are inversely related. *Am. J. Clin. Nutr.* **1992**, *55*, 1117–1119. [PubMed]

7. Musso, G.; Gambino, R.; Pacini, G.; de Michieli, F.; Cassader, M. Prolonged saturated fat-induced, glucose-dependent insulinotropic polypeptide elevation is associated with adipokine imbalance and liver injury in nonalcoholic steatohepatitis: Dysregulated enteroadipocyte axis as a novel feature of fatty liver. *Am. J. Clin. Nutr.* **2009**, *89*, 558–567. [CrossRef] [PubMed]

8. Marinou, K.; Adiels, M.; Hodson, L.; Frayn, K.N.; Karpe, F.; Fielding, B.A. Young women partition fatty acids towards ketone body production rather than VLDL-TAG synthesis, compared with young men. *Br. J. Nutr.* **2011**, *105*, 857–865. [CrossRef] [PubMed]

9. Nelson, R.H.; Basu, R.; Johnson, C.M.; Rizza, R.A.; Miles, J.M. Splanchnic spillover of extracellular lipase-generated fatty acids in overweight and obese humans. *Diabetes* **2007**, *56*, 2878–2884. [CrossRef] [PubMed]

10. Hardy, S.; El-Assaad, W.; Przybytkowski, E.; Joly, E.; Prentki, M.; Langelier, Y. Saturated fatty acid induced-apoptosis in MDA-MB-231 breast cancer cells—A role for cardiolipin. *J. Biol. Chem.* **2003**, *278*, 31861–31870. [CrossRef] [PubMed]

11. Musso, G.; Gambino, R.; Durazzo, M.; Biroli, G.; Carello, M.; Faga, E.; Pacini, G.; de Michieli, F.; Rabbione, L.; Premoli, A.; *et al.* Adipokines in NASH: Postprandial lipid metabolism as a link between adiponectin and liver disease. *Hepatology* **2005**, *42*, 1175–1183. [CrossRef] [PubMed]

12. Okere, I.; Chandler, M.; McElfresh, T.; Rennison, J.H.; Sharov, V.; Sabbah, H.N.; Tserng, K.T.; Hoit, B.D.; Ernsberger, P.; Young, M.E.; *et al.* Differential effects of saturated and unsaturated fatty acid diets on cardiomyocyte apoptosis, adipose distribution, and serum leptin. *Am. J. Physiol. Heart Circ. Physiol.* **2006**, *291*, H38–H44. [CrossRef] [PubMed]

13. Wang, D.; Wei, Y.R.; Pagliassotti, M.J. Saturated fatty acids promote endoplasmic reticulum stress and liver injury in rats with hepatic steatosis. *Endocrinology* **2006**, *147*, 943–951. [CrossRef] [PubMed]

14. Spector, A.A.; Yorek, M.A. Membrane lipid-composition and cellular function. *J. Lipid Res.* **1985**, *26*, 1015–1035. [PubMed]

15. Borradaile, N.M.; Han, X.; Harp, J.D.; Gale, S.E.; Ory, D.S.; Schaffer, J.E. Disruption of endoplasmic reticulum structure and integrity in lipotoxic cell death. *J. Lipid Res.* **2006**, *47*, 2726–2737. [CrossRef] [PubMed]

16. Satapati, S.; Sunny, N.E.; Kucejova, B.; Fu, X.; He, T.T.; Méndez-Lucas, A.; Shelton, J.M.; Perales, J.C.; Browning, J.D.; Burgess, S.C. Elevated TCA cycle function in the pathology of diet-induced hepatic insulin resistance and fatty liver. *J. Lipid Res.* **2012**, *53*, 1080–1092. [CrossRef] [PubMed]

17. Sunny, N.E.; Parks, E.J.; Browning, J.D.; Burgess, S.C. Excessive hepatic mitochondrial TCA cycle and gluconeogenesis in humans with nonalcoholic fatty liver disease. *Cell Metab.* **2011**, *14*, 804–810. [CrossRef] [PubMed]

18. Nakamura, S.; Takamura, T.; Matsuzawa-Nagata, N.; Takayama, H.; Misu, H.; Noda, H.; Nabemoto, S.; Kurita, S.; Ota, T.; Ando, H.; *et al.* Palmitate induces insulin resistance in H4IIEC3 hepatocytes through reactive oxygen species produced by mitochondria. *J. Biol. Chem.* **2009**, *284*, 14809–14818. [CrossRef] [PubMed]

19. Paumen, M.B.; Ishida, Y.; Muramatsu, M.; Yamamoto, M.; Honjo, T. Inhibition of carnitine palmitoyltransferase I augments sphingolipid synthesis and palmitate-induced apoptosis. *J. Biol. Chem.* **1997**, *272*, 3324–3329. [CrossRef] [PubMed]

20. Summers, S.A. Ceramides in insulin resistance and lipotoxicity. *Prog. Lipid Res.* **2006**, *45*, 42–72. [CrossRef] [PubMed]

21. Maeda, K.; Cao, H.; Kono, K.; Gorgun, C.Z.; Furuhashi, M.; Uysal, K.T.; Cao, Q.; Atsumi, G.; Malone, H.; Krishnan, B.; *et al.* Adipocyte/macrophage fatty acid binding proteins control integrated metabolic responses in obesity and diabetes. *Cell Metab.* **2005**, *1*, 107–119. [CrossRef] [PubMed]

22. Yli-Jama, P.; Meyer, H.E.; Ringstad, J.; Pedersen, J.I. Serum free fatty acid pattern and risk of myocardial infarction: A case-control study. *J. Intern. Med.* **2002**, *251*, 19–28. [CrossRef] [PubMed]

23. Miles, J.M.; Park, Y.S.; Walewicz, D.; Russell-Lopez, C.; Windsor, S.; Isley, W.L.; Coppack, S.W.; Harris, W.S. Systemic and forearm triglyceride metabolism: Fate of lipoprotein lipase-generated glycerol and free fatty acids. *Diabetes* **2004**, *53*, 521–527. [CrossRef] [PubMed]

24. Havel, R.J.; Hamilton, R.L. Hepatic catabolism of remnant lipoproteins: Where the action is. *Arterioscler. Thromb. Vasc. Biol.* **2004**, *24*, 213–215. [PubMed]

25. Griffiths, A.J.; Humphreys, S.M.; Clark, M.L.; Fielding, B.A.; Frayn, K.N. Immediate metabolic availability of dietary fat in combination with carbohydrate. *Am. J. Clin. Nutr.* **1994**, *59*, 53–59. [PubMed]

26. Weiss, E.P.; Fields, D.A.; Mittendorfer, B.; Dorien Haverkort, A.M.; Klein, S. Reproducibility of postprandial lipemia test and validity of an abbreviated 4-h test. *Metabolism* **2008**, *57*, 1479–1485. [CrossRef] [PubMed]

27. Musso, G.; Gambino, R.; De Michieli, F.; Cassader, M.; Rizzetto, M.; Durazzo, M.; Fagà, E.; Silli, B.; Pagano, G. Dietary habits and their relation to insulin resistance in nonalcoholic steatohepatitis. *Hepatology* **2003**, *37*, 909–916. [CrossRef] [PubMed]

28. Cassader, M.; Gambino, R.; Musso, G.; Depetris, N.; Mecca, F.; Cavallo-Perin, P.; Pacini, G.; Rizzetto, M.; Pagano, G. Postprandial triglyceride-rich lipoprotein metabolism and insulin sensitivity in nonalcoholic steatohepatitis patients. *Lipids* **2001**, *36*, 1117–1124. [CrossRef] [PubMed]

29. Ntambi, J.M.; Miyazaki, M. Regulation of stearoyl-CoA desaturases and role in metabolism. *Prog. Lipid Res.* **2004**, *43*, 91–104. [CrossRef]

30. Inagaki, K.; Aki, T.; Fukuda, Y.; Kawamoto, S.; Shigeta, S.; Ono, K.; Suzuki, O. Identification and expression of a rat fatty acid elongase involved in the biosynthesis of C18 fatty acids. *Biosci. Biotechnol. Biochem.* **2002**, *66*, 613–621. [CrossRef] [PubMed]

31. Sampath, H.; Ntambi, J.M. The fate and intermediary metabolism of stearic acid. *Lipids* **2005**, *40*, 1187–1191. [CrossRef] [PubMed]

32. Sun, Y.; Hao, M.M.; Luo, Y.; Liang, C.P.; Silver, D.L.; Cheng, C.; Maxfield, F.R.; Tall, A.R. Stearoyl-CoA desaturase inhibits ATP-binding cassette transporter A1-mediated cholesterol efflux and modulates membrane domain structure. *J. Biol. Chem.* **2003**, *278*, 5813–5820. [CrossRef] [PubMed]

33. Attie, A.D.; Krauss, R.M.; Gray-Keller, M.P.; Brownlie, A.; Miyazaki, M.; Kastelein, J.J.; Lusis, A.J.; Stalenhoef, A.F.; Stoehr, J.P.; Hayden, M.R.; *et al.* Relationship between stearoyl-CoA desaturase activity and plasma triglycerides in human and mouse hypertriglyceridemia. *J. Lipid Res.* **2002**, *43*, 1899–1907. [CrossRef] [PubMed]

34. Le, H.D.; Meisel, J.A.; de Meijer, V.E.; Gura, K.M.; Puder, M. The essentiality of arachidonic acid and docosahexaenoic acid. *Prostaglandins Leukot. Essent. Fatty Acids* **2009**, *81*, 165–170. [CrossRef] [PubMed]

35. Brenna, J.T.; Salem, N., Jr.; Sinclair, A.J.; Cunnane, S.C. α-Linolenic acid supplementation and conversion to n-3 long-chain polyunsaturated fatty acids in humans. *Prostaglandins Leukot. Essent. Fatty Acids* **2009**, *80*, 85–91. [CrossRef] [PubMed]

36. Roche, H.M.; Gibney, M.J. Effect of long-chain n-3 polyunsaturated fatty acids on fasting and postprandial triacylglycerol metabolism. *Am. J. Clin. Nutr.* **2000**, *71*, 232s–237s. [PubMed]

37. Tulk, H.; Robinson, L. Modifying the n-6/n-3 polyunsaturated fatty acid ratio of a high-saturated fat challenge does not acutely attenuate postprandial changes in inflammatory markers in men with metabolic syndrome. *Metabolism* **2009**, *58*, 1709–1716. [CrossRef] [PubMed]

38. Song, Z.; Yang, L.; Shu, G.; Lu, H.; Sun, G. Effects of the *n*-6/*n*-3 polyunsaturated fatty acids ratio on postprandial metabolism in hypertriacylglycerolemia patients. *Lipids Health Dis.* **2013**, *12*, 181–188. [CrossRef] [PubMed]

39. Warnick, G.R.; Albers, J.J. A comprehensive evolution of the heparin manganese precipitation procedure for estimating high density lipoprotein cholesterol. *J. Lipid Res.* **1978**, *29*, 65–76.

40. Gidez, L.I.; Miller, G.J.; Burnstein, M.; Slagle, S.; Eder, H.A. Separation and quantitation of subclasses of human plasma HDL by a single precipitation procedure. *J. Lipid Res.* **1982**, *23*, 1206–1216. [PubMed]

41. Katz, A.; Nambi, S.S.; Mather, K.; Baron, A.D.; Follmann, D.A.; Sullivan, G.; Quon, M.J. Quantitative insulin sensitivity check index: A simple, accurate method for assessing insulin sensitivity in humans. *J. Clin. Endocrinol. Metab.* **2000**, *85*, 2402–2410. [CrossRef] [PubMed]

42. Matthews, D.R.; Hosker, J.P.; Rudenski, A.S.; Naylor, B.A.; Treacher, D.F.; Turner, R.C. Homeostasis model assessment: Insulin resistance and β-cell function from fasting plasma glucose and insulin concentrations in man. *Diabetologia* **1985**, *28*, 412–419. [CrossRef] [PubMed]

43. Matsuzawa, T.; Mishima, K.; Nishii, M.; Ito, M. Serum fatty acids analysis by high performance liquid chromatography, after enzymatic hydrolysis and isolation by Sep-Pak C18 minicolumn. *Biochem. Int.* **1987**, *15*, 693–702. [PubMed]

6

PNPLA3 Expression is Related to Liver Steatosis in Morbidly Obese Women with Non-Alcoholic Fatty Liver Disease

Gemma Aragonès [1,†], Teresa Auguet [1,2,†], Sandra Armengol [1], Alba Berlanga [1],
Esther Guiu-Jurado [1], Carmen Aguilar [1], Salomé Martínez [3], Fátima Sabench [4],
José Antonio Porras [2], Maikel Daniel Ruiz [2], Mercé Hernández [4], Joan Josep Sirvent [3],
Daniel Del Castillo [4] and Cristóbal Richart [1,2,*]

[1]   Group de Recerca GEMMAIR (AGAUR)-Medicina Aplicada, Institut Investigació Sanitària Pere
      Virgili (IISPV), Departament de Medicina i Cirurgia, Universitat Rovira i Virgili (URV), 43007 Tarragona,
      Spain; gemma.aragones@iispv.cat (G.A.); tauguet.hj23.ics@gencat.cat (T.A.); sandra.armengol@urv.cat (S.A.);
      alba.berlanga@urv.cat (A.B.); esther.guiu@urv.cat (E.G.-J.); caguilar.hj23.ics@gencat.cat (C.A.)
[2]   Servei Medicina Interna, Hospital Universitari Joan XXIII Tarragona, Mallafré Guasch, 4, 43007 Tarragona,
      Spain; aporras.hj23.ics@gencat.cat (J.A.P.); drgorrin@yahoo.es (M.D.R.)
[3]   Servei Anatomia Patològica, Hospital Universitari Joan XXIII Tarragona, Mallafré Guasch, 4,
      43007 Tarragona, Spain; mgonzalez.hj23.ics@gencat.cat (S.M.); jsirvent.hj23.ics@gencat.cat (J.J.S.)
[4]   Servei de Cirurgia, Hospital Sant Joan de Reus, Departament de Medicina i Cirurgia,
      Universitat Rovira i Virgili (URV), IISPV, Avinguda Doctor Josep Laporte, 2, 43204 Tarragona, Spain;
      fatima.sabench@urv.cat (F.S.); mhernandezg@grupsagessa.com (M.H.);
      ddelcastillo@grupsagessa.com (D.D.C.)
*   Correspondence: crichart.hj23.ics@gencat.cat
†   These authors contributed equally to this work.

Academic Editors: Giovanni Targher and Amedeo Lonardo

Abstract: Recent reports suggest a role for the Patatin-like phospholipase domain-containing protein 3 (PNPLA3) in the pathology of non-alcoholic fatty liver disease (NAFLD). Lipid deposition in the liver seems to be a critical process in the pathogenesis of NAFLD. The aim of the present work was to evaluate the association between the liver *PNPLA3* expression, key genes of lipid metabolism, and the presence of NAFLD in morbidly obese women. We used real-time polymerase chain reaction (PCR) analysis to analyze the hepatic expression of *PNPLA3* and lipid metabolism-related genes in 55 morbidly obese subjects with normal liver histology (NL, $n = 18$), simple steatosis (SS, $n = 20$), and non-alcoholic steatohepatitis (NASH, $n = 17$). Liver biopsies were collected during bariatric surgery. We observed that liver *PNPLA3* expression was increased in NAFLD than in NL. It was also upregulated in SS than in NL. Interestingly, we found that the expression of *PNPLA3* was significantly higher in severe than mild SS group. In addition, the expression of the transcription factors *LXRα*, *PPARα*, and *SREBP2* was positively correlated with *PNPLA3* liver expression. Regarding rs738409 polymorphism, GG genotype was positive correlated with the presence of NASH. In conclusion, our results show that PNPLA3 could be related to lipid accumulation in liver, mainly in the development and progression of simple steatosis.

Keywords: PNPLA3; morbid obesity; non-alcoholic fatty liver disease; simple steatosis; fatty acid metabolism; non-alcoholic steatohepatitis

1. Introduction

Non-alcoholic fatty liver disease (NAFLD), the most common liver disease in Western countries, is characterized by the accumulation of excess triglycerides (TG) in hepatocytes and is associated with or anticipates the metabolic syndrome and its individual features, including visceral obesity, hyperlipidemia, and type 2 diabetes mellitus (T2DM) [1]. NAFLD includes a range of diseases from simple fatty infiltration (simple steatosis (SS)), fat accumulation, and inflammation (non-alcoholic steatohepatitis (NASH)) to liver fibrosis/cirrhosis [2]. General prevalence of NAFLD is 25.24%, with the highest prevalence in the Middle East and South America. This prevalence is particularly high in obese adults (80%–90%), patients with T2DM (30%–50%), and up to 90% in patients with hyperlipidemia [3]. NAFLD is usually diagnosed by abdominal ultrasonography in subjects without any apparent liver alteration who do not consume excessive alcohol [4]. Some studies have shown that insulin resistance (IR) promotes not only the recruitment of free fatty acids (FAs) in liver from the serum pool, but also the accumulation of intrahepatic FA, which indicates that IR is, among other mechanisms, crucial to the pathogenesis of NAFLD/NASH. In this regard, some authors have attempted to explain the pathophysiology of NAFLD by advancing the "multiple parallel hits hypothesis" [5]. However, the specific process responsible for the development and progression of NAFLD is still an open question. While SS is considered a relatively benign condition with little risk of progression, NASH may progress to cirrhosis and, in a small percentage of patients, to hepatocellular carcinoma (HCC) [6]. In fact, there is increasing evidence to indicate a complex interplay between environmental genetic factors that predispose the progression of NAFLD [7].

Patatin-like phospholipase domain-containing protein 3 (PNPLA3), which is also known as adiponutrin, is mainly expressed in hepatocytes but also in adipocytes [8]. The protein is one of the candidates potentially related to NAFLD susceptibility. Regarding PNPLA3 lipase activity against TG and acylglycerol transacetylase activity, its expression is responsible for energy mobilization and the storage in lipid droplets [9,10]. Additionally, it is highly modulated by nutritional stimuli at transcriptional and posttranscriptional levels [11].

In 2008, Romeo et al. [12] reported that a PNPLA3 single nucleotide polymorphism at residue 148 in the DNA sequence, resulting in a substitution of isoleucine for methionine (I148M, rs738409), was a genetic determinant of NAFLD. Since then, the correlation between the PNPLA3 148M variant and NAFLD has been investigated in considerable detail. Multiple studies have demonstrated a link between the PNPLA3 148M variant and the development and progression of NAFLD, including liver fibrosis [13–18]. Recently, it has been reported that PNPLA3 148M elevates retinyl-palmitate content in human hepatic stellate cells providing evidence for a potential link between the PNPLA3 variant, human hepatic retinoid metabolism, and chronic liver disease [19,20]. All this research indicates that this variant is a potential modifier of NAFLD. Nevertheless, its role in the NAFLD development and the specific molecular mechanisms has not been fully elucidated.

Lipid deposition in the liver seems to be a critical mechanism in the pathogenesis of NAFLD, so its regulatory processes need to be elucidated if the progression of NAFLD is to be controlled. Although these potential regulatory mechanisms are multiple, one of them affecting TG remodeling could be PNPLA3 [21–23].

On the basis of this data, the aim of our work was to study the relationship between the liver expression of PNPLA3 and the presence of NAFLD in morbidly obese women. Furthermore, as lipid metabolism seems to be involved in the pathogenesis of NAFLD, we investigated the association between the hepatic expression of PNPLA3 and the expression of the main lipid metabolism-related genes. Finally, in order to explore the impact of the PNPLA3 genetic variant on the presence of NAFLD, we determined the relationships between the rs738409 polymorphism in the PNPLA3 gene and the severity of the disease.

2. Results

2.1. General Characteristics of Cohort

Our morbidly obese women (MO) cohort was sub-classified according to liver pathology study into normal liver (NL, n = 18), simple steatosis (SS, n = 20), and non-alcoholic steatohepatitis

(NASH, n = 17) (Table 1). We found no significant differences regarding age and anthropometrical measurements between the three groups studied. With regard to biochemical analysis, glucose levels were significantly increased in the SS and NASH groups compared to the NL group (p = 0.017 and p = 0.010). Glycosylated hemoglobin (HbA1c) levels were also higher in SS than in NL (p = 0.039). Our results showed that aspartate aminotransferase (AST) and alanine aminotransferase (ALT) activity were higher in the NASH group than in the NL group (p = 0.001 and $p \leqslant$ 0.001) and that ALT was increased in NASH compared to SS (p = 0.001).

Table 1. General characteristics of the studied cohort classified according to the liver pathology.

Variables	Morbidly Obese Subjects (n = 55)		
	NL (n = 18)	SS (n = 20)	NASH (n = 17)
	Mean ± SD	Mean ± SD	Mean ± SD
Age (years)	48.6 ± 10.9	50.4 ± 11.0	47.8 ± 13.0
Weight (kg)	120.5 ± 19.3	120.4 ± 18.1	116.6 ± 15.5
BMI (kg/m^2)	50.1 ± 7.6	48.8 ± 8.5	47.0 ± 4.8
WC (cm)	130.0 ± 17.9	129.5 ± 12.9	129.4 ± 12.0
Glucose (mg/dL)	94.2 ± 22.6	133.9 ± 50.6 *	138.7 ± 49.1 *
Insulin (mUI/L)	12.1 ± 7.8	18.6 ± 12.3	20.1 ± 16.4
HbA1c (%)	5.2 ± 0.9	6.5 ± 1.7 *	6.3 ± 1.6
HOMA2-IR	1.6 ± 0.9	2.8 ± 1.4	2.8 ± 2.1
HDL-C (mg/dL)	44.5 ± 9.8	36.8 ± 11.3	37.1 ± 5.9
LDL-C (mg/dL)	99.0 ± 27.3	100.9 ± 29.3	104.4 ± 31.2
Total cholesterol (mg/dL)	173.03 ± 35.53	169.55 ± 34.04	174.81 ± 33.66
Triglycerides (mg/dL)	136.5 ± 58.4	193.1 ± 128.6	174.0 ± 81.1
AST (U/L)	23.5 ± 12.3	40.2 ± 33.9	64.9 ± 35.8 *
ALT (U/L)	22.1 ± 8.5	37.6 ± 22.9	67.0 ± 33.4 *,#
GGT (U/L)	26.6 ± 23.5	27.6 ± 14.8	53.7 ± 59.5
ALP (U/L)	61.9 ± 12.4	74.1 ± 20.3	79.9 ± 29.7

ALP: alkaline phosphatase; ALT: alanine aminotransferase; AST: aspartate aminotransferase; BMI: body mass index; GGT: gamma-glutamyltransferase; HbA1c: glycosylated hemoglobin; HDL-C: high density lipoprotein cholesterol; HOMA2-IR: homeostatic model assessment 2-insulin resistance; LDL-C: low density lipoprotein cholesterol; NASH: morbidly obese subjects with steatohepatitis; NL: morbidly obese subjects with normal liver; SS: morbidly obese subjects with simple steatosis; WC: waist circumference. One-way ANOVA with *post-hoc* Tukey test was used to compare variables between groups. * indicates statistically significant differences respect NL group (p < 0.05); # indicates statistically significant differences respect SS group (p < 0.05). Data are expressed as mean ± SD.

2.2. Determination of Patatin-Like Phospholipase Domain-Containing Protein 3 (PNPLA3) Liver Expression

We analyzed *PNPLA3* liver expression in MO women in relation to the presence of NAFLD. The results showed that *PNPLA3* expression was a significant 72% greater in MO NAFLD women than in MO women with NL (MO NAFLD: 3.6 ± 2.2 and MO NL: 2.1 ± 0.8, p = 0.001). Furthermore, when we classified the MO cohort into NL, SS, and NASH, we observed that the expression of *PNPLA3* was significantly higher in SS than in NL (p = 0.006, Figure 1A). There were no differences between NL or SS and NASH (p = 0.380 and p = 0.170, respectively). It is important to note that, in our work, any patient with steatohepatitis had fibrosis in the liver histology, so we could not perform correlations between fibrosis staging and *PNPLA3* liver expression.

In addition, in order to explore the increased expression of *PNPLA3* in simple steatosis, we classified the SS group into grades: mild (n = 9), moderate (n = 5), or severe SS (n = 6). We found that the expression of *PNPLA3* was significantly increased in the severe group compared to the mild SS group (p = 0.020, Figure 1B).

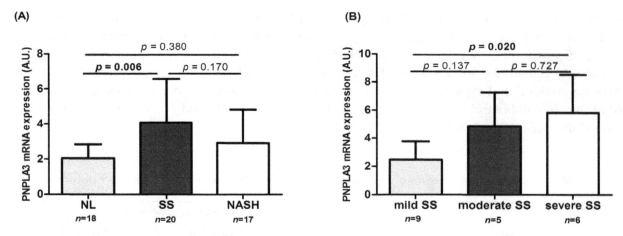

Figure 1. Hepatic expression of *PNPLA3* gene in morbidly obese women according to the liver histopathology (**A**) and subclassifying the SS group into: mild, moderate, or severe SS (**B**). A.U.: arbitrary units; NASH: morbidly obese women with steatohepatitis; NL: morbidly obese women with a normal liver; SS: morbidly obese women with simple steatosis. ANOVA test was used to determinate differences between groups. $p < 0.05$ are considered statistically significant.

2.3. Correlations between the Expression of PNPLA3 and Biochemical Variables, Histopathological Parameters and Genes Involved in Lipid Metabolism and Inflammation in Liver from Morbidly Obese Subjects

When we analyzed the associations between *PNPLA3* expression and parameters related to glucose metabolism and lipid profile, we observed a direct correlation between circulating levels of triglycerides and *PNPLA3* expression in the whole study cohort ($r = 0.272$, $p = 0.046$).

Regarding histopathological features, we only found a direct association between *PNPLA3* expression and degree of steatosis in the total MO group ($r = 0.441$, $p = 0.001$).

In order to clarify whether *PNPLA3* was associated with hepatic lipid metabolism, we studied the correlation between *PNPLA3* expression and lipid metabolism related genes in liver from the MO cohort. In the lipogenic and fatty acid oxidation pathways, hepatic liver X receptor (*LXRα*) and peroxisome-proliferator-activated receptor α (*PPARα*) expression correlated directly with PNPLA3 expression in the total morbidly obese group ($r = 0.671$, $p = 0.008$ and $r = 0.640$, $p = 0.008$; Table 2). We also showed a positive association between *PNPLA3* and both the transcription factor sterol regulatory element binding protein 2 (*SREBP2*) ($r = 0.412$, $p = 0.032$) and lipocalin 2 (*LCN2*) ($r = 0.570$, $p = 0.032$) in the whole population.

Interestingly, when we analyzed the relationship between the expression of these genes in the SS subgroup, we observed that both *LXRα* and *PPARα* correlations were stronger (*LXRα*: $r = 0.806$, $p = 0.016$; *PPARα*: $r = 0.796$, $p = 0.024$).

2.4. rs738409 Genotype Distribution in Morbidly Obese Subjects

The distribution of the studied genetic polymorphism is shown in Table 3, as are comparisons between NL, SS, and NASH patients. The G allele was more frequent (66.6%) than the C allele (33.3%) in the whole population. No individuals were homozygous for the C allele. The genotype frequencies of the rs738409 polymorphism showed significant variations between NL, SS, and NASH patients ($p = 0.021$). In addition, the GG genotype was correlated with the presence of NASH ($r = 0.382$, $p < 0.001$). However, the allele frequencies did not show statistically significant differences ($p = 0.145$). Regarding clinical and biochemical variables, the GG genotype was only associated with increased body mass index (BMI) ($r = 0.300$, $p = 0.032$). There was no association between PNPLA3 genetic variant and its hepatic expression ($p = 0.478$).

Table 2. Correlations between *PNPLA3* expression and genes related to *de novo* lipogenesis, FA oxidation, FA transport and uptake, inflammation, adipocytokines, and cholesterol metabolism in livers from MO women and those sub-classified as SS in the MO cohort.

Variables	MO PNPLA3 (n = 55)		SS PNPLA3 (n = 20)	
	r	p-Value *	r	p-Value *
De Novo Lipogenesis				
SREBP1c	−0.016	0.920	0.130	0.906
LxRα	**0.671**	**0.008**	**0.806**	**0.016**
ACC1	−0.025	0.920	0.090	0.906
FAS	−0.021	0.920	0.114	0.906
Fatty Acid Oxidation				
PPARα	**0.640**	**0.008**	**0.796**	**0.024**
CPT1α	0.134	0.576	−0.233	0.906
CROT	0.200	0.466	0.098	0.906
Cholesterol Metabolism				
ABCA1	0.016	0.920	−0.189	0.906
SREBP2	**0.412**	**0.032**	0.361	0.784
Transport and Uptake FA				
FABP4	−0.371	0.285	0.464	0.784
ABCG1	0.099	0.713	−0.074	0.906
Inflammation				
IL6	−0.379	0.285	−0.012	0.980
TNFα	0.227	0.576	0.089	0.906
LCN2	**0.570**	**0.032**	0.466	0.784
Adipokines				
RESISTIN	0.209	0.576	0.124	0.906
ADIPOR2	−0.245	0.576	0.491	0.784

ABCA1: ATP-binding cassette transporter A1; ABCG1: ATP-binding cassette transporter G1; ADIPOR2: adiponectin receptor; ACC1: acetyl-coenzyme A carboxylase 1; CROT: carnitine O-octanoyltransferase; FA: fatty acid; FABP4: fatty acid binding protein 4; FAS: fatty acid synthase; IL6: interleukin 6; LCN2: lipocalin 2; LXRα: liver X receptor; MO: morbidly obese women; PPARα: peroxisome-proliferator-activated receptor α; SREBP1c: sterol regulatory element binding protein 1c; SREBP2: sterol regulatory element binding protein 2; SS: simple steatosis; TNFα: tumor necrosis factor. Bold numbers indicate statistically significant correlations (p-value < 0.05). * p-Value adjusted by the Benjamini–Hochberg method [24].

Table 3. The distribution of rs738409 polymorphism in morbidly obese women according to liver histology.

Groups	Genotype, n (%)		Allele, n (%)	
	CG	GG	C	G
NL (n = 16)	12 (75)	4 (25)	12 (37.5)	20 (62.5)
SS (n = 18)	15 (83.3)	3 (16.6)	15 (41.7)	21 (58.3)
NASH (n = 17)	7 (41.2)	10 (58.8)	7 (20.6)	27 (79.4)

CG: individuals carrying the genotype (CG); GG: individuals carrying the genotype (GG); C: Allele C; G: Allele G; NASH: morbidly obese subjects with steatohepatitis; NL: morbidly obese subjects with normal liver; SS: morbidly obese subjects with simple steatosis.

3. Discussion

In an own previous work, we demonstrated a downregulation of the lipogenic pathway related to the severity of steatosis in a cohort of women with morbid obesity [25]. As PNPLA3 seems to be related with the accumulation of hepatic TG, in the present study, we examined the relationship between the liver expression levels of *PNPLA3*, the key lipid metabolism-related genes expression, and the clinicopathological factors in a cohort of morbidly obese women with NAFLD. In our study, 36% and 31% of morbidly obese women were diagnosed with SS and NASH, respectively, using the diagnostic *gold standard* liver biopsy. Our findings show that *PNPLA3* liver expression was increased in morbidly obese women with NAFLD. It is important to note that we have demonstrated a clear relationship between *PNPLA3* and the degrees of SS, suggesting a direct correlation between *PNPLA3* and the severity of steatosis.

Nowadays, more than 50 studies on the genotyping of *PNPLA3* have confirmed the association between the 148M variant and the full range of NAFLD, including simple steatosis, steatohepatitis, cirrhosis, and hepatocellular carcinoma. PNPLA3 148M has been shown to be related to an increased risk of NAFLD across multiple ethnic groups [26–34]. The aim of the present work was to compare the hepatic expression of *PNPLA3* in a cohort of morbidly obese women presenting a normal liver or NAFLD. We showed that the hepatic expression of PNPLA3 in morbidly obese women with NAFLD was higher than in MO women with NL. Consistent with our work, Kotronen *et al.* [8] described a direct correlation between *PNPLA3* liver expression and liver fat content measured by magnetic resonance. It is important to note that our study confirms this finding in biopsy-proven NAFLD. Regarding steatosis degree, recent studies observed that a variant of this protein has an association with moderate-to-severe steatosis [35,36]. Although these studies analyzed only a variant of PNPLA3, not its liver expression, their results are in agreement with ours. A recent interesting work by Donati *et al.* [37] has demonstrated that PNPLA3 rs2294918 E434K diminished *PNPLA3* expression and protein levels, lessening the effect of the rs738409 polymorphism on the predisposition to steatosis liver injury. Moreover, the authors suggested that this PNPLA3 variant had a codominant negative effect on TG mobilization from lipid droplets. Regarding non-alcoholic steatohepatitis, a DNA microarray study in human liver revealed an upregulation of *PNPLA3* in NASH *vs.* healthy controls [38]. Nevertheless, Kitamoto *et al.* [39] described lower *PNPLA3* mRNA levels in the liver of patients with an advanced grade of NAFLD (with fibrosis) compared with those with mild NAFLD. However, we were not able to reproduce any of these findings. Perhaps the differences in the groups studied in these works regarding age, gender, BMI, or race can explain these discrepancies.

Because PNPLA3 has previously been reported to influence lipid metabolism in animal models and in *in vitro* studies [40,41], we evaluated the interplay of *PNPLA3* liver expression with the expression of the main lipid metabolism-related genes. In the current first human study in this sense, *PNPLA3* expression positively correlated with *LXRα*, *PPARα*, and *SREBP2* liver expression. All these proteins are transcription factors that relate to response elements found in a various genes that are associated with lipid turnover including their own genes [42]. Specifically, *LXRα* belong to the nuclear hormone receptor superfamily of ligand-activated transcription factors as *SREBP1* which, in liver, serve as lipid sensors and regulate the expression of main genes which modulate the cholesterol and FA metabolism [43]. Regarding NAFLD, interaction between *LXR* and *SREBP1* is a crucial step in the molecular cascade of events characterizing steatogenesis [44]. In this regard, Huang *et al.* [41] determined that the overexpression of the three SREBP family members (*SREBP1a*, *1c*, and *2*) increases liver *PNPLA3* expression in mice. They also found that PNPLA3 expression was regulated by *SREBP1c* and *LXRα*. Similar results were described by Dubuquoy *et al.* [45], who showed that, in the mouse liver, *PNPLA3* gene expression was under the direct transcriptional control of *SREBP1c* in response to insulin. However, at variance with murine studies, we were not able to find any association with *SREBP1*, one of the key genes related to *de novo* lipogenesis. Moreover, Mancina *et al.* [34] conducted a study to evaluate the contribution of *de novo* lipogenesis to liver fat accumulation in the PNPLA3 I148M genetic variant of NAFLD. They showed a dissociation between hepatic *de novo* lipogenesis and liver fat content due to the PNPLA3 148M allele, suggesting that increased *de novo* lipogenesis is not a main feature in all subjects with steatosis. However, these authors have not studied the hepatic expression of *PNPLA3*. Regarding the positive relationship between *PPARα* and PNPLA3, it is known that *PPARα* seems to control the expression of genes regulating peroxisomal/mitochondrial β-oxidation [46]. In this context, perhaps the induction of fatty acid catabolism might act as a defense mechanism, preventing hepatocellular fat accumulation [47]; in other words, it might represent an inefficient physiological response to counteract steatosis by promoting the β-oxidation of fatty acids in the hepatocytes. In our study, the association between *PNPLA3* and *SREBP2* may suggest a novel association with cholesterol metabolism in humans. Currently, experimental and human evidence has related to altered hepatic cholesterol metabolism and free cholesterol accumulation to the pathogenesis of steatosis and liver damage [48]. Specifically, Min *et al.* [49] have demonstrated dysregulated cholesterol metabolism in NAFLD, which may contribute to disease severity through activation of SREBP2 and 3-Hydroxy-3-Methylglutaryl-CoA Reductase (HMGCR).

In the present work, we observed an interesting association between liver PNPLA3 expression and the liver expression of *LCN2* in the severely obese women group, which has not been previously described. In one of our previous studies, we described increased liver *LCN2* expression in NAFLD, and this expression positively correlated with SS [50]. Additionally, in this work, an increased regulation of *LCN2* expression was detected in *in vitro* experiments with HepG2 cells under harmful conditions. Perhaps, as some authors have suggested, *LCN2* is a protective molecule [51]—in this case, against the development of NAFLD.

Moreover, we did not find any relationship between *PNPLA3* liver expression and other adipocytokines studied, probably because the molecular function of PNPLA3 is related to cellular lipid accumulation in the liver more than with inflammation [52]. Unexpectedly, we did not find any relationship with the expression of genes related to transport and the uptake of fatty acids. Perhaps this mechanism of liver accumulation of fatty acids has a lower contribution in humans, as we and other authors have previously shown [25,38].

Finally, to explore the effect of the *PNPLA3* genetic variant with a potential impact on NAFLD, we determined the relationship between the rs738409 polymorphism in the *PNPLA3* gene and the severity of disease. In this sense, we found that the GG genotype, encoding I148M, was directly correlated with the presence of NASH. Our results are similar to recent studies that showed a relationship between this genetic variant and the severity of NAFLD [12,13,15,53]. Consistent with our results, Kotronen *et al.* [8] observed that there were no differences in the hepatic *PNPLA3* mRNA expression between different *PNPLA3* genotype carriers.

We should point out the following drawbacks of our study. The main limitation of this work is an adjusted sample size and the lack of evaluation of protein expression. Additionally, the study is cross-sectional. We could not prove a causal link between *PNPLA3* expression and NALFD development. However, our study cohort of morbidly obese women has revealed clear relationships between the expression of *PNPLA3* and NAFLD, without the interference of gender or age. Thus, our findings cannot be extrapolated to men or other obesity groups such as normal-weight or over-weight women.

4. Materials and Methods

4.1. Subjects

The study was approved by the ethics committee of the Hospital Joan XXIII (23c/2015, Tarragona, Spain), and all subjects gave written informed consent. We included 55 Caucasian MO women (BMI > 40 kg/m^2). Liver biopsies were obtained during planned laparoscopic bariatric surgery and were performed for clinical indications.

The diagnosis of NAFLD was made using the following criteria: (1) liver pathology; (2) an intake of less than 10 g of ethanol/day; and (3) appropriate exclusion of other liver diseases.

The body weight of all women had not fluctuated more than 2% for at least 3 months prior to bariatric surgery. The exclusion criteria were: (1) concurrent use of medications known to produce hepatic steatosis; (2) patients using hypolipemiant treatment; (3) diabetic subjects who were receiving insulin or on medication likely to influence endogenous insulin levels; (4) menopausal or post-menopausal women; (5) women undergoing contraceptive treatment and subjects receiving contraceptive treatment; (6) patients who had an acute illness, current evidence of acute or chronic inflammatory or infectious diseases, or malignant diseases.

4.2. Liver Pathology

Liver samples were processed by two experienced hepatopathologists using methods previously described [54,55]. Simple steatosis (SS) was graded as follows: Grade 1 or mild SS: more than 5% and less than 33% of hepatocytes affected; Grade 2 or moderate SS: 33% to 66% of hepatocytes affected; or Grade 3 or severe SS: more than 66% of hepatocytes affected. Moreover, the minimum criteria for the steatohepatitis diagnosis included the presence of either ballooning cells and lobular inflammation or perisinusoidal/pericellular fibrosis in zone 3 of the hepatic acinus.

According to liver pathology, women were sub-classified into: (1) normal liver (NL) histology ($n = 18$); (2) simple steatosis (SS) (micro/macrovesicular steatosis without inflammation or fibrosis, $n = 20$); (3) non-alcoholic steatohepatitis (NASH) (Brunt Grades 1–3, $n = 17$).

4.3. Biochemical Analyses

Each of our patients was evaluated with a complete physical, anthropometrical, and biochemical assessment. BMI was calculated as body weight divided by height squared (kg/m^2). Fasting glucose, insulin, HbA1c, HDL-C, LDL-C, TG, and transaminases were measured using a conventional automated analyzer after overnight fasting. Insulin resistance was calculated using HOMA2-IR [56].

4.4. RNA Isolation and Real-Time PCR

Liver samples were preserved in RNAlater (Sigma, Barcelona, Spain) for 24 h at 4 °C and then stored at −80 °C. Total RNA was extracted by using an RNeasy mini kit (Qiagen, Barcelona, Spain). And was reverse transcribed by the High Capacity RNA-to-cDNA Kit (Applied Biosystems, Madrid, Spain). Real-time quantitative PCR was carried out with the TaqMan Assay predesigned by Applied Biosystems for the detection of *PNPLA3* (Hs00228747_m1), *ABCA1* (Hs01059118_m1), *ABCG1* (Hs00245154_m1), *ADIPOR2* (Hs00226105_m1), *ACC1* (Hs00167385_m1), *CROT* (Hs00221733_m1), *FABP4* (Hs00609791_m1), *FAS* (Hs00188012_m1), *IL6* (Hs00985639_m1), *LCN2* (Hs00194353_m1), *LXRα* (Hs00173195_m1), *PPARα*(Hs00947538_m1), *RESISTIN* (Hs00220767_m1), *SREBP1c* (Hs01088691_m1), *SREBP2* (Hs01081784_m1), *TNFα*(Hs99999043_m1), and *18S ribosomal RNA* (4352930E), which was used as the housekeeping gene. All reactions were performed in duplicate using the 7900HT Fast Real-Time PCR systems (Applied Biosystems).

4.5. Genotyping

Subjects were genotyped for the rs738409 polymorphism using the TaqMan 5′ allelic discrimination assay (TaqMan SNP Genotyping Assay C 7241 10, Applied Biosystems,). Amplifications were carried out using the 7900HT Sequencing Detection System for continuous fluorescence monitoring.

4.6. Statistical Analysis

We used the SPSS/PC+ statistical package for Windows (version 22.0; SPSS, Chicago, IL, USA). One-way ANOVA with a *post-hoc* Tukey test was carried out to determine differences between groups. The correlations between variables was analyzed using Pearson's method (parametric variables) and Spearman's test (non-parametric variables). Allele and genotype frequencies were evaluated with the χ-squared test. *p*-Values <0.05 were considered to be statistically significant.

5. Conclusions

The main results of our study show that liver *PNPLA3* expression is increased in NAFLD patients and is particularly associated to severity of steatosis. Moreover, *PNPLA3* expression is correlated with the expression of main cholesterol and hepatic lipid metabolism-related genes. Further human studies are required to confirm these associations.

Acknowledgments: This study was supported by the Fondo de Investigación Sanitaria and Fondo Europeo de Desarrollo Regional (FEDER, grant number PI13/00468, to Teresa Auguet), by funds from Agència de Gestió d'Ajuts Universitaris de Recerca (AGAUR 2009 SGR 959 to Cristóbal Richart) and the Grup de Recerca en Medicina Aplicada-Universitat Rovira Virgili (2015 PFR-URV-B2-72 to Cristóbal Richart), and by the Fundación Biociencia.

Author Contributions: Gemma Aragonès and Teresa Auguet participated in the design of the study and in the analysis and interpretation of data and were involved in the drafting of the manuscript. Teresa Auguet reviewed/edited the manuscript. Sandra Armengol, Alba Berlanga, Esther Guiu-Jurado, and Carmen Aguilar carried out the experimental work. Salomé Martinez and Joan Josep Sirvent are the pathologists. Maikel Daniel Ruiz, Fátima Sabench, Mercé Hernández, José Antonio Porras, and Daniel Del Castillo made substantial contributions to the conception and design of the study, and to the acquisition of the samples. Cristóbal Richart revised the draft and gave the final approval for publication. The authors have all seen the final version.

Abbreviations

ABCA1	ATP-binding cassette transporter A1
ABCG1	ATP-binding cassette transporter G1
ADIPOR	adiponectin receptor
ACC1	acetyl-coenzyme A carboxylase 1
ALT	alanine aminotransaminase
AST	aspartate aminotransaminase
ALP	alkaline phosphatase
BMI	body mass index
CROT	carnitine O-octanoyltransferase
FABP4	fatty acid binding protein 4
FAS	fatty acid synthase
18S	18S ribosomal RNA
GGT	γ-glutamyl transferase
HbA1c	glycosylated hemoglobin
HDL-C	high density lipoprotein
HOMA2-IR	homeostasis model assessment of insulin resistance
IL6	interleukin 6
LDL-C	low density lipoprotein
LCN2	lipocalin 2
LXRα	liver X receptor
MO	morbidly obese
NAFLD	non-alcoholic fatty liver disease
NASH	non-alcoholic steatosis
NL	normal liver
PPARα	peroxisome-proliferator-activated receptor α
SREBP1c	sterol regulatory element binding protein 1c
SREBP2	sterol regulatory element binding protein 2
SS	simple steatosis
TG	triglycerides
TNFα	tumor necrosis factor
WC	waist circumference

References

1.   Lonardo, A.; Bellentani, S.; Argo, C.K.; Ballestri, S.; Byrne, C.D.; Caldwell, S.H.; Cortez-Pinto, H.; Grieco, A.; Machado, M.V.; Miele, L.; *et al.* Epidemiological modifiers of non-alcoholic fatty liver disease: Focus on high-risk groups. *Dig. Liver Dis.* **2015**, *47*, 997–1006. [CrossRef]

2.   Farrell, G.C.; Larter, C.Z. Nonalcoholic fatty liver disease: From steatosis to cirrhosis. *Hepatology* **2006**, *43*, S99–S112. [CrossRef]

3.   Younossi, Z.M.; Koenig, A.B.; Abdelatif, D.; Fazel, Y.; Henry, L.; Wymer, M. Global epidemiology of non-alcoholic fatty liver disease-meta-analytic assessment of prevalence, incidence and outcomes. *Hepatology* **2015**. [CrossRef]

4.   Ballestri, S.; Romagnoli, D.; Nascimbeni, F.; Francica, G.; Lonardo, A. Role of ultrasound in the diagnosis and treatment of nonalcoholic fatty liver disease and its complications. *Expert Rev. Gastroenterol. Hepatol.* **2015**, *9*, 603–627. [CrossRef]

5.   Buzzetti, E.; Pinzani, M.; Tsochatzis, E.A. The multiple-hit pathogenesis of non-alcoholic fatty liver disease (NAFLD). *Metabolism* **2016**, 1–11. [CrossRef]

6.   Vernon, G.; Baranova, A.; Younossi, Z.M. Systematic review: The epidemiology and natural history of non-alcoholic fatty liver disease and non-alcoholic steatohepatitis in adults. *Aliment. Pharmacol. Ther.* **2011**, *34*, 274–285. [CrossRef]

7.   Daly, A.K.; Ballestri, S.; Carulli, L.; Loria, P.; Day, C.P. Genetic determinants of susceptibility and severity in nonalcoholic fatty liver disease. *Expert Rev. Gastroenterol. Hepatol.* **2011**, *5*, 253–263. [CrossRef]

8.   Kotronen, A.; Johansson, L.E.; Johansson, L.M.; Roos, C.; Westerbacka, J.; Hamsten, A.; Bergholm, R.; Arkkila, P.; Arola, J.; Kiviluoto, T.; *et al.* A common variant in PNPLA3, which encodes adiponutrin, is associated with liver fat content in humans. *Diabetologia* **2009**, *52*, 1056–1060. [CrossRef]

9.   Sookoian, S.; Pirola, C.J. PNPLA3, the triacylglycerol synthesis/hydrolysis/storage dilemma, and nonalcoholic fatty liver disease. *World J. Gastroenterol.* **2012**, *18*, 6018–6026. [CrossRef]

10. Jenkins, C.M.; Mancuso, D.J.; Yan, W.; Sims, H.F.; Gibson, B.; Gross, R.W. Identification, cloning, expression, and purification of three novel human calcium-independent phospholipase A2 family members possessing triacylglycerol lipase and acylglycerol transacylase activities. *J. Biol. Chem.* **2004**, *279*, 48968–48975. [CrossRef]

11. Lake, A.C.1.; Sun, Y.; Li, J.L.; Kim, J.E.; Johnson, J.W.; Li, D.; Revett, T.; Shih, H.H.; Liu, W.; Paulsen, J.E.; *et al.* Expression, regulation, and triglyceride hydrolase activity of Adiponutrin family members. *J. Lipid Res.* **2005**, *46*, 2477–2487. [CrossRef]

12. Romeo, S.; Kozlitina, J.; Xing, C.; Pertsemlidis, A.; Cox, D.; Pennacchio, L.A.; Boerwinkle, E.; Cohen, J.C.; Hobbs, H.H. Genetic variation in PNPLA3 confers susceptibility to nonalcoholic fatty liver disease. *Nat. Genet.* **2008**, *40*, 1461–1465. [CrossRef]

13. Rotman, Y.; Koh, C.; Zmuda, J.M.; Kleiner, D.E.; Liang, T.J. The association of genetic variability in patatin-like phospholipase domain-containing protein 3 (PNPLA3) with histological severity of nonalcoholic fatty liver disease. *Hepatology* **2010**, *52*, 894–903. [CrossRef]

14. Valenti, L.; Alisi, A.; Galmozzi, E.; Bartuli, A.; Del Menico, B.; Alterio, A.; Dongiovanni, P.; Fargion, S.; Nobili, V. I148M patatin-like phospholipase domain-containing 3 gene variant and severity of pediatric nonalcoholic fatty liver disease. *Hepatology* **2010**, *52*, 1274–1280. [CrossRef]

15. Sookoian, S.; Pirola, C.J. Meta-analysis of the influence of I148M variant of patatin-like phospholipase domain containing 3 gene (*PNPLA3*) on the susceptibility and histological severity of nonalcoholic fatty liver disease. *Hepatology* **2011**, *53*, 1883–1894. [CrossRef]

16. Krawczyk, M.; Grünhage, F.; Zimmer, V.; Lammert, F. Variant adiponutrin (PNPLA3) represents a common fibrosis risk gene: Non-invasive elastography-based study in chronic liver disease. *J. Hepatol.* **2011**, *55*, 299–306. [CrossRef]

17. Valenti, L.; Al-Serri, A.; Daly, A.K.; Galmozzi, E.; Rametta, R.; Dongiovanni, P.; Nobili, V.; Mozzi, E.; Roviaro, G.; Vanni, E.; *et al.* Homozygosity for the patatin-like phospholipase-3/adiponutrin I148M polymorphism influences liver fibrosis in patients with nonalcoholic fatty liver disease. *Hepatology* **2010**, *51*, 1209–1217. [CrossRef]

18. Zain, S.M.; Mohamed, R.; Mahadeva, S.; Cheah, P.L.; Rampal, S.; Basu, R.C.; Mohamed, Z. A multi-ethnic study of a *PNPLA3* gene variant and its association with disease severity in non-alcoholic fatty liver disease. *Hum. Genet.* **2012**, *131*, 1145–1152. [CrossRef] [PubMed]

19. Kovarova, M.; Königsrainer, I.; Königsrainer, A.; Machicao, F.; Häring, H.-U.; Schleicher, E.; Peter, A. The genetic variant I148M in *PNPLA3* is associated with increased hepatic retinyl-palmitate storage in humans. *J. Clin. Endocrinol. Metab.* **2015**, *100*, E1568–E1574. [CrossRef] [PubMed]

20. Pirazzi, C.; Valenti, L.; Motta, B.M.; Pingitore, P.; Hedfalk, K.; Mancina, R.M.; Burza, M.A.; Indiveri, C.; Ferro, Y.; Montalcini, T.; *et al.* PNPLA3 has retinyl-palmitate lipase activity in human hepatic stellate cells. *Hum. Mol. Genet.* **2014**, *23*, 4077–4085. [CrossRef] [PubMed]

21. Chamoun, Z.; Vacca, F.; Parton, R.G.; Gruenberg, J. PNPLA3/adiponutrin functions in lipid droplet formation. *Biol. Cell* **2013**, *105*, 219–233. [CrossRef] [PubMed]

22. Ruhanen, H.; Perttilä, J.; Hölttä-Vuori, M.; Zhou, Y.; Yki-Järvinen, H.; Ikonen, E.; Käkelä, R.; Olkkonen, V.M. PNPLA3 mediates hepatocyte triacylglycerol remodelling. *J. Lipid Res.* **2014**, *55*, 739–746. [CrossRef] [PubMed]

23. Min, H.-K.; Sookoian, S.; Pirola, C.J.; Cheng, J.; Mirshahi, F.; Sanyal, A.J. Metabolic profiling reveals that PNPLA3 induces widespread effects on metabolism beyond triacylglycerol remodeling in Huh-7 hepatoma cells. *Am. J. Physiol. Gastrointest. Liver Physiol.* **2014**, *307*, G66–G76. [CrossRef] [PubMed]

24. Benjamini, Y.; Hochberg, Y. Controlling the false discovery rate: A practical and powerful approach to multiple testing. *J. R. Stat. Soc. B* **1995**, *57*, 289–300.

25. Auguet, T.; Berlanga, A.; Guiu-Jurado, E.; Martinez, S.; Porras, J.A.; Aragonès, G.; Sabench, F.; Hernandez, M.; Aguilar, C.; Sirvent, J.J.; *et al.* Altered fatty acid metabolism-related gene expression in liver from morbidly obese women with non-alcoholic fatty liver disease. *Int. J. Mol. Sci.* **2014**, *15*, 22173–22187. [CrossRef] [PubMed]

26. Lin, Y.-C.; Chang, P.-F.; Chang, M.-H.; Ni, Y.-H. Genetic variants in GCKR and PNPLA3 confer susceptibility to nonalcoholic fatty liver disease in obese individuals. *Am. J. Clin. Nutr.* **2014**, *99*, 869–874. [CrossRef] [PubMed]

27. Wu, P.; Shu, Y.; Guo, F.; Luo, H.; Zhang, G.; Tan, S. [Association between patatin-like phospholipase domain-containing protein 3 gene rs738409 polymorphism and non-alcoholic fatty liver disease susceptibility: A meta-analysis]. *Zhonghua Liu Xing Bing Xue Za Zhi* **2015**, *36*, 78–82. [PubMed]

28. Xu, R.; Tao, A.; Zhang, S.; Deng, Y.; Chen, G. Association between patatin-like phospholipase domain containing 3 gene (PNPLA3) polymorphisms and nonalcoholic fatty liver disease: A HuGE review and meta-analysis. *Sci. Rep.* **2015**, *5*, 9284. [CrossRef] [PubMed]

29. Zhang, L.; You, W.; Zhang, H.; Peng, R.; Zhu, Q.; Yao, A.; Li, X.; Zhou, Y.; Wang, X.; Pu, L.; *et al.* PNPLA3 polymorphisms (rs738409) and non-alcoholic fatty liver disease risk and related phenotypes: A meta-analysis. *J. Gastroenterol. Hepatol.* **2015**, *30*, 821–829. [CrossRef] [PubMed]

30. León-Mimila, P.; Vega-Badillo, J.; Gutiérrez-Vidal, R.; Villamil-Ramírez, H.; Villareal-Molina, T.; Larrieta-Carrasco, E.; López-Contreras, B.E.; Kauffer, L.R.M.; Maldonado-Pintado, D.G.; Méndez-Sánchez, N.; *et al.* A genetic risk score is associated with hepatic triglyceride content and non-alcoholic steatohepatitis in Mexicans with morbid obesity. *Exp. Mol. Pathol.* **2015**, *98*, 178–183. [CrossRef] [PubMed]

31. Zhang, Y.; Cai, W.; Song, J.; Miao, L.; Zhang, B.; Xu, Q.; Zhang, L.; Yao, H. Association between the PNPLA3 I148M polymorphism and non-alcoholic fatty liver disease in the Uygur and Han ethnic groups of northwestern China. *PLoS ONE* **2014**, *9*, e108381. [CrossRef] [PubMed]

32. Tai, C.-M.; Huang, C.-K.; Tu, H.-P.; Hwang, J.-C.; Chang, C.-Y.; Yu, M.-L. PNPLA3 genotype increases susceptibility of nonalcoholic steatohepatitis among obese patients with nonalcoholic fatty liver disease. *Surg. Obes. Relat. Dis.* **2014**, *11*, 888–894. [CrossRef] [PubMed]

33. Lee, S.S.; Byoun, Y.-S.; Jeong, S.-H.; Woo, B.H.; Jang, E.S.; Kim, J.-W.; Kim, H.Y. Role of the PNPLA3 I148M polymorphism in nonalcoholic fatty liver disease and fibrosis in Korea. *Dig. Dis. Sci.* **2014**, *59*, 2967–2974. [CrossRef] [PubMed]

34. Margherita Mancina, R.; Matikainen, N.; Maglio, C.; Söderlund, S.; Lundbom, N.; Hakkarainen, A.; Rametta, R.; Mozzi, E.; Fargion, S.; Valenti, L.; *et al.* Paradoxical dissociation between hepatic fat content and *de novo* lipogenesis due to PNPLA3 sequence variant. *J. Clin. Endocrinol. Metab.* **2015**, *100*, E821–E825. [CrossRef] [PubMed]

35. Shang, X.R.; Song, J.Y.; Liu, F.H.; Ma, J.; Wang, H.J. GWAS-identified common variants with nonalcoholic fatty liver disease in chinese children. *J. Pediatr. Gastroenterol. Nutr.* **2015**, *60*, 669–674. [CrossRef] [PubMed]

36. Nobili, V.; Liccardo, D.; Bedogni, G.; Salvatori, G.; Gnani, D.; Bersani, I.; Alisi, A.; Valenti, L.; Raponi, M. Influence of dietary pattern, physical activity, and I148M PNPLA3 on steatosis severity in at-risk adolescents. *Genes Nutr.* **2014**, *9*, 392. [CrossRef] [PubMed]

37. Donati, B.; Motta, B.M.; Pingitore, P.; Meroni, M.; Pietrelli, A.; Alisi, A.; Petta, S.; Xing, C.; Dongiovanni, P.; del Menico, B.; *et al.* The rs2294918 E434K variant modulates patatin-like phospholipase domain-containing 3 expression and liver damage. *Hepatology* **2016**, *63*, 787–798. [CrossRef] [PubMed]

38. Arendt, B.M.; Comelli, E.M.; Ma, D.W.L.; Lou, W.; Teterina, A.; Kim, T.; Fung, S.K.; Wong, D.K.H.; McGilvray, I.; Fischer, S.E.; *et al.* Altered hepatic gene expression in nonalcoholic fatty liver disease is associated with lower hepatic n-3 and n-6 polyunsaturated fatty acids. *Hepatology* **2015**, *61*, 1565–1578. [CrossRef]

39. Kitamoto, T.; Kitamoto, A.; Ogawa, Y.; Honda, Y.; Imajo, K.; Saito, S.; Yoneda, M.; Nakamura, T.; Nakajima, A.; Hotta, K. Targeted-bisulfite sequence analysis of the methylation of CpG islands in genes encoding PNPLA3, SAMM50, and PARVB of patients with non-alcoholic fatty liver disease. *J. Hepatol.* **2015**, *63*, 494–502. [CrossRef] [PubMed]

40. Hao, L.; Ito, K.; Huang, K.H.; Sae-tan, S.; Lambert, J.D.; Ross, A.C. Shifts in dietary carbohydrate-lipid exposure regulate expression of the non-alcoholic fatty liver disease-associated gene PNPLA3/adiponutrin in mouse liver and HepG2 human liver cells. *Metabolism* **2014**, *63*, 1352–1362. [CrossRef] [PubMed]

41. Huang, Y.; He, S.; Li, J.Z.; Seo, Y.-K.; Osborne, T.F.; Cohen, J.C.; Hobbs, H.H. A feed-forward loop amplifies nutritional regulation of PNPLA3. *Proc. Natl. Acad. Sci. USA* **2010**, *107*, 7892–7897. [CrossRef] [PubMed]

42. Bechmann, L.P.; Hannivoort, R.A.; Gerken, G.; Hotamisligil, G.S.; Trauner, M.; Canbay, A. The interaction of hepatic lipid and glucose metabolism in liver diseases. *J. Hepatol.* **2012**, *56*, 952–964. [CrossRef] [PubMed]

43. Zhang, X.; Liu, J.; Su, W.; Wu, J.; Wang, C.; Kong, X.; Gustafsson, J.-Å.; Ding, J.; Ma, X.; Guan, Y. Liver X receptor activation increases hepatic fatty acid desaturation by the induction of SCD1 expression through an LXRα-SREBP1c-dependent mechanism. *J. Diabetes* **2014**, *6*, 212–220. [CrossRef] [PubMed]

44. Ballestri, S.; Nascimbeni, F.; Romagnoli, D.; Baldelli, E.; Lonardo, A. The role of nuclear receptors in the pathophysiology, natural course, and drug treatment of NAFLD in humans. *Adv. Ther.* **2016**, *33*, 291–319. [CrossRef] [PubMed]

45. Dubuquoy, C.; Robichon, C.; Lasnier, F.; Langlois, C.; Dugail, I.; Foufelle, F.; Girard, J.; Burnol, A.F.; Postic, C.; Moldes, M. Distinct regulation of adiponutrin/PNPLA3 gene expression by the transcription factors ChREBP and SREBP1c in mouse and human hepatocytes. *J. Hepatol.* **2011**, *55*, 145–153. [CrossRef] [PubMed]

46. Pawlak, M.; Lefebvre, P.; Staels, B. Molecular mechanism of PPARα action and its impact on lipid metabolism, inflammation and fibrosis in non-alcoholic fatty liver disease. *J. Hepatol.* **2015**, *62*, 720–733. [CrossRef] [PubMed]

47. Dongiovanni, P.; Valenti, L. Peroxisome proliferator-activated receptor genetic polymorphisms and nonalcoholic Fatty liver disease: Any role in disease susceptibility? *PPAR Res.* **2013**, *2013*, 452061. [CrossRef] [PubMed]

48. Musso, G.; Gambino, R.; Cassader, M. Cholesterol metabolism and the pathogenesis of non-alcoholic steatohepatitis. *Prog. Lipid Res.* **2013**, *52*, 175–191. [CrossRef] [PubMed]

49. Min, H.-K.; Kapoor, A.; Fuchs, M.; Mirshahi, F.; Zhou, H.; Maher, J.; Kellum, J.; Warnick, R.; Contos, M.J.; Sanyal, A.J. Increased hepatic synthesis and dysregulation of cholesterol metabolism is associated with the severity of nonalcoholic fatty liver disease. *Cell Metab.* **2012**, *15*, 665–674. [CrossRef] [PubMed]

50. Auguet, T.; Terra, X.; Quintero, Y.; Martínez, S.; Manresa, N.; Porras, J.A.; Aguilar, C.; Orellana-Gavaldà, J.M.; Hernández, M.; Sabench, F.; *et al.* Liver lipocalin 2 expression in severely obese women with non alcoholic fatty liver disease. *Exp. Clin. Endocrinol. Diabetes* **2013**, *121*, 119–124. [CrossRef] [PubMed]

51. Lee, E.-K.; Kim, H.-J.; Lee, K.-J.; Lee, H.-J.; Lee, J.-S.; Kim, D.-G.; Hong, S.-W.; Yoon, Y.; Kim, J.-S. Inhibition of the proliferation and invasion of hepatocellular carcinoma cells by lipocalin 2 through blockade of JNK and PI3K/Akt signaling. *Int. J. Oncol.* **2011**, *38*, 325–333. [CrossRef] [PubMed]

52. Kumari, M.; Schoiswohl, G.; Chitraju, C.; Paar, M.; Rangrez, A.Y.; Wongsiriroj, N.; Nagy, H.M.; Pavlina, T.; Scott, S.A.; Knittelfelder, O.; *et al.* Adiponutrin functions as a nutritionally regulated lysophosphatidic acid acyltransferase. *Cell Metab.* **2012**, *15*, 691–702. [CrossRef] [PubMed]

53. Chen, L.Z.; Xin, Y.N.; Geng, N.; Jiang, M.; Zhang, D.D.; Xuan, S.Y. PNPLA3 I148M variant in nonalcoholic fatty liver disease: Demographic and ethnic characteristics and the role of the variant in nonalcoholic fatty liver fibrosis. *World J. Gastroenterol.* **2015**, *21*, 794–802. [PubMed]

54. Kleiner, D.E.; Brunt, E.M.; Van Natta, M.; Behling, C.; Contos, M.J.; Cummings, O.W.; Ferrell, L.D.; Liu, Y.-C.; Torbenson, M.S.; Unalp-Arida, A.; *et al.* Design and validation of a histological scoring system for nonalcoholic fatty liver disease. *Hepatology* **2005**, *41*, 1313–1321. [CrossRef] [PubMed]
55. Brunt, E.M.; Janney, C.G.; Di Bisceglie, A.M.; Neuschwander-Tetri, B.A.; Bacon, B.R. Nonalcoholic steatohepatitis: A proposal for grading and staging the histological lesions. *Am. J. Gastroenterol.* **1999**, *94*, 2467–2474. [CrossRef] [PubMed]
56. Terra, X.; Quintero, Y.; Auguet, T.; Porras, J.A.; Hernández, M.; Sabench, F.; Aguilar, C.; Luna, A.M.; Del Castillo, D.; Richart, C. FABP 4 is associated with inflammatory markers and metabolic syndrome in morbidly obese women. *Eur. J. Endocrinol.* **2011**, *164*, 539–547. [CrossRef] [PubMed]

7

Role of Hedgehog Signaling Pathway in NASH

Mariana Verdelho Machado [1,2,*] and Anna Mae Diehl [1,*]

[1]   Division of Gastroenterology, Department of Medicine, Duke University Medical Center, Durham, NC 27710, USA

[2]   Gastroenterology Department, Hospital de Santa Maria, Centro Hospitalar Lisboa Norte (CHLN), Lisboa 1649-035, Portugal

*   Correspondence: mverdelhomachado@gmail.com (M.V.M.); diehl004@mc.duke.edu or annamae.diehl@dm.duke.edu (A.M.D.)

Academic Editors: Amedeo Lonardo and Giovanni Targher

Abstract: Non-alcoholic fatty liver disease (NAFLD) is the number one cause of chronic liver disease in the Western world. Although only a minority of patients will ultimately develop end-stage liver disease, it is not yet possible to efficiently predict who will progress and, most importantly, effective treatments are still unavailable. Better understanding of the pathophysiology of this disease is necessary to improve the clinical management of NAFLD patients. Epidemiological data indicate that NAFLD prognosis is determined by an individual's response to lipotoxic injury, rather than either the severity of exposure to lipotoxins, or the intensity of liver injury. The liver responds to injury with a synchronized wound-healing response. When this response is abnormal, it leads to pathological scarring, resulting in progressive fibrosis and cirrhosis, rather than repair. The hedgehog pathway is a crucial player in the wound-healing response. In this review, we summarize the pre-clinical and clinical evidence, which demonstrate the role of hedgehog pathway dysregulation in NAFLD pathogenesis, and the preliminary data that place the hedgehog pathway as a potential target for the treatment of this disease.

Keywords: nonalcoholic fatty liver disease; hedgehog pathway; wound-healing response

1. Introduction

Nonalcoholic fatty liver disease (NAFLD), the ectopic accumulation of fat in the liver that is unrelated to excessive alcohol consumption, is the liver pandemic of our century. NAFLD affects roughly one billion subjects worldwide [1]. When steatosis is accompanied by cell death and inflammation it is dubbed nonalcoholic steatohepatitis (NASH). The main risk factors for NAFLD/NASH are obesity and its associated metabolic disorders, such as type 2 diabetes mellitus and the metabolic syndrome [2]. Energy surplus overcomes the reservoir capacity of the adipose tissue, leading to ectopic accumulation of fat in the cardiovascular system, the pancreas and the liver [3]. The majority of individuals affected with NAFLD have non-progressive, isolated steatosis; about a quarter will develop NASH, and fewer than 10% will progress to liver cirrhosis and end-stage liver disease [4]. However, due to the high prevalence of NAFLD, it is already the second cause of liver transplantation in the US [5], and the most rapidly growing cause of liver transplantation in patients with hepatocellular carcinoma [6]. These epidemiological data have huge implications for the management of NAFLD: To follow and/or treat all individuals with NAFLD would be impractical and pointless. On the other hand, we clearly need to identify those at risk for severe liver-related morbidity and mortality. Our aim should be to identify this high-risk subpopulation in an effective, non-invasive, simple, and inexpensive way. Ideally, we should also have an effective treatment to apply. Recent epidemiological studies have demonstrated that neither the severity of steatosis, nor the presence of hepatocellular injury (*i.e.*, NASH), independently predict which NAFLD patients will develop bad liver outcomes [7–9]. On the other hand, NAFLD prognosis strongly correlates with the presence and severity of liver fibrosis [7,8]. Liver fibrosis is a manifestation of defective regeneration and thus, whether or not liver injury is repaired effectively is a better determinant of liver outcome than the severity of the insult (steatosis), or the severity of the injury (hepatocellular ballooning and NASH), *per se*. Lipotoxic insults that damage the liver trigger a wound-healing response to regenerate normal hepatic architecture and function. This process involves coordinated actions of different cell types, such as epithelial cells, progenitor cells, matrix-producing cells, endothelial cells and inflammatory cells, which collaborate to restrain toxicity and match the increased metabolic demands required to remodel the matrix, replace lost liver cells, and regenerate functional liver mass. Inability to assemble a wound-healing response may lead to liver failure. However, an overly exuberant response leads to excessive fibrogenesis and promotes scarring that may progress to cirrhosis and its complications. In fact, a study evaluating hepatic gene expression in patients with NAFLD showed that the most important difference between patients with mild NAFLD and NAFLD with advanced fibrosis was up-regulation of several genes in tissue repair and regeneration [10]. Therefore, understanding the mechanisms governing the wound-healing response is critical to develop therapeutic strategies that optimize liver repair to permit full recovery from fatty liver damage. The hedgehog pathway is a pivotal maestro of the wound-healing response, and its actions are conserved across different organs, including the skin [11], lung [12], kidney [13], pancreas [14] and liver [15]. Because hedgehog is the best characterized pathway that mediates liver fibrosis in NAFLD, we will summarize the role of hedgehog in the pathogenesis and progression of NAFLD, in this review.

2. The Hedgehog Signaling Pathway

The hedgehog (Hh) pathway was first identified by Nüsslein-Volhard and Wirschaus, in a genetic screen in *Drosophila melanogaster* [16]. Flies deficient in Hh had developmental defects in the cuticle, displaying a layer of disorganized hair-liked bristles that resembled the mammal hedgehog. Hh is a morphogen, and as such, its effect on cell fate depends on its local concentration. Hh diffuses to the extracellular matrix and thus, cells closer to the Hh-producing cells are exposed to high concentrations of Hh ligands [17]. Hh ligands (Sonic hedgehog, Shh; Indian hedgehog, Ihh; and Desert hedgehog, Dhh) are produced as 45 kDa precursor proteins, and undergo autocatalytic cleavage. The resultant N-terminal fragment has intrinsic cholesterol transferase activity, which promotes cholesterol lipidation of the active N-terminal fragment. Cholesterol modification is very important for Hh activity, promoting its retention in plasma membrane lipid rafts where Hh ligands interact with other lipids. A member of the membrane-bound O-acyltransferase (MBOAT) protein family, skinny hedgehog (SKI), mediates a second lipidation with palmitic acid. Palmitoylation is necessary for full ligand activity, as well as for long-distance movement [18]. Release of Hh from producing cells occurs in one of three ways: a process facilitated by the protein Dispatched, through assembly in very low-density lipoproteins (VLDL), or through exosomes [18].

All three mammalian Hh ligands have similar affinity for Hh binding proteins. They are equipotent in some but not all cell types, denoting overlap but also some specificity in their action [19]. Shh and Ihh are expressed widely, though Shh is the predominant ligand in the proximal gut, and Ihh in the hindgut. Dhh expression, however, is restricted to the nervous tissue and testis [20].

The cellular receptor for Hh is the 12-transmembranar protein Patched (Ptch). Ptch exists in two isoforms: Ptch-1, which is the one definitely involved in the activation of the Hh pathway, and Ptch-2, which seems to be expressed independently of pathway activity [21]. Three co-receptors enhance ligand-receptor interaction: CAM-related down-regulated by oncogenes (Cdo), brother of Cdo (Boc), and growth arrest-specific (GAS)-1 [17].

Cells in the resting state express Ptch that exerts a repressing effect on Smoothened (Smo). When Hh ligand binds to Ptch, it eliminates the repressing effect on Smo, allowing activation of the hedgehog pathway, through regulation of the processing and stability of Gli transcription factors. In short, when Smo is inactive, Gli factors are either degraded or processed in inactive forms. In contrast, when Smo is active, full-length Gli factors (or processed active forms) are stabilized and can accumulate/translocate to the nucleus, where they act as transcription factors.

In the absence of Hh ligand, Gli couples to a suppressor protein complex composed by fused kinase (Fu), suppressor of Fused (Sufu) and Costal-2 (Cos) [20,22]. This complex sequesters Gli in the cytoplasm promoting its sequential serine phosphorylations by protein kinase A (PKA), glycogen synthase kinase (GSK)-3β, and members of casein kinase-1 (CK1) family. Phosphorylation enhances binding of Gli to β-transducin repeat-containing protein (βTrCp), which targets Gli for ubiquitination and subsequent proteasome degradation. Partial degradation generates an inhibitor Gli-peptide that can translocate to the nucleus and repress transcription. Active Smo allows dissociation of Sufu from Gli [23]. Full-length Gli-protein can then translocate to the nucleus, where it acts as a transcription factor. Important known target genes are: vascular endothelial growth factor (VEGF), angiopoietin-1 and -2 (in endothelial cells); snail, twist-2, FoxF1, α-smooth muscle actin (α-SMA), vimentin, interleukin (IL)-6 (in fibroblasts/myofibroblasts); and Sox-2, Sox-9 and Nanog (in stem/progenitor cells) [20].

Gli proteins belong to the Kruppel-like family of transcription factors with highly conserved zinc finger DNA-binding domain [21]. Mammals have three Gli proteins: Gli-1, Gli-2 and Gli-3, which behave differently. Gli-1 and Gli-2 transcription profiles overlap, but are not identical [21]. Unlike the other Gli factors, Gli-1 is not proteolytically processed to a repressor form. Gli-1 is also a direct transcriptional target of Gli-2 [24]. Gli-3 acts mainly as a transcription repressor, with very efficient proteolytic processing, whereas Gli-2 acts mainly as a transcription activator, with an extremely inefficient proteolytic processing [25].

The activation of Hh signaling through Smo seems to require the presence of primary cilia. Primary cilia are small, immotile cilia, elaborated in interphase by most quiescent, differentiated cells [26]. Primary cilia are made of polymerized tubulin, and consist of the basal body (that derives from the mother centriole at the end of cell division), and the filamentous axoneme that protrudes into the extracellular space.

In resting cells, Smo resides in intracytoplasmic vesicles outside of the primary cilia. Hh binding removes Ptch from the primary cilia, allowing Smo to accumulate in the cilia membrane. Smo can then move along the cilia from the base to the tip, in a kinesin motor protein-based transport system, which is facilitated by the ciliary Bardet-Biedl syndrome proteins (BBS) and intraflagellar transport proteins (IFP). At the tip of the cilia, Smo enables removal of Gli from the inhibitor complex with Sufu. Free Gli then moves along the cilia in a retrograde fashion via a dynein motor protein-based transport system, which is facilitated by BBS, IFP and Kif7. Full length Gli ultimately translocates from the cytoplasm to the nucleus, where it acts as a transcription factor [20] (Figure 1).

The Hh pathway has several intrinsic mechanisms of negative regulation that limit sustained activation. For example, Gli, the main effector in the Hh pathway, increases the expression of important inhibitors of the pathway. In fact, three direct Gli-target genes are Ptch, hedgehog-interacting protein (Hip) and Foxa2, all of them can inhibit Hh pathway activity. Ptch constitutively suppresses Smo, Hip binds to Hh and prevents ligand from engaging Ptch so that Smo cannot be de-repressed; and Foxa2 suppresses Gli-2 transcription, thereby depleting cells of the factor that drives transcription of Gli-1, the main activator of Hh target gene expression [27].

In addition to the aforementioned "canonical" Hh signaling pathway, two types of non-canonical Hh signaling have been described: type 1 is Ptch-dependent (but Smo-independent) and type 2 is Smo-dependent (but does not require Hh interaction with Ptch) [21,22]. In type 1 signaling, binding of Hh ligand to Ptch prevents Ptch from directly interacting with, and activating, caspases [28], and thus has an anti-apoptotic effect. In addition, the interaction promotes proliferation by preventing Ptch from blocking cyclin B translocation into the nucleus [29,30]. In type 2 signaling, Smo behaves as a 7-transmembrane protein that has a G-protein-coupled receptor (GPCR)-like function and acts independently of Gli and of the primary cilia [31]. The GPCR-like functions of Smo engage a calcium-AMP kinase axis that induces a Warburg-like glycolytic metabolic reprogramming in muscle and adipose tissue [32]. Smo GPCR-like activity also stimulates small GTPases that promote cytoskeletal rearrangement allowing migration of fibroblasts, and tubulogenesis in endothelial cells [33–35].

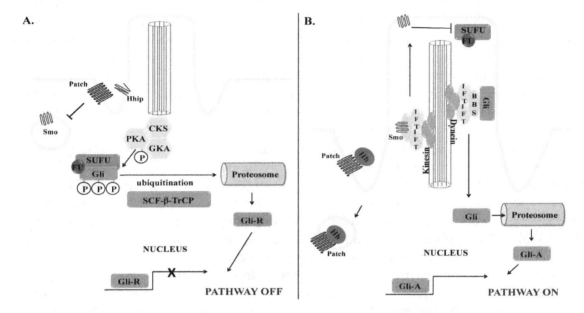

Figure 1. Hedgehog signaling pathway and the primary cilia. **(A)** In the absence of Hedgehog (Hh) ligand, Gli localizes in the cytoplasm as part of an inhibitory complex with Fused kinase (Fu) and Suppressor of Fused (SuFu), which allows the sequential phosphorylation by several kinases: Protein kinase A (PKA), glycogen synthase-3β (GSK3β) and casein kinase-1 (CK1). Thereafter, ubiquitination by Skip-Cullin-F-box (SCF) protein/β-Transducing repeat Containing Protein (TrCP) primes the phosphorylated Gli to limited proteosomic degradation, exposing the N-terminal repressor domain (GliR), which translocates to the nucleus and represses; **(B)** When Hh ligand binds to Ptch, it releases the inhibitory effect of Ptch on Smo that localizes in cytoplasmic vesicles. Smo then undergoes anterograde movement along the cilia, directed by kinesin and facilitated by the ciliary proteins Bardet-Biedl syndrome proteins (BBS) and intraflagellar transport proteins (IFP). At the tip of the cilia, Smo releases Gli from the suppressor complex, allowing it to move along the cilia, directed by dynein proteins. Unphosphorylated Gli undergoes limited proteosomal degradation, exposing the C-terminal activator domain (GliA), which translocates to the nucleus promoting gene transcription.

Finally, Gli-2 transcription/activation can be induced by Hedgehog-ligand independent pathways, including transforming growth factor (TGF)-β, phosphatydilinositol 3-kinase (PI3K)/AKT, Ras and mitogen-activated protein kinases (MAPK)/extracellular signal-regulated kinases (ERK) [22]. Osteopontin, besides being a target gene of Gli, also inhibits GSK3β, thereby promoting Gli activation [36].

3. Hedgehog Pathway and the Wound Healing Response

The Hh pathway is a recognized maestro of the wound healing response [37]. The wound-healing response is a coordinated reaction to liver injury that aims to overcome the loss of hepatic structure and function that results when liver cells die. Injured or fatty hepatocytes cannot mount an adequate proliferative response to replace these cells [38], and hence progenitor cells are crucial for sick livers to regenerate. Progenitors in the liver (similar to other populations of stem/progenitor cells [39]) are sensitive to Hh [40–43]. Indeed, Hh activation enhances progenitor cell viability and proliferation, whereas Hh inhibition promotes progenitor differentiation or cell death by apoptosis [40,44]. Another conserved wound healing response that occurs after liver injury is the development of an inflammatory reaction, which is also strongly regulated by the Hh pathway. For example, hepatic NKT cells respond to Hh with improved viability and proliferation, and acquire a profibrogenic phenotype that includes up-regulating their expression of IL-13 [45]. Hh also directly induces M2 pro-fibrogenic polarization of macrophages/Kupffer cells, further crafting a pro-fibrogenic liver microenvironment [46]. Another important player in the wound healing response is the hepatic stellate cell (HSC), the main source of myofibroblasts in the liver [47]. HSC not only produce the extracellular matrix necessary to maintain hepatic architecture during injury, they are a rich source of paracrine trophic substances that act on all other cell types involved in the healing response [37], and have recently been shown to function as progenitor cells themselves [48]. Excessive HSC activation may lead to anomalous matrix deposition that causes progressive fibrosis. Hh enhances HSC survival by inhibiting apoptosis, promotes HSC proliferation, and stimulates HSC to undergo an epithelial to mesenchymal-like transition in order to acquire a myofibroblastic phenotype [49]. Lastly, liver sinusoidal endothelial cells respond to Hh with capillarisation of hepatic sinusoids and vascular remodeling; perpetuation of this response favors the development of portal hypertension [50].

Whereas in the healthy liver the expression of Hh ligands is barely detected [40], Hh pathway activation increases proportionally to the severity and duration of the liver insult [42,51]. During injury, several cell types up-regulate expression of Hh ligands. For example, Hh production is virtually absent in healthy hepatocytes, but injured ballooned hepatocytes are a major source of Hh ligands in NAFLD [51–53]. Other sources of Hh ligands during a regenerative/repair response in the liver are inflammatory cells [45,46], activated ductular/progenitor cells [54] and HSC [49,55,56].

Although the hedgehog pathway seems important in wound-healing response/regeneration in different systems besides the liver, such as kidney, skin, cardiovascular system [57], a recent report in the lung showed that the hedgehog pathway may be important in maintaining adult lung quiescence and is down-regulated in response to epithelial injury [58]. These data demonstrate how complex this exciting pathway is, and further research is needed to clarify its function in liver health and repair.

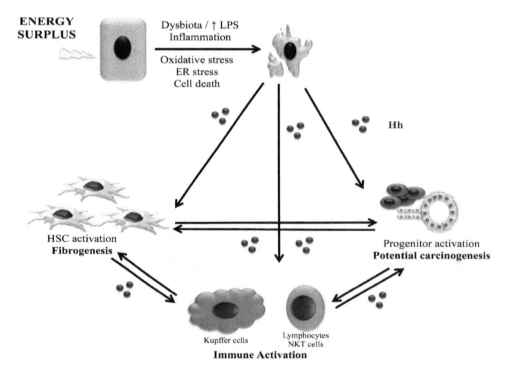

Figure 2. The role of Hedgehog on the wound-healing response. Energy surplus leads to fat accumulation in the hepatocytes, which promote oxidative stress, endoplasmic reticulum (ER) stress and cell death. The injury of hepatocytes is promoted by an inflammatory state, among other factors, favored by a deregulated gut microbiota and increase in lipopolysaccharide (LPS). Injured and dying hepatocytes release hedgehog ligands (Hh) that act on the immune system increasing inflammation, in stellate cells and progenitors cells activating them and inducing fibrogenesis and pathways of hepatocarcinogenesis. Once started, the regenerative/repair response perpetuates through crosstalk between the different cell types involved.

In summary, the wound-healing response depends on coordinated cross-talk among different cell types. Injured hepatocytes produce Hh ligands that attract and activate inflammatory cells. Infiltrating inflammatory cells, in turn, up-regulate their expression of Hh ligands and begin to produce profibrogenic cytokines, such as IL-13 and transforming growth factor (TGF)-β. These factors, not only activate myofibroblasts, but also are toxic to hepatocytes, further increasing hepatocyte injury and Hh ligand production [43]. Hh ligands also activate progenitor cells, inducing a ductular reaction. Activated ductular/progenitor cells up-regulate expression of chemokines/cytokines such as CXCL16 and platelet-derived growth factor (PDGF), which recruit more inflammatory cells and promote accumulation of myofibroblasts [59,60]. Hh ligands also activate HSC, causing their transdifferentiation into myofibroblasts and thus, promoting a fibrogenic response. If this initially adaptive response is not appropriately constrained, excessive activation of HSC/myofibroblasts promotes progressive fibrosis, and excessive proliferation of relatively immature liver epithelial cells represses regeneration of fully functional hepatocytes, leading to liver failure and carcinogenesis (Figure 2).

4. The Role of Hedgehog in Animal Models of NASH

Activation of the Hh pathway is a conserved feature of chronic liver disease, and NAFLD/NASH is no exception. Different rodent animal models of NAFLD show activation of the Hh pathway, demonstrated by increased expression of Hh ligands and Hh-producing cells, with accumulation of nuclear Gli-2 positive cells and increased expression of Gli-target genes such as osteopontin [42,53,61–65]. Furthermore, the activation of the Hh pathway is proportional to liver injury, namely to hepatocyte injury/apoptosis, ductular reaction and, most importantly, fibrosis [42,53,65].

Lipotoxic dying hepatocytes are a main source of Hh ligands that can trigger the repair response during NAFLD/NASH. *In vitro* models of lipotoxicity demonstrated up-regulation of Hh ligands in hepatocytes incubated with saturated fatty acids and lysophospholipid [65,66]. The mechanism leading to Hh ligand expression has not been clearly demonstrated. However, agents that can induce endoplasmic reticulum stress or activation of the NFkB pathway mimic the lipotoxic phenotype [52,67].

In animal models of NASH, the Hh-responsive progenitor population expands, and Hh-stimulated HSC undergo epithelial-to-mesenchymal transdifferentiation into myofibroblasts acquiring a pro-fibrogenic phenotype [42,61]. Activated ductular progenitor cells and myofibroblasts, in turn, up-regulate their production of Hh ligands, and release pro-inflammatory and chemotactic cytokines, such as osteopontin and CXCL-16 [60,63]. Immune cells are recruited, namely NKT cells, which have a pivotal role in NASH pathogenesis. Active NKT cells, in its turn, secrete more Hh ligands and profibrogenic cytokines, such as IL-13, perpetuating the disease progression [62,68].

Genetically modified mice, with heterozygous deficiency of Ptch (Ptch[+/−]), which display an overly active Hh pathway, develop worse liver disease when submitted to a NASH-inducing diet [61–63]. In contrast, genetically modified mice with conditional liver-specific inhibition of Smo, were protected from liver injury and liver fibrosis in different dietary models of NASH, despite similar accumulation of ectopic fat in the liver [37,69]. A recent study took advantage of a transgenic mouse with transposon encoding Shh hydrodinamically delivered to the liver to extend knowledge about hedgehog's role in NASH progression. Although this approach achieve expression of Shh in only 2%–5% of hepatocytes, it was sufficient to induce spontaneous liver fibrosis after 6 months and hepatocellular carcinoma after 13 months [70]. Hh ligands stimulate and increase proliferation of progenitor cells, as well as immune cells and hepatic stellate cells. As such, ductular progenitor cells, immune and hepatic stellate cells are Gli-2-positive (*i.e.*, Hh-responsive). Remarkably, 30%–50% of hepatocytes also exhibited nuclear Gli-2 expression. This finding challenges current dogma in the field, which posits that healthy hepatocytes cannot respond to Hh because they do not express primary cilia.

Different laboratories, studying different rodent models of diet-induced NASH, showed that pharmacological inhibition of Smo (vismodebig or LDE225) decreased activation of hedgehog pathway and consistently improved liver inflammation and fibrosis [61,69,71]. Those results place the Hh pathway as a potential therapeutic target in NASH.

5. The Hegdehog Pathway in Human NASH

The prevalence of human NAFLD is increasing worldwide in association with globalization of western lifestyles characterized by physical inactivity and overfeeding with predilection to sugar and fat enriched food. Roughly one fourth of the U.S. population has hepatic steatosis, however only a minority (2%–5%) will progress to NAFLD-related liver cirrhosis and end-stage liver disease [4]. Importantly, we still lack an effective treatment for this disease, which explains why NASH-related cirrhosis has become the second leading cause for liver transplantation in the US [5]. Liver prognosis is dictated by the fidelity of the wound healing response, with deregulated wound-healing promoting development of progressive fibrosis [7,8]. Hh is a crucial factor involved in this abnormal response to injury. Not only is Hh the best characterized fibrogenic pathway in animal models of NASH, but there is also strong human data that highlight its role in the pathogenesis of human cirrhosis.

Although isolated steatosis does not stimulate Hh pathway activation, steatohepatitis-related hepatocyte injury triggers Hh ligand production, and in human NASH the intensity of activation of the Hh pathway parallels the severity of liver disease. Hh pathway activity has been demonstrated to correlate with portal inflammation, hepatocellular ballooning, and markers of liver repair (e.g., numbers of hepatic progenitor cells and myofibroblasts) in NAFLD patients. More importantly, Hh activation correlates with the severity of fibrosis [51,61]. The major source of Hh ligands seems to be injured ballooned hepatocytes. In fact, the number of Shh expressing ballooned hepatocytes strongly correlates with fibrosis severity [51,72]. Furthermore, the number of Shh expressing ballooned hepatocytes also correlates with the severity of the ductular reaction, which strongly associates with fibrogenesis and carcinogenesis [73,74].

In the pediatric population, NAFLD can occur with a similar histology as in adults, or it can present a unique histology that is characterized by less hepatocellular ballooning but a predominantly portal phenotype, i.e., intense ductular proliferation, portal inflammation and fibrosis. A tremendous increase in the number of portal Gli-2 positive cells has been demonstrated in this pediatric pattern of NASH [75] and it occurs most often in pre-pubertal children, paralleling the kinetics of hepatic Hh expression, which is high in children and falls after adolescence [76].

Recently, a *post hoc* evaluation of the PIVENS (Pioglitazone, Vitamin E for Non-alcoholic Steatohepatitis) trial, analyzed pre- and post-treatment liver biopsies from 30 patients randomized to vitamin E and 29 to placebo [77]. Loss of Shh expressing hepatocytes strongly correlated with treatment response in terms of aminotransferases levels, hepatocyte ballooning, ductular reaction, presence of NASH and, most importantly, fibrosis stage [77]. This evidence linking reduced Hh activity with improvement of NASH in humans complements and extends the aforementioned work in preclinical models which showed that pharmacological strategies that directly decreased Hh activity abrogated NASH progression.

The roles of canonical and non-canonical pathways in liver disease in general and NASH in particular is still a matter of debate. Whereas progenitor cells clearly express primary cilia and thus can engage the canonical Hh pathway, it has been suggested that HSC, immune cells and hepatocytes do not express primary cilia, and hence Gli-2 activation/Gli-1 expression would be the result of non-canonical pathways [78,79]. In addition, type 2 non-canonical Smo-dependent RhoA/Rho kinase activation of HSC has been suggested to play a role in hepatic fibrogenesis [80]. Further research is needed to clarify the relevance of these different signaling cascades to better delineate a treatment strategy. To date, the most studied inhibitors of the Hh pathway *in vitro* and in animal models of NASH are cyclopamine and vismodegib, both strong Smo antagonists, which bind Smo and inhibit of its ciliary localization [81]. Interestingly, although HSC are sensitive to factors that induce non-canonical Hh pathway activation, they are also highly responsive to Hh ligands, antibodies against Hh and to both cyclopamine and vismodegib [49,55,56]. Furthermore, while healthy hepatocytes do not respond to cyclopamine, murine hepatocytes isolated after partial hepatectomy respond to cyclopamine with increased proliferation [82]. This suggests that the presence of a primary cilium may be a dynamic event, depending on the cell cycle phase and maybe in response to injury [83].

The aggregate data in animal models and human NASH strongly suggest that modulation of the Hh pathway may be a treatment for NASH that prevents fibrosis progression. As such, patients that would most benefit from treatment would be the ones that already have liver fibrosis to prevent progression to cirrhosis and its complications. This approach is particularly appealing because several Hh inhibitors have already been approved by the FDA to treat other diseases such as basal cell carcinoma [84] and, thus, the time lag between preclinical/clinical research and treatment of actual NASH patients should be short.

6. Conclusions

NASH-associated cirrhosis occurs when the liver reacts to lipotoxicity with a deregulated wound-healing response that is maladaptive. The liver must repair and regenerate when confronted with injury or death will ensue, just as Prometheus' survival depended upon his liver's ability to regenerate after being eaten by Zeus' eagle. When the eagle repeatedly eats the liver or when the repair/regenerative response cannot be shut down even when the satiated eagle stops eating the liver, the protracted wound-healing response leads to progressive fibrosis and carcinogenesis. The Hh pathway is a known maestro orchestrating an integrated regenerative response by the different cellular players involved in wound-healing. The Hh pathway is hibernating in the normal liver, but it wakens during injury, and the intensity of its activation is a reflection of the severity of liver injury. Data from animal models and human NASH have consistently confirmed that Hh pathway activation correlates with the severity of liver disease. More importantly, direct pharmacological inhibition of the Hh pathway prevents disease progression in different rodent models of NASH and Hh pathway activity decreases with improvement of NASH in humans. These findings position the Hh pathway as a potential therapeutic target in NASH, the hepatic pandemic of our century for which development of an effective treatment is a priority for hepatologists worldwide.

Acknowledgments: This research is supported by NIH DK0077794, DK053792 and R37 AA010154 (Diehl A.M.), and Duke Endowment: The Florence McAlister Professorship (Diehl A.M.).

Author Contributions: Mariana Verdelho Machado and Anna Mae Diehl wrote the paper.

Abbreviations

BBS	Bardet-Biedl syndrome proteins
Boc	brother of Cdo
Cdo	CAM-related downregulated by oncogenes
Cos	Costal-2
CK1	casein kinase-1
Dhh	Desert hedgehog
Fu	fused kinase
GAS-1	growth arrest-specific-1
GPCR	G-protein-coupled receptor
GSK	glycogen synthase kinase
Hh	hedgehog
Hip	hedgehog-interacting protein
HSC	hepatic stellate cell
IFP	intraflagellar transport proteins
Ihh	Indian hedgehog
IL	interleukin
MBOAT	membrane-bound O-acyltransferase
NAFLD	nonalcoholic fatty liver disease
NASH	nonalcoholic steatohepatitis
PDGF	platelet-derived growth factor
PKA	protein kinase A
Ptch	Ptched
Shh	Sonic hedgehog
SKI	skinny hedgehog

SMA	smooth muscle actin
Smo	smoothened
Sufu	suppressor of fused
TGF	transforming growth factor
TrCp	transducing repeat-containing protein
VEGF	vascular endothelial growth factor
VLDL	very low-density lipoproteins

References

1.   Loomba, R.; Sanyal, A.J. The global nafld epidemic. *Nat. Rev. Gastroenterol. Hepatol.* **2013**, *10*, 686–690. [CrossRef] [PubMed]

2.   Lonardo, A.; Bellentani, S.; Argo, C.K.; Ballestri, S.; Byrne, C.D.; Caldwell, S.H.; Cortez-Pinto, H.; Grieco, A.; Machado, M.V.; Miele, L.; *et al.* Epidemiological modifiers of non-alcoholic fatty liver disease: Focus on high-risk groups. *Dig. Liver Dis.* **2015**, *47*, 997–1006. [CrossRef] [PubMed]

3.   Machado, M.V.; Diehl, A.M. Pathogenesis of nonalcoholic steatohepatitis. *Gastroenterology* **2006**, *40*, S17–S29. [CrossRef] [PubMed]

4.   Machado, M.V.; Cortez-Pinto, H. Non-alcoholic fatty liver disease: What the clinician needs to know. *World J. Gastroenterol.* **2014**, *20*, 12956–12980. [CrossRef] [PubMed]

5.   Wong, R.J.; Aguilar, M.; Cheung, R.; Perumpail, R.B.; Harrison, S.A.; Younossi, Z.M.; Ahmed, A. Nonalcoholic steatohepatitis is the second leading etiology of liver disease among adults awaiting liver transplantation in the united states. *Gastroenterology* **2015**, *148*, 547–555. [CrossRef] [PubMed]

6.   Wong, R.J.; Cheung, R.; Ahmed, A. Nonalcoholic steatohepatitis is the most rapidly growing indication for liver transplantation in patients with hepatocellular carcinoma in the U.S. *Hepatology* **2014**, *59*, 2188–2195. [CrossRef] [PubMed]

7.   Angulo, P.; Kleiner, D.E.; Dam-Larsen, S.; Adams, L.A.; Bjornsson, E.S.; Charatcharoenwitthaya, P.; Mills, P.R.; Keach, J.C.; Lafferty, H.D.; Stahler, A.; *et al.* Liver fibrosis, but no other histologic features, is associated with long-term outcomes of patients with nonalcoholic fatty liver disease. *Gastroenterology* **2015**, *149*, 389–397.e10. [CrossRef] [PubMed]

8.   Ekstedt, M.; Hagstrom, H.; Nasr, P.; Fredrikson, M.; Stal, P.; Kechagias, S.; Hultcrantz, R. Fibrosis stage is the strongest predictor for disease-specific mortality in nafld after up to 33 years of follow-up. *Hepatology* **2015**, *61*, 1547–1554. [CrossRef] [PubMed]

9.   Singh, S.; Allen, A.M.; Wang, Z.; Prokop, L.J.; Murad, M.H.; Loomba, R. Fibrosis progression in nonalcoholic fatty liver vs nonalcoholic steatohepatitis: A systematic review and meta-analysis of paired-biopsy studies. *Clin. Gastroenterol. Hepatol.* **2015**, *13*, 643–654, e641–649; quiz e639–640. [CrossRef] [PubMed]

10. Moylan, C.A.; Pang, H.; Dellinger, A.; Suzuki, A.; Garrett, M.E.; Guy, C.D.; Murphy, S.K.; Ashley-Koch, A.E.; Choi, S.S.; Michelotti, G.A.; *et al.* Hepatic gene expression profiles differentiate presymptomatic patients with mild *versus* severe nonalcoholic fatty liver disease. *Hepatology* **2014**, *59*, 471–482. [CrossRef] [PubMed]

11. Horn, A.; Palumbo, K.; Cordazzo, C.; Dees, C.; Akhmetshina, A.; Tomcik, M.; Zerr, P.; Avouac, J.; Gusinde, J.; Zwerina, J.; *et al.* Hedgehog signaling controls fibroblast activation and tissue fibrosis in systemic sclerosis. *Arthritis Rheum.* **2012**, *64*, 2724–2733. [CrossRef] [PubMed]

12. Kugler, M.C.; Joyner, A.L.; Loomis, C.A.; Munger, J.S. Sonic hedgehog signaling in the lung. From development to disease. *Am. J. Respir. Cell Mol. Biol.* **2015**, *52*, 1–13. [CrossRef] [PubMed]

13. Fabian, S.L.; Penchev, R.R.; St-Jacques, B.; Rao, A.N.; Sipila, P.; West, K.A.; McMahon, A.P.; Humphreys, B.D. Hedgehog-gli pathway activation during kidney fibrosis. *Am. J. Pathol.* **2012**, *180*, 1441–1453. [CrossRef] [PubMed]

14. Wang, L.W.; Lin, H.; Lu, Y.; Xia, W.; Gao, J.; Li, Z.S. Sonic hedgehog expression in a rat model of chronic pancreatitis. *World J. Gastroenterol.* **2014**, *20*, 4712–4717. [CrossRef] [PubMed]

15. Choi, S.S.; Omenetti, A.; Syn, W.K.; Diehl, A.M. The role of hedgehog signaling in fibrogenic liver repair. *Int. J. Biochem. Cell Biol.* **2011**, *43*, 238–244. [CrossRef] [PubMed]

16. Nusslein-Volhard, C.; Wieschaus, E. Mutations affecting segment number and polarity in drosophila. *Nature* **1980**, *287*, 795–801. [CrossRef] [PubMed]

17. Briscoe, J.; Therond, P.P. The mechanisms of hedgehog signalling and its roles in development and disease. *Nat. Rev. Mol. Cell Biol.* **2013**, *14*, 416–429. [CrossRef] [PubMed]

18. Farzan, S.F.; Singh, S.; Schilling, N.S.; Robbins, D.J. The adventures of sonic hedgehog in development and repair. III. Hedgehog processing and biological activity. *Am. J. Physiol. Gastrointest. Liver Physiol.* **2008**, *294*, G844–G849. [CrossRef] [PubMed]

19. Pathi, S.; Pagan-Westphal, S.; Baker, D.P.; Garber, E.A.; Rayhorn, P.; Bumcrot, D.; Tabin, C.J.; Blake Pepinsky, R.; Williams, K.P. Comparative biological responses to human sonic, indian, and desert hedgehog. *Mech. Dev.* **2001**, *106*, 107–117. [CrossRef]

20. Merchant, J.L.; Saqui-Salces, M. Inhibition of hedgehog signaling in the gastrointestinal tract: Targeting the cancer microenvironment. *Cancer Treat. Rev.* **2014**, *40*, 12–21. [CrossRef] [PubMed]

21. Hu, L.; Lin, X.; Lu, H.; Chen, B.; Bai, Y. An overview of hedgehog signaling in fibrosis. *Mol. Pharmacol.* **2015**, *87*, 174–182. [CrossRef] [PubMed]

22. Teperino, R.; Aberger, F.; Esterbauer, H.; Riobo, N.; Pospisilik, J.A. Canonical and non-canonical hedgehog signalling and the control of metabolism. *Semin. Cell Dev. Biol.* **2014**, *33*, 81–92. [CrossRef] [PubMed]

23. Jia, J.; Kolterud, A.; Zeng, H.; Hoover, A.; Teglund, S.; Toftgard, R.; Liu, A. Suppressor of fused inhibits mammalian hedgehog signaling in the absence of cilia. *Dev. Biol.* **2009**, *330*, 452–460. [CrossRef] [PubMed]

24. Ikram, M.S.; Neill, G.W.; Regl, G.; Eichberger, T.; Frischauf, A.M.; Aberger, F.; Quinn, A.; Philpott, M. Gli2 is expressed in normal human epidermis and bcc and induces Gli1 expression by binding to its promoter. *J. Investig. Dermatol.* **2004**, *122*, 1503–1509. [CrossRef] [PubMed]

25. Pan, Y.; Bai, C.B.; Joyner, A.L.; Wang, B. Sonic hedgehog signaling regulates Gli2 transcriptional activity by suppressing its processing and degradation. *Mol. Cell. Biol.* **2006**, *26*, 3365–3377. [CrossRef] [PubMed]

26. Roy, S. Cilia and hedgehog: When and how was their marriage solemnized? *Differentiation* **2012**, *83*, S43–S48. [CrossRef] [PubMed]

27. Peterson, K.A.; Nishi, Y.; Ma, W.; Vedenko, A.; Shokri, L.; Zhang, X.; McFarlane, M.; Baizabal, J.M.; Junker, J.P.; van Oudenaarden, A.; *et al.* Neural-specific Sox2 input and differential Gli-binding affinity provide context and positional information in Shh-directed neural patterning. *Genes Dev.* **2012**, *26*, 2802–2816. [CrossRef] [PubMed]

28. Chinchilla, P.; Xiao, L.; Kazanietz, M.G.; Riobo, N.A. Hedgehog proteins activate pro-angiogenic responses in endothelial cells through non-canonical signaling pathways. *Cell Cycle* **2010**, *9*, 570–579. [CrossRef] [PubMed]

29. Pasca di Magliano, M.; Hebrok, M. Hedgehog signalling in cancer formation and maintenance. *Nat. Rev. Cancer* **2003**, *3*, 903–911. [CrossRef] [PubMed]

30. Barnes, E.A.; Kong, M.; Ollendorff, V.; Donoghue, D.J. Patched1 interacts with cyclin B1 to regulate cell cycle progression. *EMBO J.* **2001**, *20*, 2214–2223. [CrossRef] [PubMed]

31. Polizio, A.H.; Chinchilla, P.; Chen, X.; Manning, D.R.; Riobo, N.A. Sonic hedgehog activates the gtpases rac1 and rhoa in a Gli-independent manner through coupling of smoothened to G_i proteins. *Sci. Signal.* **2011**, *4 Pt 7*. [CrossRef] [PubMed]

32. Teperino, R.; Amann, S.; Bayer, M.; McGee, S.L.; Loipetzberger, A.; Connor, T.; Jaeger, C.; Kammerer, B.; Winter, L.; Wiche, G.; *et al.* Hedgehog partial agonism drives warburg-like metabolism in muscle and brown fat. *Cell* **2012**, *151*, 414–426. [CrossRef] [PubMed]

33. Bijlsma, M.F.; Borensztajn, K.S.; Roelink, H.; Peppelenbosch, M.P.; Spek, C.A. Sonic hedgehog induces transcription-independent cytoskeletal rearrangement and migration regulated by arachidonate metabolites. *Cell Signal.* **2007**, *19*, 2596–2604. [CrossRef] [PubMed]

34. Polizio, A.H.; Chinchilla, P.; Chen, X.; Kim, S.; Manning, D.R.; Riobo, N.A. Heterotrimeric G_i proteins link hedgehog signaling to activation of rho small gtpases to promote fibroblast migration. *J. Biol. Chem.* **2011**, *286*, 19589–19596. [CrossRef] [PubMed]

35. Razumilava, N.; Gradilone, S.A.; Smoot, R.L.; Mertens, J.C.; Bronk, S.F.; Sirica, A.E.; Gores, G.J. Non-canonical hedgehog signaling contributes to chemotaxis in cholangiocarcinoma. *J. Hepatol.* **2014**, *60*, 599–605. [CrossRef] [PubMed]

36. Das, S.; Samant, R.S.; Shevde, L.A. Nonclassical activation of hedgehog signaling enhances multidrug resistance and makes cancer cells refractory to smoothened-targeting hedgehog inhibition. *J. Biol. Chem.* **2013**, *288*, 11824–11833. [CrossRef] [PubMed]

37. Michelotti, G.A.; Xie, G.; Swiderska, M.; Choi, S.S.; Karaca, G.; Kruger, L.; Premont, R.; Yang, L.; Syn, W.K.; Metzger, D.; *et al.* Smoothened is a master regulator of adult liver repair. *J. Clin. Investig.* **2013**, *123*, 2380–2394. [CrossRef] [PubMed]

38. Sommerfeld, A.; Reinehr, R.; Haussinger, D. Free fatty acids shift insulin-induced hepatocyte proliferation towards CD95-dependent apoptosis. *J. Biol. Chem.* **2015**, *290*, 4398–4409. [CrossRef] [PubMed]

39. Mooney, C.J.; Hakimjavadi, R.; Fitzpatrick, E.; Kennedy, E.; Walls, D.; Morrow, D.; Redmond, E.M.; Cahill, P.A. Hedgehog and resident vascular stem cell fate. *Stem Cells Int.* **2015**, *2015*, 468428. [CrossRef] [PubMed]

40. Sicklick, J.K.; Li, Y.X.; Melhem, A.; Schmelzer, E.; Zdanowicz, M.; Huang, J.; Caballero, M.; Fair, J.H.; Ludlow, J.W.; McClelland, R.E.; *et al.* Hedgehog signaling maintains resident hepatic progenitors throughout life. *Am. J. Physiol. Gastrointest. Liver Physiol.* **2006**, *290*, G859–G870. [CrossRef] [PubMed]

41. Jung, Y.; Witek, R.P.; Syn, W.K.; Choi, S.S.; Omenetti, A.; Premont, R.; Guy, C.D.; Diehl, A.M. Signals from dying hepatocytes trigger growth of liver progenitors. *Gut* **2010**, *59*, 655–665. [CrossRef] [PubMed]

42. Fleig, S.V.; Choi, S.S.; Yang, L.; Jung, Y.; Omenetti, A.; VanDongen, H.M.; Huang, J.; Sicklick, J.K.; Diehl, A.M. Hepatic accumulation of hedgehog-reactive progenitors increases with severity of fatty liver damage in mice. *Lab. Investig.* **2007**, *87*, 1227–1239. [CrossRef] [PubMed]

43. Jung, Y.; Brown, K.D.; Witek, R.P.; Omenetti, A.; Yang, L.; Vandongen, M.; Milton, R.J.; Hines, I.N.; Rippe, R.A.; Spahr, L.; *et al.* Accumulation of hedgehog-responsive progenitors parallels alcoholic liver disease severity in mice and humans. *Gastroenterology* **2008**, *134*, 1532–1543. [CrossRef] [PubMed]

44. Hirose, Y.; Itoh, T.; Miyajima, A. Hedgehog signal activation coordinates proliferation and differentiation of fetal liver progenitor cells. *Exp. Cell Res.* **2009**, *315*, 2648–2657. [CrossRef] [PubMed]

45. Syn, W.K.; Witek, R.P.; Curbishley, S.M.; Jung, Y.; Choi, S.S.; Enrich, B.; Omenetti, A.; Agboola, K.M.; Fearing, C.M.; Tilg, H.; *et al.* Role for hedgehog pathway in regulating growth and function of invariant NKT cells. *Eur. J. Immunol.* **2009**, *39*, 1879–1892. [CrossRef] [PubMed]

46. Pereira, T.A.; Xie, G.; Choi, S.S.; Syn, W.K.; Voieta, I.; Lu, J.; Chan, I.S.; Swiderska, M.; Amaral, K.B.; Antunes, C.M.; *et al.* Macrophage-derived hedgehog ligands promotes fibrogenic and angiogenic responses in human schistosomiasis mansoni. *Liver Int.* **2013**, *33*, 149–161. [CrossRef] [PubMed]

47. Iwaisako, K.; Brenner, D.A.; Kisseleva, T. What's new in liver fibrosis? The origin of myofibroblasts in liver fibrosis. *J. Gastroenterol. Hepatol.* **2012**, *27* (Suppl. 2), 65–68. [CrossRef] [PubMed]

48. Swiderska-Syn, M.; Syn, W.K.; Xie, G.; Kruger, L.; Machado, M.V.; Karaca, G.; Michelotti, G.A.; Choi, S.S.; Premont, R.T.; Diehl, A.M. Myofibroblastic cells function as progenitors to regenerate murine livers after partial hepatectomy. *Gut* **2013**. [CrossRef] [PubMed]

49. Yang, L.; Wang, Y.; Mao, H.; Fleig, S.; Omenetti, A.; Brown, K.D.; Sicklick, J.K.; Li, Y.X.; Diehl, A.M. Sonic hedgehog is an autocrine viability factor for myofibroblastic hepatic stellate cells. *J. Hepatol.* **2008**, *48*, 98–106. [CrossRef] [PubMed]

50. Xie, G.; Choi, S.S.; Syn, W.K.; Michelotti, G.A.; Swiderska, M.; Karaca, G.; Chan, I.S.; Chen, Y.; Diehl, A.M. Hedgehog signalling regulates liver sinusoidal endothelial cell capillarisation. *Gut* **2013**, *62*, 299–309. [CrossRef] [PubMed]

51. Guy, C.D.; Suzuki, A.; Zdanowicz, M.; Abdelmalek, M.F.; Burchette, J.; Unalp, A.; Diehl, A.M.; Nash, C.R.N. Hedgehog pathway activation parallels histologic severity of injury and fibrosis in human nonalcoholic fatty liver disease. *Hepatology* **2012**, *55*, 1711–1721. [CrossRef] [PubMed]

52. Rangwala, F.; Guy, C.D.; Lu, J.; Suzuki, A.; Burchette, J.L.; Abdelmalek, M.F.; Chen, W.; Diehl, A.M. Increased production of sonic hedgehog by ballooned hepatocytes. *J. Pathol.* **2011**, *224*, 401–410. [CrossRef] [PubMed]

53. Machado, M.V.; Michelotti, G.A.; Pereira Tde, A.; Boursier, J.; Kruger, L.; Swiderska-Syn, M.; Karaca, G.; Xie, G.; Guy, C.D.; Bohinc, B.; *et al.* Reduced lipoapoptosis, hedgehog pathway activation and fibrosis in caspase-2 deficient mice with non-alcoholic steatohepatitis. *Gut* **2015**, *64*, 1148–1157. [CrossRef] [PubMed]

54. Omenetti, A.; Porrello, A.; Jung, Y.; Yang, L.; Popov, Y.; Choi, S.S.; Witek, R.P.; Alpini, G.; Venter, J.; Vandongen, H.M.; *et al.* Hedgehog signaling regulates epithelial-mesenchymal transition during biliary fibrosis in rodents and humans. *J. Clin. Investig.* **2008**, *118*, 3331–3342. [CrossRef] [PubMed]

55. Sicklick, J.K.; Li, Y.X.; Choi, S.S.; Qi, Y.; Chen, W.; Bustamante, M.; Huang, J.; Zdanowicz, M.; Camp, T.; Torbenson, M.S.; *et al.* Role for hedgehog signaling in hepatic stellate cell activation and viability. *Lab. Investig.* **2005**, *85*, 1368–1380. [CrossRef] [PubMed]

56. Lin, N.; Tang, Z.; Deng, M.; Zhong, Y.; Lin, J.; Yang, X.; Xiang, P.; Xu, R. Hedgehog-mediated paracrine interaction between hepatic stellate cells and marrow-derived mesenchymal stem cells. *Biochem. Biophys. Res. Commun.* **2008**, *372*, 260–265. [CrossRef] [PubMed]

57. Kramann, R.; Schneider, R.K.; DiRocco, D.P.; Machado, F.; Fleig, S.; Bondzie, P.A.; Henderson, J.M.; Ebert, B.L.; Humphreys, B.D. Perivascular Gli1$^+$ progenitors are key contributors to injury-induced organ fibrosis. *Cell Stem Cell* **2015**, *16*, 51–66. [CrossRef] [PubMed]

58. Peng, T.; Frank, D.B.; Kadzik, R.S.; Morley, M.P.; Rathi, K.S.; Wang, T.; Zhou, S.; Cheng, L.; Lu, M.M.; Morrisey, E.E. Hedgehog actively maintains adult lung quiescence and regulates repair and regeneration. *Nature* **2015**, *526*, 578–582. [CrossRef] [PubMed]

59. Omenetti, A.; Popov, Y.; Jung, Y.; Choi, S.S.; Witek, R.P.; Yang, L.; Brown, K.D.; Schuppan, D.; Diehl, A.M. The hedgehog pathway regulates remodelling responses to biliary obstruction in rats. *Gut* **2008**, *57*, 1275–1282. [CrossRef] [PubMed]

60. Omenetti, A.; Syn, W.K.; Jung, Y.; Francis, H.; Porrello, A.; Witek, R.P.; Choi, S.S.; Yang, L.; Mayo, M.J.; Gershwin, M.E.; *et al.* Repair-related activation of hedgehog signaling promotes cholangiocyte chemokine production. *Hepatology* **2009**, *50*, 518–527. [CrossRef] [PubMed]

61. Syn, W.K.; Jung, Y.; Omenetti, A.; Abdelmalek, M.; Guy, C.D.; Yang, L.; Wang, J.; Witek, R.P.; Fearing, C.M.; Pereira, T.A.; *et al.* Hedgehog-mediated epithelial-to-mesenchymal transition and fibrogenic repair in nonalcoholic fatty liver disease. *Gastroenterology* **2009**, *137*, 1478–1488.e8. [CrossRef] [PubMed]

62. Syn, W.K.; Oo, Y.H.; Pereira, T.A.; Karaca, G.F.; Jung, Y.; Omenetti, A.; Witek, R.P.; Choi, S.S.; Guy, C.D.; Fearing, C.M.; *et al.* Accumulation of natural killer T cells in progressive nonalcoholic fatty liver disease. *Hepatology* **2010**, *51*, 1998–2007. [CrossRef] [PubMed]

63. Syn, W.K.; Choi, S.S.; Liaskou, E.; Karaca, G.F.; Agboola, K.M.; Oo, Y.H.; Mi, Z.; Pereira, T.A.; Zdanowicz, M.; Malladi, P.; *et al.* Osteopontin is induced by hedgehog pathway activation and promotes fibrosis progression in nonalcoholic steatohepatitis. *Hepatology* **2011**, *53*, 106–115. [CrossRef] [PubMed]

64. Pazzaglia, S.; Cifaldi, L.; Saran, A.; Nobili, V.; Fruci, D.; Alisi, A. Hedgehog/hyaluronic acid interaction network in nonalcoholic fatty liver disease, fibrosis, and hepatocellular carcinoma. *Hepatology* **2012**, *56*, 1589. [CrossRef] [PubMed]

65. Machado, M.V.; Michelotti, G.A.; Xie, G.; Almeida Pereira, T.; Boursier, J.; Bohnic, B.; Guy, C.D.; Diehl, A.M. Mouse models of diet-induced nonalcoholic steatohepatitis reproduce the heterogeneity of the human disease. *PLoS ONE* **2015**, *10*, e0127991. [CrossRef] [PubMed]

66. Kakisaka, K.; Cazanave, S.C.; Werneburg, N.W.; Razumilava, N.; Mertens, J.C.; Bronk, S.F.; Gores, G.J. A hedgehog survival pathway in 'undead' lipotoxic hepatocytes. *J. Hepatol.* **2012**, *57*, 844–851. [CrossRef] [PubMed]

67. Nakashima, H.; Nakamura, M.; Yamaguchi, H.; Yamanaka, N.; Akiyoshi, T.; Koga, K.; Yamaguchi, K.; Tsuneyoshi, M.; Tanaka, M.; Katano, M. Nuclear factor-kappab contributes to hedgehog signaling pathway activation through sonic hedgehog induction in pancreatic cancer. *Cancer Res.* **2006**, *66*, 7041–7049. [CrossRef] [PubMed]

68. Syn, W.K.; Agboola, K.M.; Swiderska, M.; Michelotti, G.A.; Liaskou, E.; Pang, H.; Xie, G.; Philips, G.; Chan, I.S.; Karaca, G.F.; *et al.* Nkt-associated hedgehog and osteopontin drive fibrogenesis in non-alcoholic fatty liver disease. *Gut* **2012**, *61*, 1323–1329. [CrossRef] [PubMed]

69. Kwon, H.; Song, K.; Han, C.; Chen, W.; Wang, Y.; Dash, S.; Lim, K.; Wu, T. Inhibition of hedgehog signaling ameliorates hepatic inflammation in mice with nonalcoholic fatty liver disease. *Hepatology* **2015**. [CrossRef] [PubMed]

70. Chung, S.I.; Moon, H.; Ju, H.L.; Cho, K.J.; Kim, D.Y.; Han, K.H.; Eun, J.W.; Nam, S.W.; Ribback, S.; Dombrowski, F.; *et al.* Hepatic expression of sonic hedgehog induces liver fibrosis and promotes hepatocarcinogenesis in a transgenic mouse model. *J. Hepatol.* **2015**, *64*, 618–627. [CrossRef] [PubMed]

71. Hirsova, P.; Ibrahim, S.H.; Bronk, S.F.; Yagita, H.; Gores, G.J. Vismodegib suppresses trail-mediated liver injury in a mouse model of nonalcoholic steatohepatitis. *PLoS ONE* **2013**, *8*, e70599. [CrossRef] [PubMed]

72. Machado, M.V.; Michelotti, G.A.; Pereira, T.A.; Xie, G.; Premont, R.; Cortez-Pinto, H.; Diehl, A.M. Accumulation of duct cells with activated yap parallels fibrosis progression in non-alcoholic fatty liver disease. *J. Hepatol.* **2015**, *63*, 962–970. [CrossRef] [PubMed]

73. Richardson, M.M.; Jonsson, J.R.; Powell, E.E.; Brunt, E.M.; Neuschwander-Tetri, B.A.; Bhathal, P.S.; Dixon, J.B.; Weltman, M.D.; Tilg, H.; Moschen, A.R.; *et al.* Progressive fibrosis in nonalcoholic steatohepatitis: Association with altered regeneration and a ductular reaction. *Gastroenterology* **2007**, *133*, 80–90. [CrossRef] [PubMed]

..

74. Ye, F.; Jing, Y.Y.; Guo, S.W.; Yu, G.F.; Fan, Q.M.; Qu, F.F.; Gao, L.; Yang, Y.; Wu, D.; Meng, Y.; *et al.* Proliferative ductular reactions correlate with hepatic progenitor cell and predict recurrence in hcc patients after curative resection. *Cell Biosci.* **2014**, *4*, 50. [CrossRef] [PubMed]

75. Swiderska-Syn, M.; Suzuki, A.; Guy, C.D.; Schwimmer, J.B.; Abdelmalek, M.F.; Lavine, J.E.; Diehl, A.M. Hedgehog pathway and pediatric nonalcoholic fatty liver disease. *Hepatology* **2013**, *57*, 1814–1825. [CrossRef] [PubMed]

76. Omenetti, A.; Bass, L.M.; Anders, R.A.; Clemente, M.G.; Francis, H.; Guy, C.D.; McCall, S.; Choi, S.S.; Alpini, G.; Schwarz, K.B.; *et al.* Hedgehog activity, epithelial-mesenchymal transitions, and biliary dysmorphogenesis in biliary atresia. *Hepatology* **2011**, *53*, 1246–1258. [CrossRef] [PubMed]

77. Guy, C.D.; Suzuki, A.; Abdelmalek, M.F.; Burchette, J.L.; Diehl, A.M.; NASH CRN. Treatment response in the pivens trial is associated with decreased hedgehog pathway activity. *Hepatology* **2015**, *61*, 98–107. [CrossRef] [PubMed]

78. Grzelak, C.A.; Martelotto, L.G.; Sigglekow, N.D.; Patkunanathan, B.; Ajami, K.; Calabro, S.R.; Dwyer, B.J.; Tirnitz-Parker, J.E.; Watkins, D.N.; Warner, F.J.; *et al.* The intrahepatic signalling niche of hedgehog is defined by primary cilia positive cells during chronic liver injury. *J. Hepatol.* **2014**, *60*, 143–151. [CrossRef] [PubMed]

79. Matz-Soja, M.; Gebhardt, R. The many faces of hedgehog signalling in the liver: Recent progress reveals striking cellular diversity and the importance of microenvironments. *J. Hepatol.* **2014**, *61*, 1449–1450. [CrossRef] [PubMed]

80. Uschner, F.E.; Ranabhat, G.; Choi, S.S.; Granzow, M.; Klein, S.; Schierwagen, R.; Raskopf, E.; Gautsch, S.; van der Ven, P.F.; Furst, D.O.; *et al.* Statins activate the canonical hedgehog-signaling and aggravate non-cirrhotic portal hypertension, but inhibit the non-canonical hedgehog signaling and cirrhotic portal hypertension. *Sci. Rep.* **2015**, *5*, 14573. [CrossRef] [PubMed]

81. Corbit, K.C.; Aanstad, P.; Singla, V.; Norman, A.R.; Stainier, D.Y.; Reiter, J.F. Vertebrate smoothened functions at the primary cilium. *Nature* **2005**, *437*, 1018–1021. [CrossRef] [PubMed]

82. Ochoa, B.; Syn, W.K.; Delgado, I.; Karaca, G.F.; Jung, Y.; Wang, J.; Zubiaga, A.M.; Fresnedo, O.; Omenetti, A.; Zdanowicz, M.; *et al.* Hedgehog signaling is critical for normal liver regeneration after partial hepatectomy in mice. *Hepatology* **2010**, *51*, 1712–1723. [CrossRef] [PubMed]

83. Lim, Y.C.; McGlashan, S.R.; Cooling, M.T.; Long, D.S. Culture and detection of primary cilia in endothelial cell models. *Cilia* **2015**, *4*, 11. [CrossRef] [PubMed]

84. Guha, M. Hedgehog inhibitor gets landmark skin cancer approval, but questions remain for wider potential. *Nat. Rev. Drug Discov.* **2012**, *11*, 257–258. [CrossRef] [PubMed]

8

Pathophysiology of Non-Alcoholic Fatty Liver Disease

Salvatore Petta [1], Amalia Gastaldelli [2], Eleni Rebelos [3], Elisabetta Bugianesi [4], Piergiorgio Messa [5], Luca Miele [6], Gianluca Svegliati-Baroni [7], Luca Valenti [8] and Ferruccio Bonino [3,9,*]

[1]   Gastroenterology, Di.Bi.M.I.S Policlinic Paolo Giaccone Hospital, University of Palermo, PC 90127 Palermo, Italy; petsa@inwind.it
[2]   Cardiometabolic Risk Unit—Institute of Clinical Physiology, CNR, PC 56124 Pisa, Italy; amalia@ifc.cnr.it
[3]   Department of Clinical and Experimental Medicine, University of Pisa, PC 56122 Pisa, Italy; elenirebelos@gmail.com
[4]   Gastroenterology and Hepatology, Department of Medical Sciences, Città della, Salute e della Scienza di Torino Hospital, University of Turin, PC 10122 Turin, Italy; ebugianesi@yahoo.it
[5]   Department of Nephrology, Urology and Renal Transplant—Fondazione IRCCS Ca', Granda, PC 20122 Milano, Italy; pmessa@policlinico.mi.it
[6]   Institute of Internal Medicine, Gastroenterology and Liver Diseases Unit, Fondazione Policlinico Gemelli, Catholic University of Rome, PC 00168 Rome, Italy; luca.miele@policlinicogemelli.it
[7]   Department of Gastroenterology 1 and Obesity 2, Polytechnic University of Marche, PC 60121 Ancona, Italy; gsvegliati@gmail.com
[8]   Metabolic Liver Diseases—Università degli Studi Milano-Fondazione IRCCS Ca', Granda via F Sforza 35, PC 20122 Milano, Italy; luca.valenti@unimi.it
[9]   Institute for Health, PC 53042 Chianciano Terme, Italy
*   Correspondence: ferruccio.bonino@unipi.it

Academic Editors: Amedeo Lonardo and Giovanni Targher

Abstract: The physiopathology of fatty liver and metabolic syndrome are influenced by diet, life style and inflammation, which have a major impact on the severity of the clinicopathologic outcome of non-alcoholic fatty liver disease. A short comprehensive review is provided on current knowledge of the pathophysiological interplay among major circulating effectors/mediators of fatty liver, such as circulating lipids, mediators released by adipose, muscle and liver tissues and pancreatic and gut hormones in relation to diet, exercise and inflammation.

Keywords: fatty liver; insulin resistance; free fatty acids; cholesterol; adiponectin; leptin; insulin; glucagon; glucagon-like peptide 1; ghrelin; irisin; selenoprotein P

1. Introduction

Nonalcoholic fatty liver disease (NAFLD) is associated with a wide pathological spectrum, ranging from indolent liver fat storage, associated with an asymptomatic benign clinical course, to progressive cardiovascular, metabolic and/or liver and kidney diseases with higher cancer risks. Insulin resistance (IR) plays a pivotal role in the pathogenic switch of fatty liver. IR as a hallmark of metabolic syndrome stems from the complex dimensional interplay among inflammation and key circulating mediators, organs and tissues, genetic background and major conditioning factors, such as lifestyle (i.e., diet and physical activity). Here, we review the current knowledge on the dynamics of major circulating effectors/mediators of fatty liver, such as circulating lipids, released compounds from adipose, muscle and liver tissues and pancreatic and gut hormones in relation to lifestyle (i.e., diet and exercise) and inflammation. As renal function is frequently altered in patients with NAFLD, contributing to organ damage progression, the interplay with renal pathophysiology has also been addressed for circulating effectors/mediators other than pancreatic hormones.

2. Circulating Lipids

2.1. Free Fatty Acids (FFA)

Circulating FFA, which represent the major source of hepatic fat accumulation in patients with NAFLD, are mainly derived from adipose tissue lipolysis and partly from lipoprotein spill over and are the major fuel substrate for all tissues, except brain during fasting. Thus, their plasma levels are high during fasting and decline after feeding because of the anti-lipolytic action of insulin. In the presence of adipose tissue insulin resistance, FFA levels are high, despite high levels of circulating insulin, because of the resistance to the anti-lipolytic action of this hormone [1,2]. FFAs are involved in the pathogenesis of different metabolic disorders associated with insulin resistance, and different forms of FFA have different implications in cardio-metabolic disorders, ranging from protective to harmful effects [3–7]. Plasma FFAs are reabsorbed in various organs where, if not oxidized, they accumulate under the form of triglycerides within intra-cytoplasmic lipid droplets, and some lipid intermediates, such as or diacyl-glycerols (DAG), promote cell lipotoxicity and mitochondrial dysfunction (Figure 1). Hepatic FFAs can be exported as very low density lipoproteins (VLDL), which can contribute to high circulating triglycerides and low density lipoproteins (LDL), reduced high density lipoproteins (HDL) and an increased risk of atherosclerosis [8].

2.1.1. FFA and Diet

Consistent with the above evidence is that a higher saturated fatty acid (SFA) intake was associated with increased cardiovascular risk [9], whereas a higher intake of polyunsaturated fatty acids (PUFA) showed a protective effect [10], even if contradictory data arose from studies assessing the impact of PUFA supplementation on cardiovascular outcomes [11]. From a practical point of view, a recommended diet should be rich in PUFA and low in SFA.

2.1.2. FFA and Exercise

FFA mobilization and oxidation are higher during low and prolonged versus short and high intensity exercise [12]. In fact, during high intensity exercise, most energy is derived from glucose, while the highest use of FFA as a substrate occurs during low intensity exercise (25% of VO_2 max).

2.1.3. FFA and Inflammation

Elevated plasma FFA levels, affected also by diet and exercise and resulting from obesity or high-fat feeding, can cause insulin resistance, as well as low-grade inflammation [13]. Recently, the activation of the c-Jun terminal kinase (JNK) pathway by SFA was demonstrated in in vivo investigations [14], contributing to the development of hepatic steatosis and insulin resistance, as well as activation of pro-inflammatory M1 macrophages. Other in vitro studies showed that palmitate may induce endoplasmatic reticulum (ER) and oxidative stress in hepatocytes [15] and trigger the inflammasome via the activation of macrophages through TLR2/1 dimerization [16]. On the contrary, the contribution of unsaturated fatty acids (e.g., oleate, linoleate) to insulin resistance is still debated; they seem unable to affect the cell, but can impact TG storage [17]. Finally, FFAs are the source of diacyl glycerol (DAG), triglycerides and other metabolites, such as ceramides, which are synthesized in the ER of hepatocytes from long-chain SFA, as a substrate [18]. Ceramides were shown to be lipotoxic to pancreatic cells and involved in hepatic insulin resistance [19], but direct evidence of their pro-apoptotic role on hepatocytes is missing [20]. Increased hepatic ceramides and saturated TG and FFA were found in patients with NAFLD [21]. ER stress contributes to NASH progression, and saturated FFAs were shown to induce an ER stress response in hepatocytes and increased levels of ER stress in patients with NAFLD/NASH [22].

2.1.4. FFA and Nonalcoholic Fatty Liver Disease (NAFLD)

The above-mentioned effect of FFA on insulin resistance and low grade inflammation can explain the link between FFA and NAFLD/NASH. Recent in vitro and in vivo studies support the hypothesis that FFAs, which are not esterified and compartmentalized in lipid droplets, may induce irreversible cell damage and trigger pro-inflammatory signaling pathways (lipotoxicity), either alone or in combination with other lipid metabolites [23–25]. In addition, other in vitro and in vivo studies have shown that inhibiting hepatic TG synthesis results in an amelioration of hepatic steatosis, but exacerbates liver cell damage due to an increased intra-hepatic accumulation of FFAs [26]. All together, these observations suggest a possible protective role for increased hepatic TG synthesis against FFA-mediated cell toxicity.

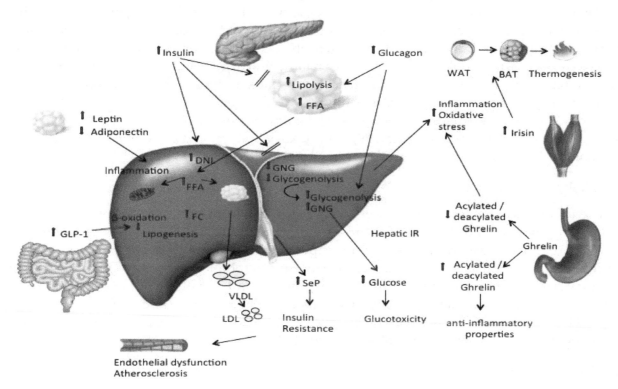

Figure 1. The key metabolic players and the major pathogenic pathways involved in NAFLD. Fatty liver is considered to be the hepatic component of metabolic syndrome. Systemic insulin resistance reduces adiponectin and increases leptin concentrations, while adipose tissue lipolysis is not suppressed (as shown with the "//" symbol), despite high circulating insulin levels, and plasma FFA concentration is increased. Increased glucagon levels have also been reported in NAFLD patients. The altered insulin/glucagon ratio promotes DNL, glycogenolysis and gluconeogenesis in the liver, thus increasing hepatic glucose production and hepatic insulin resistance. Several hormones secreted by the gastrointestinal tract regulate glucose/lipid metabolism, as well as food intake and, thus, might be implicated in the development of NAFLD. Impaired GLP-1 secretion and decreased levels of GLP-1 receptors have been reported in the liver of subjects with NAFLD, which further impair hepatic glucose and lipid metabolism. Ghrelin modulates appetite and insulin secretion, and an increased acylated/deacylated ghrelin ratio exerts anti-inflammatory properties. The liver secretes several hepatokines, including SeP, which further enhance insulin resistance, increase the production of small LDL particles that induce atherosclerosis and promote oxidative stress. Adipose tissues secrete adipokine-like leptin and adiponectin that are involved in the modulation of inflammation, fatty acid oxidation and energy expenditure, insulin resistance and insulin secretion. Myokines can also affect glucose and lipid metabolism, e.g., irisin, of which secretion is stimulated by exercise and induces thermogenesis, although its role has not yet been completely elucidated. Small red arrows versus the top: indicate increased concentrations; small red arrows versus the bottom: indicate reduced concentrations.

2.1.5. FFA and Kidney

The same mechanisms advocating FFA in the pathogenesis of NAFLD/NASH could also be involved in chronic kidney disease (CKD), where the lipotoxicity of FFAs in kidney cells, and in particular on podocytes [27], via ER stress, could explain the pathogenic role of obesity in CKD. Additionally in CKD, although polyunsaturated FAs (such as linoleic acid) probably play a protective role on the kidneys, saturated FFAs, such as palmitic acid, are responsible for intracellular lipotoxicity [28,29].

2.2. Cholesterol

Cholesterol is a major lipotoxic molecule, critical in the development of experimental and human metabolic disorders, such as atherosclerosis [30,31]. Different lines of evidence have reported that the accumulation of LDL in vessels make macrophages and smooth muscle cells able to convert esterified cholesterol into cholesterol [31–33]. When intra- and extra-cellular accumulation of cholesterol cannot be removed HDL mediated mechanisms, this leads to the generation of cholesterol crystals that, in turn, promote cell death, intima injury and atherosclerotic plaque destabilization [31]. The Seven Countries Study clearly reported a strong link between circulating total cholesterol levels, cardiovascular mortality and diet, with a higher intake of both refined sugar and fat being associated with poor outcomes [31], while dietary fibers have a protective effect [33,34].

2.2.1. Cholesterol and Diet

The influence of cholesterol-free diets on cholesterol serum levels is controversial, in spite of the very large number of different cholesterol-free diet programs [35]. One major reason for this may be the fact that the impact of different diet components on plasma lipid composition is mediated by gut microbiota [36]. The interactions between gut microbiota and dietary lipids in regulating liver and plasma lipid composition, liver gene expression and hepatic cholesterol metabolism were recently shown in germ-free and normally-raised mice [36]. In a study on mice fed lard, gut microbiota increased hepatic, but not serum, levels of cholesterol and cholesteryl esters, while, in mice fed fish oil, neither hepatic nor serum levels of cholesterol and cholesteryl esters were affected [36].

2.2.2. Cholesterol and Exercise

Considering the effect of exercise on cholesterol levels [37], available evidence suggests the particular effectiveness of higher-intensity aerobic exercise [38] and moderate-intensity resistance training [39], with a dose-response relationship between activity levels and increases in HDL cholesterol. However, in order to observe a reduction in plasma cholesterol with exercise training, a reduction in caloric intake and dietary fat during the exercise training program, resulting in a decrease in body weight/body fat, is important [40].

2.2.3. Cholesterol and Inflammation

Cholesterol accumulation in macrophages leads to the induction and secretion of two major inflammatory cytokines, tumor necrosis factor-α (TNF-α) and interleukin-6 (IL-6), which induce inflammation via NLRP3 (nucleotide-binding domain, leucine-rich-containing family, pyrin domain-containing-3) activation and the production of IL1-β and C-reactive protein, suggesting that excess ER cholesterol triggers endogenous cellular events. This proinflammatory activity can explain the link between high cholesterol levels, cholesterol deposition in atherosclerotic plaques and vascular damage [41].

2.2.4. Cholesterol and NAFLD

Lipidomic analyses of NAFLD have demonstrated that, apart from triglycerides, there is also an accumulation of free cholesterol (FC) without a similar increase in cholesterol esters (CE) in both

NAFLD and NASH [42] (Figure 1). Again, the above-mentioned cholesterol-related proinflammatory mechanisms, involved in vascular damage, have been also linked to cholesterol-mediated liver damage in NASH [31–33]. Along this line, multiple and complex alterations occur in the pathways of cholesterol homeostasis in both NAFLD and NASH [43]. Consistently, statin use has been associated with possible protection from hepatic damage and fibrosis in NAFLD [44].

2.2.5. Cholesterol and Kidney

Several findings suggest the role of systemic and renal lipids in kidney disease development and progression [45]. In fact, lipid loaded cells (i.e., foam cells) are frequently observed in many progressive nephropathies, such as in experimental diabetic kidney disease (DKD) and in focal segmental glomerular sclerosis (FSGS) or minimal change nephropathy in humans [46–48]. Secondly, the high prevalence, in African American subjects, of genetic variants of the APOL1 gene, encoding apolipoprotein L1 (a component of HDL), may explain the high susceptibility to nephropathy, in particular to FSGS, of this ethnic group [49]. Finally, some interventions that interfere with lipid accumulation in glomerular cells (podocytes) are effective in reducing kidney damage in some experimental kidney diseases [50]. Although no clear benefit of statin use on chronic kidney disease (CKD) occurrence and/or progression has been demonstrated in a clinical setting [51], the mechanism(s) by which cholesterol might play a causal role in CKD may be more complex than that which is only related to serum cholesterol concentration; again, involving its ability to activate pro-inflammatory mechanisms already involved in atherosclerosis and NASH [45].

3. Adipose Tissue Released Compounds

3.1. Adiponectin

Adiponectin is a cytokine that is mostly produced by adipocytes, its expression being primarily determined by adipocyte size and insulin sensitivity, with larger, insulin-resistant adipocytes being less productive [52,53]. It is a "protective" adipocytokine, involved in the regulation of glucose and lipid metabolism, as well as in inflammation inhibiting NF-κB and TNF-α production in macrophages; consistent with these data, its serum concentrations are inversely related to obesity and diabetes [54]. Adiponectin levels are inversely related to insulin resistance and are lower in obese subjects and patients with established insulin resistance, e.g., in type 2 diabetes, NAFLD/NASH and hypertension.

3.1.1. Adiponectin and Diet

High-fat, but not low fat, diets were associated with increased adiponectin levels, whereas a modest increase was reported with n-3 polyunsaturated fatty acids (PUFA) supplementation [55]; however, on the contrary, conjugated linoleic acid supplementation showed a reduction in adiponectin levels [55]. In mice, a high-carbohydrate diet was shown to increase adiponectin levels [56], and in humans, Rezvani et al. reported a significant increase of adiponectin levels during the consumption of glucose, but not fructose [57]. Some evidence suggests that adiponectin production by adipocytes is regulated via insulin-stimulated glucose utilization [58].

3.1.2. Adiponectin and Exercise

Mild or moderate physical activity does not change adiponectin levels, though a positive effect was reported with longer exercise [59]. Consistently, increased serum adiponectin levels paralleled the improvement of carotid vascular function in obese individuals undergoing intense exercise and moderate caloric restriction [60].

3.1.3. Adiponectin and Inflammation

While the impact of diet and exercise on adiponectin is controversial, the anti-inflammatory activity of this adipokine, able to inhibit NF-κB and TNF-α production in macrophages, is well established (Figure 1); consistent with these data, its serum concentrations are inversely related to obesity and chronic metabolic disorders, such as insulin resistance and diabetes. In contrast, adiponectin levels are elevated in classic chronic inflammatory/autoimmune diseases unrelated to increased adipose tissue, such as rheumatoid arthritis, systemic lupus erythematosus (SEL), inflammatory bowel disease, type 1 diabetes (T1D) and cystic fibrosis [61].

3.1.4. Adiponectin and NAFLD

Due to the above-mentioned insulin sensitizing and anti-inflammatory activity of adiponectin, its plasma levels are decreased in patients with NAFLD and are associated with fat content [62]. After treatment with thiazolidinediones, adiponectin values increase in NASH as a sign of improvement of hepatic steatosis, necroinflammation and, most importantly, fibrosis [63].

3.1.5. Adiponectin and Kidney

Adiponectin, due to its insulin sensitizing and anti-inflammatory activities, has a protective role on the kidney [64]. In fact, low adiponectin levels were associated with increased albumin urinary excretion and histological evidence of kidney damage, both in experimental and clinical studies [65–67]. At odds with these findings, in CKD, the levels of adiponectin are often increased. Whether this finding represents a compensatory phenomenon or just the consequence of the reduced renal clearance of a relatively small molecule (30 kD) and/or of an altered signaling at cellular levels is still a matter of debate [68–70].

3.2. Leptin

Leptin is a cytokine that is primarily secreted from adipose tissue, with a critical role in the regulation of body weight and fat mass. In obese mice, leptin causes weight loss, increasing energy expenditure and fatty acid oxidation, reducing appetite and triglyceride synthesis and counteracting the lipogenic action of insulin [71]. Its role in humans is less clear-cut; only patients with lipodystrophy have a beneficial effect when treated with leptin, while obese subjects do not lose weight. Circulating leptin is strongly associated with both subcutaneous and visceral fat [72], and different studies have hypothesized that obesity might induce a state of leptin resistance. High leptin levels are associated with reduced insulin secretion, increased gluconeogenesis and reduced glucose uptake, leading to hyperglycemia and ultimately contributing to increased insulin resistance [73–75] (Figure 1). Leptin may negatively affect the cardiovascular system by exerting potential atherogenic, thrombotic and angiogenic activities, as well as, even if with contrasting data, leading to cardiac hypertrophy [76].

3.2.1. Leptin and Diet

A higher energy storage is directly related to serum leptin levels [71]. Considering different types of fatty acids: SFAs are associated with increased leptin levels, whereas MUFA and PUFA have an opposite effect [71]. Finally, fiber and higher protein intake increase leptin sensitivity, which induces central satiety [71].

3.2.2. Leptin and Exercise

Available evidence suggests that, while acute and short-term physical activity do not affect leptin levels, longer exercise (at least 60 min) is associated with increased energy expenditure that could lead to leptin decrease [59]. Accordingly, the adiponectin/leptin ratio results as an independent predictor of carotid intima-media thickness (CIMT) alterations [77].

3.2.3. Leptin and Inflammation

Leptin may exert pro-inflammatory activity by the impairment of NO-related vassal relaxation, via increased oxidative stress, and by increased endothelin expression [54,78], by potentiating the effect of angiotensin II, which, in turn, increases leptin synthesis by inducing pro-inflammatory cytokines (e.g., TNF-α, IL-6 and MCP-1 receptor) by increasing the expression of adhesion molecules (e.g., VCAM-1, ICAM-1 and E-selectin). These features could explain why hyperleptinemia is observed in many chronic inflammatory diseases [79,80], such as atherosclerosis, and how it can participate in damage.

3.2.4. Leptin and NAFLD

A recent meta-analysis indicates that circulating leptin levels are higher in patients with NAFLD than in controls, and higher serum leptin levels were associated with an increased severity of NAFLD [81]. This is in agreement with the above-mentioned evidence of inflammatory-mediated damage related to leptin and potential involvement in NASH pathogenesis.

3.2.5. Leptin and Kidney

Leptin is cleared from circulation by glomerular filtration and metabolic degradation in renal tubules, which accounts for the elevated levels of leptin in CKD patients [79]. Given its anoxygenic and pro-inflammatory activities, leptin might contribute to malnutrition and inflammation, often observed in CKD patients, and a consistently higher risk of cardio-vascular morbidity and mortality [80,82,83]. Again, common inflammatory pathways could account for the role of leptin in kidney damage.

4. Pancreatic Hormones and NAFLD

4.1. Insulin

Insulin is secreted by the pancreas in response to changes in glucose concentrations that occur after a meal or after hormone release, such as catecholamines or glucagon [2]. Insulin tightly regulates glucose metabolism and plasma concentrations, on the one hand, by promoting glucose uptake in skeletal muscle and liver (for glucose oxidation or glycogen storage), in adipose tissue (where glucose is utilized for triglyceride synthesis) and, on the other hand, by suppressing hepatic glucose production. Insulin also acts on lipid metabolism, as it promotes fatty acid re-esterification into triglycerides in adipose tissue and liver, but also inhibits peripheral adipose tissue lipolysis (Figure 1). Thus, the role of insulin in the development of NAFLD is crucial. In the presence of insulin resistance, the pancreas is stimulated to increase insulin secretion to overcome the defect in peripheral glucose uptake and to decrease hepatic glucose production. Since the pancreas releases secreted insulin into the portal vein and the liver clears most of it, the amount of insulin that reaches the liver is much higher than in the periphery. Thus, when hepatic glucose production rates are high in the presence of high insulin values, it is recognized as a sign of hepatic insulin resistance [84]. Insulin mainly acts in suppressing hepatic glycogenolysis, rather than gluconeogenesis; however, until "hepatic autoregulation" is maintained, fasting glucose concentrations remain within normal ranges (Figure 1). When hepatic autoregulation is lost, both components of hepatic glucose production (i.e., glycogenolysis and gluconeogenesis) are increased and assist in the development of fasting hyperglycemia and type 2 diabetes [85]. Finally, different evidence supports a bidirectional link between insulin resistance and chronic inflammation. However, this topic is not the main goal of the present paper, while being the object of a huge debate in the literature, as reported in different reviews [86–88].

4.1.1. Insulin and Diet

A carbohydrate-rich diet (with a high glycemic index) determines higher glucose excursion and triggers a higher insulin secretion rate. Moreover, both lipids and amino acids determine increased insulin secretion; oral amino acids elicit a stronger and sustained insulin secretion, as compared to amino acids given intravenously [89]. In addition, lipids have an incretin effect, and a diet high in saturated fats determines insulin resistance and a higher glucose-stimulated insulin secretion (GSIS) [90]. A sustained increase in plasma free fatty acids by long-term intralipid infusion increases GSIS, but this response was found to be impaired in non-diabetic subjects, genetically predisposed to develop type 2 diabetes [91].

4.1.2. Insulin and NAFLD

Insulin promotes de novo lipogenesis (DNL) and glyceroneogenesis [25] (Figure 1). Both pathways are increased in NAFLD, even in non-diabetic patients, contributing to the synthesis of hepatic triglycerides and the promotion of hepatic steatosis [92]. In addition, patients with NAFLD have increased hepatic synthesis of palmitate through DNL, and this increases the risk of lipotoxicity and cell damage [25,93]. Finally, insulin, in the context of insulin resistance, prompts fibrogenesis by stellate cells [94,95]. Most patients with NAFLD have normal fasting glucose concentrations, but high levels of fasting insulin and high hepatic insulin resistance. Thus, it is not surprising that NAFLD is a major risk factor for the development of type 2 diabetes.

4.1.3. Insulin and Exercise

Exercise increases the demand of glucose in the periphery (muscle), and thus, there is a demand for increased endogenous glucose production (EGP). However, since glucose is immediately used by the muscle to produce ATP, glucose concentrations are usually stable, and thus, there is no stimulus for an increase in insulin secretion. However, other hormones, such as glucagon and catecholamine, are increased during exercise and stimulate EGP [12,96].

4.2. Glucagon

Glucagon is produced and secreted from alpha cells located in clusters of endocrine cells, in the islets of Langerhans, distributed throughout the pancreas [97]. Glucagon secretion is found to be increased, not only in diabetes, but also in several insulin resistant states, including NAFLD [98]. The role of glucagon is opposite that of insulin (Figure 1); glucagon stimulates glucose production via activation of hepatic glycogenolysis and gluconeogenesis by inhibition of glycolysis [98]. It also regulates fatty acid metabolism via stimulation of peripheral lipolysis, reduction of malonyl-CoA and stimulation of fatty acid oxidation [99]. However, the most recent data indicate that glucagon is also involved in amino acid metabolism, both because amino acids can stimulate glucagon secretion and because glucagon can stimulate protein metabolism [98].

4.2.1. Glucagon and Diet

Glucose is the most important regulator of pancreatic glucagon secretion. In normal glucose tolerant (NGT) subjects, when glucose concentrations are high, glucagon secretion is suppressed, and when there are low glucose concentrations, glucagon secretion is increased, securing an essential supply of energy (i.e., glucose) to the central nervous system and muscles. In patients with diabetes, glucagon concentrations are elevated in the fasting state and fail to decrease appropriately, or even increase, during an oral glucose tolerance test (OGTT) or after ingestion of a mixed meal [100–102]. Certain amino acids, such as glutamine, alanine and arginine, are also important glucagon secretors, with the latter being the most potent stimulatory amino acid [103,104]. Fat intake also increases glucagon secretion [105].

4.2.2. Glucagon and NAFLD

Since glucagon stimulates lipolysis and reduces lipogenesis [99], glucagon was proposed as a therapy option for hepatic steatosis [106]. Similarly, it was thought that the reduction of glucagon signaling, i.e., via the use of glucagon receptor antagonists, might lead to the accumulation of lipids in the liver [107]. However, more recent studies [108] have shown that glucagon receptor knockout mice have reduced hepatic lipid contents compared with wild-type mice. The impact of glucagon on NAFLD has not been elucidated. Junker and colleagues [109] have shown that patients with NAFLD have fasting hyperglucagonemia, independent of their glucose tolerance status. According to the authors, this finding suggests that NAFLD might be involved in the generation of hyperglucagonemia in T2D, which is supported by several animal studies [110].

4.2.3. Glucagon and Exercise

Exercise induces an increase in glucagon secretion in order to increase hepatic glucose production and gluconeogenesis. However, although pancreatic hormones are important in the stimulation of EGP during low or moderate intensity exercise, during strenuous exercise (i.e., 80% VO_2 max), EGP is increased, mainly because of increased catecholamine, while changes in glucagon and insulin are not necessary to stimulate the increase in Ra [96].

4.2.4. Glucagon and Inflammation

Patients with trauma, burns or sepsis normally exhibit increased plasma levels of glucagon, in order to promote gluconeogenesis, increase circulating glucose and compensate for the energetic demand of the body during these extreme situations [111]. Interestingly, significant increases of both glucagon and inflammatory mediators occur after a high fat high carbohydrate meal, as compared with an American Heart Association-recommended meal [112]. Plasma IL-6, a pro-inflammatory cytokine, is elevated in physiological and pathophysiological settings where glucagon is also elevated, such as exercise [113], diabetes [114] and inflammatory stress [115]. Tweedell et al. have demonstrated that IL-6-deficient (IL-6-KO) mice have a blunted glucagon response to acute inflammation compared with their wild-type littermates, while glucagon response is completely rescued by intravenous replacement of IL-6 [116]. Consistent with this, Ortega and colleagues demonstrated that, in patients with altered glucose tolerance, but not in NGT subjects, circulating glucagon levels were associated with inflammatory mediators, such as IL-6 [111].

5. Gut Released Hormones

5.1. GLP-1

Glucagon-like peptide 1 (GLP-1) is an incretin hormone produced mainly by the L-cells of the gut in response to food intake. GLP-1 has an important role in the regulation of glucose metabolism, since it potentiates insulin secretion and inhibits glucagon release [117,118] (Figure 1). GLP-1 exerts its effect through binding to GLP-1 receptors, which are mainly expressed in the pancreas and brain, but also in the heart, liver, colon and kidney [117]. Other effects of GLP-1 include the central suppression of appetite and the induction of satiety by delaying gastric emptying [117,119]. Other than these classical activities, GLP-1 seems to be able to modulate the function of different key organs by interacting with GLP-1 receptors present in the lung, stomach, liver, colon, kidney and heart. Consistent with these data, growing evidence suggests a direct protective effect of GLP-1 on the cardiovascular system [117,119].

5.1.1. GLP-1 and Diet

GLP-1 release can be stimulated by mixed meals or individual nutrients, including glucose and other sugars, fatty acids, essential amino acids and dietary fiber. Oral, but not intravenous, glucose administration stimulates GLP-1 secretion in humans [120].

5.1.2. GLP-1 and Exercise

Exercise-related studies have shown that healthy people have increased levels of incretin hormones, such as GLP-1, after physical activity [121]. Lee et al. showed higher GLP-1 levels after high intensity vs. low intensity exercise, with matched energy expenditures [122].

5.1.3. GLP-1 and Inflammation

GLP-1 receptor agonists (GLP-1RAS) have anti-inflammatory effects in different cell types, including human umbilical vein endothelial cells, glomerular endothelial cells, monocytes and macrophages [123,124]. GLP-1 levels decreased for a mean duration of 7.5 months in a retrospective analysis of 110 obese patients with T2D who were treated with liraglutide [125]. Consistently, TNF-α induced systemic inflammation and reduced GLP-1 concentrations, thereby reducing the suppression of endogenous glucose production (EGP) during GLP-1 infusion [126].

5.1.4. GLP-1 and NAFLD

In vitro studies have shown that human hepatocytes express the GLP-1 receptor [127,128]. In liver tissue, the expression of GLP-1 receptors is controversial [117], but Svegliati-Baroni was able to demonstrate that, in human livers of subjects with NASH, both the expression and protein content of GLP-1R were decreased compared to subjects without NASH [128]. In subjects with hepatic steatosis, open-label studies have shown that exenatide may improve liver enzymes and decrease steatosis when assessed by magnetic resonance spectroscopy (MRS) [129,130] and even improve histology [131]. A recent study by Armstrong et al. has shown that, after 48 months of double blind treatment with liraglutide vs. placebo (the LEAN study), 39% of patients receiving liraglutide vs. 9% of those receiving placebo had a resolution of definite non-alcoholic steatohepatitis with no worsening in fibrosis [132]. Among the mechanisms that lead to the improvement in liver histology were significant weight loss, reduced FFA flux to the liver, reduced de novo hepatic DNL and the above-mentioned anti-inflammatory activities [133] (Figure 1). All in all, these findings qualify GLP-1RA as a potential candidate for the treatment of NAFLD.

5.1.5. GLP-1 and Kidney

The effects of GLP-1 on glucose metabolism and inflammation, again, can indirectly benefit the kidney. Furthermore, incretin may also have direct renal effects, since its specific receptors have been described both in renal tubular and in glomerular cells [123,134]. One potential mechanism by which GLP-1 may play a nephro-protective role is its natriuretic activity, due to the direct inhibition of two key sodium transporters (Na-hydrogen exchanger-3 and sodium-glucose co-transporter-2) at the tubular level [124]. Furthermore, GLP-1 might also have a positive hemodynamic effect on the kidney by its stimulating and inhibitory effects on atrial natriuretic peptide (ANP) and angiotensin 2, respectively [125].

5.2. Ghrelin

Ghrelin is a hormone that is mainly derived from the stomach and duodenum, with a key role in growth hormone release and in food intake control by inducing appetite and controlling energy expenditure [135]. Ghrelin molecules are present as two major endogenous forms, an acylated form, which is the biologically-active form of ghrelin (AG), and a de-acylated form (DeAG) that does not bind to ghrelin receptors [136]. AG is secreted before a meal and disappears more rapidly from plasma than total ghrelin, with an elimination half-life of 9–13 vs. 27–31 min. The main organ that secretes ghrelin is the stomach, where 65%–90% of the circulating ghrelin is synthesized, followed by the small bowel, and in small amounts by other organs, including liver, pancreas, hypothalamus, kidney, liver, fat, muscle and heart (Figure 1). Ghrelin O-acyltransferase (GOAT), the enzyme responsible for acylation, was found to be involved in glucose metabolism, insulin resistance, lipid metabolism dysfunction and inflammation [137,138]. GOAT is expressed in several organs, mainly in the gastrointestinal tract, but also in the central nervous system, pancreas, heart, kidney, muscle, tongue, testis, thymus and adipose tissue, but not in the liver.

5.2.1. Ghrelin and Diet

Ghrelin levels (both AG and DeAG) increase with prolonged food deprivation and prior to meal time, while decreases in weight gain, adiposity and in the post-prandial phase with a magnitude proportional to caloric intake and macronutrient content [135,139,140]. GOAT expression and activity and, thus, the availability of AG are modified by dietary lipids, in particular by the availability of short and medium chain fatty acids [138]. Specifically, in a trial using isocaloric beverages, mostly containing fat or carbohydrates or proteins, the lipid drink was the least effective, and the protein drink was the most effective in lowering ghrelin levels, while the carbohydrate drink induced the largest drop in ghrelin levels and was then followed by a significant rebound [141]. Van Name et al. studied the AG response to glucose and fructose beverage in lean and obese adolescents (IS or IR). They found that AG levels were suppressed after either glucose or fructose consumption in lean subjects. In obese IS subjects, AG suppression was higher after glucose as compared to fructose consumption, whereas in obese IR subjects, suppression of AG was blunted following fructose consumption [142]. Thus, it would appear that, in addition to obesity in adolescents, the presence of insulin resistance further limits the capacity of fructose to suppress this key orexigenic hormone and may continue to promote hunger and overconsumption of fructose (or other calories), particularly in obese adolescents who are insulin resistant.

5.2.2. Ghrelin and Exercise

Contradictory results exist on the effect of physical activity on ghrelin levels. Short-term running, cycling or rowing exercise do not alter plasma total ghrelin [143–145]. On the other hand, Mackelvie et al. showed that daily exercise for five consecutive days (1-h sessions of aerobic exercise) is associated with an increase in plasma concentrations of AG, independent of the acute effect of exercise and from changes in weight or markers of insulin sensitivity. In addition, the increase in AG was more pronounced in normal weights compared with overweight subjects and was associated with an increase in markers of appetite [146]. However, Shiiya et al. report that plasma AG, but not DeAG levels, are suppressed during acute moderate exercise (cycle exercise for 60 minutes at 50% of VO_2 max) [146]. From a clinical point of view, this seems more reasonable since exercise increases appetite and exercise is associated with an increase in ghrelin levels (total or acylated form). However, more studies are needed to address the links between different forms of exercise, type, intensity and duration and ghrelin yield.

5.2.3. Ghrelin and Inflammation

Ghrelin, and especially AG, exert anti-inflammatory activity by reducing the production of pro-inflammatory cytokines, such as IL-1, IL-6 and TNF-α, via suppression of NF-κB [137]. The anti-inflammatory properties of ghrelin are consistent with the evidence from murine models that ghrelin prevents diabetes [139] and has a protective cardiovascular effect. These anti-inflammatory properties of ghrelin prompt the ghrelin-GOAT system as a promising new target for the treatment of NASH [137]. AG can improve cardiac function by increasing cardiac output, ameliorating cardiac contractility, acting on cardiac remodeling, reducing pulmonary hypertension, reducing fatal arrhythmia after myocardial infarction and leading to vasodilation [139,147–150].

5.2.4. Ghrelin and NAFLD

Whether ghrelin levels are altered in NAFLD is still controversial, as Marchesini et al. [151] reported low total ghrelin levels, while Mykhalchyshyn et al. [152] found high serum levels of AG in NAFLD compared to controls. However, the above-mentioned effects of ghrelin on energy and lipid metabolism, IR, inflammation and apoptotic cell death, which are common to both obesity and NAFLD, highly suggest its interplay with NAFLD/NASH pathogenesis [137].

5.2.5. Ghrelin and Kidney

In CKD, increased levels of total ghrelin, but not of AG, are frequently observed, due to the reduced metabolic clearance of the total (mainly DeAG) by failed kidneys. The consequently-reduced AG/DeAG ratio might contribute to inflammatory and malnutrition status, which is typical in many CKD patients [153,154].

6. Muscle Released Compounds

6.1. Irisin

Irisin is a recently-discovered myokine, encoded by the *FNDC5* gene; it is implicated in the regulation of energy homeostasis and metabolism and the interactions between skeletal muscle and other tissues (Figure 1). Irisin can induce the differentiation of white adipose into brown adipocytes, along with upregulation of uncoupling protein 1 (UCP1) expression and an increase in heat production [155,156]. Accordingly, circulating irisin can increase total energy expenditure, thus reducing obesity and insulin resistance [155,156].

6.1.1. Irisin and Diet

Results of studies on the effect of diet on irisin concentrations are not unanimous. Some studies report that irisin is not affected by food intake [157], while others indicate that irisin levels are positively associated with increasing fruit intake and negatively associated with meat consumption [158]. Finally, an inverse association between irisin and higher caloric intake has been shown [159].

6.1.2. Irisin and Exercise

The reported relationship between irisin and exercise are also contradictory. Some reports have claimed increased irisin serum levels in subjects who exercise [156], while a recent meta-analysis reported that chronic exercise training leads to significantly-decreased circulating irisin levels in randomized controlled trials only, with evidence remaining inconclusive in some other studies [160].

6.1.3. Irisin, NAFLD and Inflammation

To the best of our knowledge, there is only one study in which lower irisin levels were independently associated with higher intrahepatic triglyceride content, as assessed by 1H magnetic resonance spectroscopy [161]. However, in a recent study by Polyzos and colleagues [162], irisin levels were slightly higher in patients with NAFLD and significantly higher in NAFLD patients with portal inflammation, as compared to those without portal inflammation. Contrasting data on higher or lower serum irisin levels in relation with metabolic disorders, diet and exercise are worth further investigation and could be mostly due to the inaccuracy and lack of standardization of commercially-available ELISA assays. Mechanisms underlying the protective metabolic effects of irisin are not well understood and seem to be mostly related to higher induced energy expenditure and not to anti-inflammatory activities, such as NF-κB inactivation [157–159].

6.1.4. Irisin and Kidney

CKD patients have been reported to have lower, normal or higher energy expenditures than normal healthy people. The discrepancy among the different studies may be due to many factors related to the type of CKD stage, different therapies and also other, as of yet, unrecognized factors [163,164]. In this complex picture, a recent paper reported an inverse relationship between serum irisin levels and intima-media thickness in dialysis patients [165]. It is also well known that malnourished CKD patients have a worse outcome compared, not only with normally-nourished, but even obese CKD patients. Irisin levels have been found to be lower in CKD patients, and its concentrations were directly dependent on renal function and were related to the components of metabolic syndrome [166,167]. Furthermore, higher irisin levels were associated with sarcopenia in peritoneal dialysis patients [165]. On the basis of these considerations, irisin has been suggested as a candidate for the malnutrition status, often found in the more advanced stages of CKD. However, as for liver diseases, the role and the mechanisms by which irisin affects CKD remain to be further investigated.

7. Liver-Released Compounds

7.1. Selenoprotein P

Selenoprotein P (SeP; encoded by *SEPP1* in humans) is a secretory protein produced mainly by the liver [168,169] that functions as a selenium transporter from the liver to the rest of the body [170,171]. SeP functions as a hepatokine that contributes to insulin resistance in type 2 diabetes [172] (Figure 1). Importantly, the RNA interference-mediated knockdown of SeP improves insulin resistance and hyperglycemia in a mouse model of type 2 diabetes, suggesting the suppression of SeP production in the liver [173].

7.1.1. Selenoprotein P and Diet

SeP serum levels are directly correlated with the selenium (Se) diet supply (up to 0.1 mg/kg), and Se plays a pivotal role in homeostasis, with its inextricable U-shaped link with health status. Additional selenium intake may benefit people with low levels, whereas it may adversely affect those with adequate-to-high selenium levels. Individuals with serum or plasma selenium concentration of 122 μg/L or higher should not be supplemented with selenium [174].

7.1.2. Selenoprotein P and Exercise

SeP serum levels represent the biologically-active body Se-pool that was shown to slowly decrease during basic training in both trained and untrained individuals [175].

7.1.3. Selenoprotein P and Inflammation

SeP acts as an intracellular antioxidant in phagocytes, modulating inflammatory response via switching macrophage differentiation from M1 to M2 and, of consequence, limiting pathogenicity and oxidative damage [176,177]. On the other hand, SeP serum levels were shown to be lowered by acute-phase inflammatory response [178,179]. A systemic inflammatory response produces cytokines, inhibiting the expression of SEPP1 and reducing selenium levels; pro-inflammatory cytokines, downregulating the SELP promoter in vitro, can, overall, reduce the anti-inflammatory effects of SeP [180]. The interplay between SeP and inflammation may be the link of such a molecule with atherosclerosis, and some controversial epidemiologic data in type 2 diabetes exist [181]. Higher serum levels, inversely related to adiponectin and hepatic SeP concentrations, were reported in patients with type 2 diabetes, with a direct and independent link between SeP and both serum C-reactive protein levels and carotid intima-media thickness, while lower SeP expression was observed in murine adipocytes [173,182,183]. Differences in diabetes-related inflammation and the U-shaped association between SeP and type 2 diabetes risk, mimicking the U-shaped link of Se with health status, might explain some of the apparently contradictory epidemiologic findings. All of these data are worthy of further studies and validation, but indicate the key role of SeP in inflammatory-related cardiovascular alterations.

7.1.4. Selenoprotein P and NAFLD

SeP was found to be increased in NAFLD patients after correction for confounding factors [184]. However, the role of SeP in NAFLD remains to be well elucidated, even if they are able to act, as mentioned earlier, by their ability to modulate inflammatory response and insulin resistance.

In addition, different evidence suggests that metformin improves systemic insulin sensitivity through the regulation of SeP production, suggesting a novel potential therapeutic approach to treating type 2 diabetes [185].

7.1.5. Selenoprotein P and Kidney

SeP is the major carrier transporting selenium to target tissues and organs, including kidneys, were it is taken up by mechanisms, which are dependent, by specific receptor-related proteins [186]. According to Reinhardt and colleagues, in patients with CKD, SeP concentrations increase with impaired renal function (even after correction for age and CRP concentrations), whereas SeP concentrations are significantly lower in dialysis patients [187]. The reasons for the discrepant SeP concentrations among the stages of chronic renal failure are not yet completely defined, though the increased inflammatory status in dialysis patients [188] could play an important pathogenic role.

7.2. Fetuin-A

Human Fetuin-A/a2-Heremans-Schmid glycoprotein is an abundant 59-kDa serum glycoprotein, produced principally by the liver (thus, it can be classified as a "hepatokine"), and adipose tissue [189]. It works as a natural inhibitor of insulin receptors in the liver and skeletal muscle [190] and also exerts pro-adipogenic effects and suppresses adiponectin release [191]. Deletion of Fetuin-A improves insulin resistance and dyslipidemia and enhances glucose clearance in mice [192], whereas with genetic variants in humans, Fetuin-A has been associated with type 2 diabetes [193] and is linked with insulin action in adipocytes [194]. Serum Fetuin-A levels have been shown to correlate with metabolic syndrome and its main features [191].

7.2.1. Fetuin-A and Diet

In the general population, circulating Fetuin-A was decreased by alcohol intake and milk/dairy product intake, whereas meat and fish had no effect [195]. Resveratrol and curcumin intake may decrease Fetuin-A release [196].

7.2.2. Fetuin-A and Exercise

Short-term exercise training has been shown to reduce Fetuin-A levels, contributing to improvement in hepatic insulin sensitivity, especially in patients with NAFLD [197], although evidence concerning other exercise regimens is still controversial [198].

7.2.3. Fetuin-A and Inflammation

Fetuin-A does not seem to be directly regulated by inflammation, and no correlation was observed between hepatic inflammation and serum levels in patients with NAFLD [199].

7.2.4. Fetuin-A and NAFLD

Increased Fetuin-A has been reported in obese children and lean adults with NAFLD [199,200]. In patients with NAFLD, Fetuin-A levels were associated with the severity of steatosis, were influenced by genetic risk factors for hepatic fat accumulation and also correlated with insulin resistance and metabolic syndrome features [199]. Consistent with the above-mentioned lack of interplay between Fetuin-A and inflammatory response, no correlation was observed between hepatic inflammation and serum Fetuin-A levels in patients with NAFLD [189]. Fetuin-A could affect NAFLD/NASH because it is implicated in the development of insulin resistance and accelerated atherogenesis associated with fatty liver [199,201].

7.2.5. Fetuin-A and Kidney

Fetuin-A is also an inhibitor of vascular calcification, is progressively reduced in patients with renal failure and may modulate the progression of atherosclerosis in patients with chronic kidney disease [202].

8. Conclusions

Recent years have brought a great deal of new insights into the complex and dynamic interplay among the multiple effectors/mediators of fatty liver disease. Genomic, meta-genomic and metabolic profiling technologies and other top-down systems biology approaches are well suited for studies of metabolic syndrome and fatty liver disease. The appropriate analysis and interpretation of the physiopathological signatures require a new system of approaches to study and stratify the multifaceted clinical profiles of fatty liver and metabolic syndromes. Bio-statistical modeling will help to identify and combine genomic and meta-genomic determinants of the metabolic pathways and protein interaction networks. Similarly, the systems approach will help to stratify and re-define clinical phenotypes assessing the multiple nature of disease susceptibility and progression. The integration of metabolomic with genomic and meta-genomic markers will improve the understanding of metabolic syndrome and fatty liver disease, and the combined molecular and clinic-pathologic stratification of individuals with metabolic syndrome will allow redefining risks and prognoses, as well as identifying new diagnostic criteria, new markers of disease progression and new endpoints of clinical trials for specific groups of individuals with fatty liver.

Author Contributions: All authors contributed in preparing the draft; All authors revised the draft; All authors approved the final version of the manuscript.

Abbreviations

AG	acylated ghrelin
AMPK	adenosine monophosphate-activated protein kinase
ANP	atrial natriuretic peptide
BAT	brown adipose tissue
BMI	body mass index
CIMT	carotid intima-media thickness
CKD	chronic kidney disease
CRP	C-reactive protein
DAG	diacyl glycerol
DeAG	des-acylated ghrelin
DKD	diabetic kidney disease
DNL	de novo lipogenesis
ELISA	enzyme-linked immunosorbent assay
FC	free cholesterol
FFA	free fatty acid
FNDC5	fibronectin type III domain-containing protein 5
FoxO3a	forkhead box O3a
FSGS	focal segmental glomerular sclerosis
GLP-1	glucagon-like peptide 1
GLP-1R	glucagon-like peptide 1 receptor
GNG	gluconeogenesis
GOAT	ghrelin-ghrelin O-acyltransferase
(Oct)-1	organic cation transporter
IR	insulin resistance
IS	insulin sensitive
JNK	c-Jun terminal kinase
LDL	low density lipoprotein
MRS	magnetic resonance spectroscopy
MS	metabolic syndrome
MUFA	monounsaturated fatty acids
NAFLD	non-alcoholic fatty liver disease
NASH	non-alcoholic steatohepatitis

NF-κB	nuclear factor kappa-light-chain-enhancer of activated B cells
NGT	normal glucose tolerance
NLRP3	nucleotide-binding domain, leucine-rich-containing family, pyrin domain-containing-3
NO	nitric oxide
OGTT	oral glucose tolerance test
PUFA	polyunsaturated fatty acids
SC	subcutaneous
Se	selenium
SeP	selenoprotein P
SEPP1	selenoprotein P, plasma 1
SFA	saturated fatty acids
T2D	type 2 diabetes
TLR	toll like receptors
TNF-α	tumor necrosis factor-α
UCP1	uncoupling protein 1
VS	visceral
VLDL	very low density lipoprotein
WAT	white adipose tissue

References

1.   Groop, L.C.; Bonadonna, R.C.; DelPrato, S.; Ratheiser, K.; Zyck, K.; Ferrannini, E.; DeFronzo, R.A. Glucose and free fatty acid metabolism in non-insulin-dependent diabetes mellitus. Evidence for multiple sites of insulin resistance. *J. Clin. Investig.* **1989**, *84*, 205–213. [CrossRef] [PubMed]

2.   Bugianesi, E.; Gastaldelli, A.; Vanni, E.; Gambino, R.; Cassader, M.; Baldi, S.; Ponti, V.; Pagano, G.; Ferrannini, E.; Rizzetto, M. Insulin resistance in non-diabetic patients with non-alcoholic fatty liver disease: Sites and mechanisms. *Diabetologia* **2005**, *48*, 634–642. [CrossRef] [PubMed]

3.   Lafontan, M.; Langin, D. Lipolysis and lipid mobilization in human adipose tissue. *Prog. Lipid Res.* **2009**, *48*, 275–297. [CrossRef] [PubMed]

4.   Ferrannini, E.; Camastra, S.; Coppack, S.W.; Fliser, D.; Golay, A.; Mitrakou, A. Insulin action and non-esterified fatty acids. The European Group for the Study of Insulin Resistance (EGIR). *Proc. Nutr. Soc.* **1997**, *56*, 753–761. [CrossRef] [PubMed]

5.   Legrand-Poels, S.; Esser, N.; L'Homme, L.; Scheen, A.; Paquot, N.; Piette, J. Free fatty acids as modulators of the NLRP3 inflammasome in obesity/type 2 diabetes. *Biochem. Pharmacol.* **2014**, *92*, 131–141. [CrossRef] [PubMed]

6.   Rocha, D.M.; Caldas, A.P.; Oliveira, L.L.; Bressan, J.; Hermsdorff, H.H. Saturated fatty acids trigger TLR4-mediated inflammatory response. *Atherosclerosis* **2016**, *244*, 211–215. [CrossRef] [PubMed]

7.   Moreira, A.P.; Texeira, T.F.; Ferreira, A.B.; Peluzio Mdo, C.; Alfenas Rde, C. Influence of a high-fat diet on gut microbiota, intestinal permeability and metabolic endotoxaemia. *Br. J. Nutr.* **2012**, *108*, 801–809. [CrossRef] [PubMed]

8.   Mittendorfer, B.; Yoshino, M.; Patterson, B.W.; Klein, S. VLDL triglyceride kinetics in lean, overweight, and obese men and women. *J. Clin. Endocrinol. Metab.* **2016**, *101*, 4151–4160. [CrossRef] [PubMed]

9.   De Souza, R.J.; Mente, A.; Maroleanu, A.; Cozma, A.I.; Ha, V.; Kishibe, T.; Uleryk, E.; Budylowski, P.; Schunemann, H.; Beyene, J.; et al. Intake of saturated and trans unsaturated fatty acids and risk of all cause mortality, cardiovascular disease, and type 2 diabetes: Systematic review and meta-analysis of observational studies. *BMJ* **2015**, *351*, h3978. [CrossRef] [PubMed]

10.   Patterson, E.; Wall, R.; Fitzgerald, G.F.; Ross, R.P.; Stanton, C. Health implications of high dietary omega-6 polyunsaturated Fatty acids. *J. Nutr. Metab.* **2012**, *2012*, 539426. [CrossRef] [PubMed]

11.   Maehre, H.K.; Jensen, I.J.; Elvevoll, E.O.; Eilertsen, K.E. Omega-3 fatty acids and cardiovascular diseases: Effects, mechanisms and dietary relevance. *Int. J. Mol. Sci.* **2015**, *16*, 22636–22661. [CrossRef] [PubMed]

12.   Romijn, J.A.; Coyle, E.F.; Sidossis, L.S.; Gastaldelli, A.; Horowitz, J.F.; Endert, E.; Wolfe, R.R. Regulation of endogenous fat and carbohydrate metabolism in relation to exercise intensity and duration. *Am. J. Physiol.* **1993**, *265*, E380–E391. [PubMed]

13.   Boden, G. Fatty acid-induced inflammation and insulin resistance in skeletal muscle and liver. *Curr. Diabetes Rep.* **2006**, *6*, 177–181. [CrossRef]

14. Gadang, V.; Kohli, R.; Myronovych, A.; Hui, D.Y.; Perez-Tilve, D.; Jaeschke, A. MLK3 promotes metabolic dysfunction induced by saturated fatty acid-enriched diet. *Am. J. Physiol. Endocrinol. Metab.* **2013**, *305*, E549–E556. [CrossRef] [PubMed]

15. Leamy, A.K.; Egnatchik, R.A.; Shiota, M.; Ivanova, P.T.; Myers, D.S.; Brown, H.A.; Young, J.D. Enhanced synthesis of saturated phospholipids is associated with ER stress and lipotoxicity in palmitate treated hepatic cells. *J. Lipid Res.* **2014**, *55*, 1478–1488. [CrossRef] [PubMed]

16. Snodgrass, R.G.; Huang, S.; Choi, I.W.; Rutledge, J.C.; Hwang, D.H. Inflammasome-mediated secretion of IL-1β in human monocytes through TLR2 activation; modulation by dietary fatty acids. *J. Immunol.* **2013**, *191*, 4337–4347. [CrossRef] [PubMed]

17. Das, S.K.; Mondal, A.K.; Elbein, S.C. Distinct gene expression profiles characterize cellular responses to palmitate and oleate. *J. Lipid Res.* **2010**, *51*, 2121–2131. [CrossRef] [PubMed]

18. Yang, G.; Badeanlou, L.; Bielawski, J.; Roberts, A.J.; Hannun, Y.A.; Samad, F. Central role of ceramide biosynthesis in body weight regulation, energy metabolism, and the metabolic syndrome. *Am. J. Physiol. Endocrinol. Metab.* **2009**, *297*, E211–E224. [CrossRef] [PubMed]

19. Ussher, J.R.; Koves, T.R.; Cadete, V.J.; Zhang, L.; Jaswal, J.S.; Swyrd, S.J.; Lopaschuk, D.G.; Proctor, S.D.; Keung, W.; Muoio, D.M.; et al. Inhibition of de novo ceramide synthesis reverses diet-induced insulin resistance and enhances whole-body oxygen consumption. *Diabetes* **2010**, *59*, 2453–2464. [CrossRef] [PubMed]

20. Wei, Y.; Wang, D.; Topczewski, F.; Pagliassotti, M.J. Saturated fatty acids induce endoplasmic reticulum stress and apoptosis independently of ceramide in liver cells. *Am. J. Physiol. Endocrinol. Metab.* **2006**, *291*, E275–E281. [CrossRef] [PubMed]

21. Luukkonen, P.K.; Zhou, Y.; Sadevirta, S.; Leivonen, M.; Arola, J.; Oresic, M.; Hyotylainen, T.; Yki-Jarvinen, H. Hepatic ceramides dissociate steatosis and insulin resistance in patients with non-alcoholic fatty liver disease. *J. Hepatol.* **2016**, *64*, 1167–1175. [CrossRef] [PubMed]

22. Gregor, M.F.; Yang, L.; Fabbrini, E.; Mohammed, B.S.; Eagon, J.C.; Hotamisligil, G.S.; Klein, S. Endoplasmic reticulum stress is reduced in tissues of obese subjects after weight loss. *Diabetes* **2009**, *58*, 693–700. [CrossRef] [PubMed]

23. Mantzaris, M.D.; Tsianos, E.V.; Galaris, D. Interruption of triacylglycerol synthesis in the endoplasmic reticulum is the initiating event for saturated fatty acid-induced lipotoxicity in liver cells. *FEBS J.* **2011**, *278*, 519–530. [CrossRef] [PubMed]

24. Listenberger, L.L.; Han, X.; Lewis, S.E.; Cases, S.; Farese, R.V., Jr.; Ory, D.S.; Schaffer, J.E. Triglyceride accumulation protects against fatty acid-induced lipotoxicity. *Proc. Natl. Acad. Sci. USA* **2003**, *100*, 3077–3082. [CrossRef] [PubMed]

25. Saponaro, C.; Gaggini, M.; Carli, F.; Gastaldelli, A. The subtle balance between lipolysis and lipogenesis: A critical point in metabolic homeostasis. *Nutrients* **2015**, *7*, 9453–9474. [CrossRef] [PubMed]

26. Yamaguchi, K.; Yang, L.; McCall, S.; Huang, J.; Yu, X.X.; Pandey, S.K.; Bhanot, S.; Monia, B.P.; Li, Y.X.; Diehl, A.M. Inhibiting triglyceride synthesis improves hepatic steatosis but exacerbates liver damage and fibrosis in obese mice with nonalcoholic steatohepatitis. *Hepatology* **2007**, *45*, 1366–1374. [CrossRef] [PubMed]

27. Sieber, J.; Jehle, A.W. Free fatty acids and their metabolism affect function and survival of podocytes. *Front. Endocrinol.* **2014**, *5*, 186. [CrossRef] [PubMed]

28. Lennon, R.; Pons, D.; Sabin, M.A.; Wei, C.; Shield, J.P.; Coward, R.J.; Tavare, J.M.; Mathieson, P.W.; Saleem, M.A.; Welsh, G.I. Saturated fatty acids induce insulin resistance in human podocytes: Implications for diabetic nephropathy. *Nephrol. Dial. Transplant.* **2009**, *24*, 3288–3296. [CrossRef] [PubMed]

29. Sieber, J.; Lindenmeyer, M.T.; Kampe, K.; Campbell, K.N.; Cohen, C.D.; Hopfer, H.; Mundel, P.; Jehle, A.W. Regulation of podocyte survival and endoplasmic reticulum stress by fatty acids. *Am. J. Physiol. Ren. Physiol.* **2010**, *299*, F821–F829. [CrossRef] [PubMed]

30. Ioannou, G.N. The role of cholesterol in the pathogenesis of NASH. *Trends Endocrinol. Metab.* **2016**, *27*, 84–95. [CrossRef] [PubMed]

31. Janoudi, A.; Shamoun, F.E.; Kalavakunta, J.K.; Abela, G.S. Cholesterol crystal induced arterial inflammation and destabilization of atherosclerotic plaque. *Eur. Heart J.* **2016**, *37*, 1959–1967. [CrossRef] [PubMed]

32. Tall, A.R.; Yvan-Charvet, L. Cholesterol, inflammation and innate immunity. *Nat. Rev. Immunol.* **2015**, *15*, 104–116. [CrossRef] [PubMed]

33. Keys, A. Coronary heart disease, serum cholesterol, and the diet. *Acta Med. Scand.* **1980**, *207*, 153–160. [CrossRef] [PubMed]

34. Franklin, B.A.; Durstine, J.L.; Roberts, C.K.; Barnard, R.J. Impact of diet and exercise on lipid management in the modern era. *Best Pract. Res. Clin. Endocrinol. Metab.* **2014**, *28*, 405–421. [CrossRef] [PubMed]

35. Virtanen, J.K.; Mursu, J.; Virtanen, H.E.; Fogelholm, M.; Salonen, J.T.; Koskinen, T.T.; Voutilainen, S.; Tuomainen, T.P. Associations of egg and cholesterol intakes with carotid intima-media thickness and risk of incident coronary artery disease according to apolipoprotein E phenotype in men: The Kuopio Ischaemic Heart Disease Risk Factor Study. *Am. J. Clin. Nutr.* **2016**, *103*, 895–901. [CrossRef] [PubMed]

36. Caesar, R.; Nygren, H.; Oresic, M.; Backhed, F. Interaction between dietary lipids and gut microbiota regulates hepatic cholesterol metabolism. *J. Lipid Res.* **2016**, *57*, 474–481. [CrossRef] [PubMed]

37. Mann, S.; Beedie, C.; Jimenez, A. Differential effects of aerobic exercise, resistance training and combined exercise modalities on cholesterol and the lipid profile: Review, synthesis and recommendations. *Sports Med.* **2014**, *44*, 211–221. [CrossRef] [PubMed]

38. O'Donovan, G.; Owen, A.; Bird, S.R.; Kearney, E.M.; Nevill, A.M.; Jones, D.W.; Woolf-May, K. Changes in cardiorespiratory fitness and coronary heart disease risk factors following 24 wk of moderate- or high-intensity exercise of equal energy cost. *J. Appl. Physiol.* **2005**, *98*, 1619–1625. [CrossRef] [PubMed]

39. Lira, F.S.; Yamashita, A.S.; Uchida, M.C.; Zanchi, N.E.; Gualano, B.; Martins, E., Jr.; Caperuto, E.C.; Seelaender, M. Low and moderate, rather than high intensity strength exercise induces benefit regarding plasma lipid profile. *Diabetol. Metab. Syndr.* **2010**, *2*, 31. [CrossRef] [PubMed]

40. Katzmarzyk, P.T.; Leon, A.S.; Rankinen, T.; Gagnon, J.; Skinner, J.S.; Wilmore, J.H.; Rao, D.C.; Bouchard, C. Changes in blood lipids consequent to aerobic exercise training related to changes in body fatness and aerobic fitness. *Metabolism* **2001**, *50*, 841–848. [CrossRef] [PubMed]

41. Li, Y.; Schwabe, R.F.; Devries-Seimon, T.; Yao, P.M.; Gerbod-Giannone, M.C.; Tall, A.R.; Davis, R.J.; Flavell, R.; Brenner, D.A.; Tabas, I. Free cholesterol-loaded macrophages are an abundant source of tumor necrosis factor-α and interleukin-6: Model of NF-κB and map kinase-dependent inflammation in advanced atherosclerosis. *J. Biol. Chem.* **2005**, *280*, 21763–21772. [CrossRef] [PubMed]

42. Puri, P.; Baillie, R.A.; Wiest, M.M.; Mirshahi, F.; Choudhury, J.; Cheung, O.; Sargeant, C.; Contos, M.J.; Sanyal, A.J. A lipidomic analysis of nonalcoholic fatty liver disease. *Hepatology* **2007**, *46*, 1081–1090. [CrossRef] [PubMed]

43. Min, H.K.; Kapoor, A.; Fuchs, M.; Mirshahi, F.; Zhou, H.; Maher, J.; Kellum, J.; Warnick, R.; Contos, M.J.; Sanyal, A.J. Increased hepatic synthesis and dysregulation of cholesterol metabolism is associated with the severity of nonalcoholic fatty liver disease. *Cell Metab.* **2012**, *15*, 665–674. [CrossRef] [PubMed]

44. Dongiovanni, P.; Petta, S.; Maglio, C.; Fracanzani, A.L.; Pipitone, R.; Mozzi, E.; Motta, B.M.; Kaminska, D.; Rametta, R.; Grimaudo, S.; et al. Transmembrane 6 superfamily member 2 gene variant disentangles nonalcoholic steatohepatitis from cardiovascular disease. *Hepatology* **2015**, *61*, 506–514. [CrossRef] [PubMed]

45. Wahl, P.; Ducasa, G.M.; Fornoni, A. Systemic and renal lipids in kidney disease development and progression. *Am. J. Physiol. Ren. Physiol.* **2016**, *310*, F433–F445. [CrossRef] [PubMed]

46. Lee, H.S.; Kruth, H.S. Accumulation of cholesterol in the lesions of focal segmental glomerulosclerosis. *Nephrology* **2003**, *8*, 224–223. [CrossRef] [PubMed]

47. Fornoni, A.; Merscher, S.; Kopp, J.B. Lipid biology of the podocyte—New perspectives offer new opportunities. *Nat. Rev. Nephrol.* **2014**, *10*, 379–388. [CrossRef] [PubMed]

48. Wang, X.X.; Jiang, T.; Shen, Y.; Caldas, Y.; Miyazaki-Anzai, S.; Santamaria, H.; Urbanek, C.; Solis, N.; Scherzer, P.; Lewis, L.; et al. Diabetic nephropathy is accelerated by farnesoid X receptor deficiency and inhibited by farnesoid X receptor activation in a type 1 diabetes model. *Diabetes* **2010**, *59*, 2916–2927. [CrossRef] [PubMed]

49. Kopp, J.B.; Smith, M.W.; Nelson, G.W.; Johnson, R.C.; Freedman, B.I.; Bowden, D.W.; Oleksyk, T.; McKenzie, L.M.; Kajiyama, H.; Ahuja, T.S.; et al. MYH9 is a major-effect risk gene for focal segmental glomerulosclerosis. *Nat. Genet.* **2008**, *40*, 1175–1184. [CrossRef] [PubMed]

50. Kiss, E.; Kranzlin, B.; Wagenblabeta, K.; Bonrouhi, M.; Thiery, J.; Grone, E.; Nordstrom, V.; Teupser, D.; Gretz, N.; Malle, E.; et al. Lipid droplet accumulation is associated with an increase in hyperglycemia-induced renal damage: Prevention by liver X receptors. *Am. J. Pathol.* **2013**, *182*, 727–741. [CrossRef] [PubMed]

51. Agarwal, R. Effects of statins on renal function. *Am. J. Cardiol.* **2006**, *97*, 748–755. [CrossRef] [PubMed]

52. Nigro, E.; Scudiero, O.; Monaco, M.L.; Palmieri, A.; Mazzarella, G.; Costagliola, C.; Bianco, A.; Daniele, A. New insight into adiponectin role in obesity and obesity-related diseases. *BioMed Res. Int.* **2014**, *2014*, 658913. [CrossRef] [PubMed]

53. Scherer, P.E. The multifaceted roles of adipose tissue-therapeutic targets for diabetes and beyond: The 2015 banting lecture. *Diabetes* **2016**, *65*, 1452–1461. [CrossRef] [PubMed]

54. Freitas Lima, L.C.; Braga, V.A.; do Socorro de Franca Silva, M.; Cruz, J.C.; Sousa Santos, S.H.; de Oliveira Monteiro, M.M.; Balarini, C.M. Adipokines, diabetes and atherosclerosis: An inflammatory association. *Front. Physiol.* **2015**, *6*, 304. [CrossRef] [PubMed]

55. Von Frankenberg, A.D.; Silva, F.M.; de Almeida, J.C.; Piccoli, V.; do Nascimento, F.V.; Sost, M.M.; Leitao, C.B.; Remonti, L.L.; Umpierre, D.; Reis, A.F.; et al. Effect of dietary lipids on circulating adiponectin: A systematic review with meta-analysis of randomised controlled trials. *Br. J. Nutr.* **2014**, *112*, 1235–1250. [CrossRef] [PubMed]

56. Kamari, Y.; Grossman, E.; Oron-Herman, M.; Peleg, E.; Shabtay, Z.; Shamiss, A.; Sharabi, Y. Metabolic stress with a high carbohydrate diet increases adiponectin levels. *Horm. Metab. Res.* **2007**, *39*, 384–388. [CrossRef] [PubMed]

57. Rezvani, R.; Cianflone, K.; McGahan, J.P.; Berglund, L.; Bremer, A.A.; Keim, N.L.; Griffen, S.C.; Havel, P.J.; Stanhope, K.L. Effects of sugar-sweetened beverages on plasma acylation stimulating protein, leptin and adiponectin: Relationships with metabolic outcomes. *Obesity* **2013**, *21*, 2471–2480. [CrossRef] [PubMed]

58. Swarbrick, M.M.; Havel, P.J. Physiological, pharmacological, and nutritional regulation of circulating adiponectin concentrations in humans. *Metab. Syndr. Relat. Disord.* **2008**, *6*, 87–102. [CrossRef] [PubMed]

59. Golbidi, S.; Laher, I. Exercise induced adipokine changes and the metabolic syndrome. *J. Diabetes Res.* **2014**, *2014*, 726861. [CrossRef] [PubMed]

60. Ahmadi, N.; Eshaghian, S.; Huizenga, R.; Sosnin, K.; Ebrahimi, R.; Siegel, R. Effects of intense exercise and moderate caloric restriction on cardiovascular risk factors and inflammation. *Am. J. Med.* **2011**, *124*, 978–982. [CrossRef] [PubMed]

61. Fantuzzi, G. Adiponectin and inflammation: Consensus and controversy. *J. Allergy Clin. Immunol.* **2008**, *121*, 326–330. [CrossRef] [PubMed]

62. Bugianesi, E.; Pagotto, U.; Manini, R.; Vanni, E.; Gastaldelli, A.; de Iasio, R.; Gentilcore, E.; Natale, S.; Cassader, M.; Rizzetto, M.; et al. Plasma adiponectin in nonalcoholic fatty liver is related to hepatic insulin resistance and hepatic fat content, not to liver disease severity. *J. Clin. Endocrinol. Metab.* **2005**, *90*, 3498–3504. [CrossRef] [PubMed]

63. Gastaldelli, A.; Harrison, S.; Belfort-Aguiar, R.; Hardies, J.; Balas, B.; Schenker, S.; Cusi, K. Pioglitazone in the treatment of NASH: The role of adiponectin. *Aliment. Pharmacol. Ther.* **2010**, *32*, 769–775. [CrossRef] [PubMed]

64. Kadowaki, T.; Yamauchi, T. Adiponectin and adiponectin receptors. *Endocr. Rev.* **2005**, *26*, 439–451. [CrossRef] [PubMed]

65. Yano, Y.; Hoshide, S.; Ishikawa, J.; Hashimoto, T.; Eguchi, K.; Shimada, K.; Kario, K. Differential impacts of adiponectin on low-grade albuminuria between obese and nonobese persons without diabetes. *J. Clin. Hypertens.* **2007**, *9*, 775–782. [CrossRef]

66. Ohashi, K.; Iwatani, H.; Kihara, S.; Nakagawa, Y.; Komura, N.; Fujita, K.; Maeda, N.; Nishida, M.; Katsube, F.; Shimomura, I.; et al. Exacerbation of albuminuria and renal fibrosis in subtotal renal ablation model of adiponectin-knockout mice. *Arterioscler. Thromb. Vasc. Biol.* **2007**, *27*, 1910–1917. [CrossRef] [PubMed]

67. Sharma, K.; Ramachandrarao, S.; Qiu, G.; Usui, H.K.; Zhu, Y.; Dunn, S.R.; Ouedraogo, R.; Hough, K.; McCue, P.; Chan, L.; et al. Adiponectin regulates albuminuria and podocyte function in mice. *J. Clin. Investig.* **2008**, *118*, 1645–1656. [CrossRef] [PubMed]

68. Iwashima, Y.; Horio, T.; Kumada, M.; Suzuki, Y.; Kihara, S.; Rakugi, H.; Kawano, Y.; Funahashi, T.; Ogihara, T. Adiponectin and renal function, and implication as a risk of cardiovascular disease. *Am. J. Cardiol.* **2006**, *98*, 1603–1608. [CrossRef] [PubMed]

69. Ignacy, W.; Chudek, J.; Adamczak, M.; Funahashi, T.; Matsuzawa, Y.; Kokot, F.; Wiecek, A. Reciprocal association of plasma adiponectin and serum C-reactive protein concentration in haemodialysis patients with end-stage kidney disease—A follow-up study. *Nephron Clin. Pract.* **2005**, *101*, c18–c24. [CrossRef] [PubMed]

70. Marchlewska, A.; Stenvinkel, P.; Lindholm, B.; Danielsson, A.; Pecoits-Filho, R.; Lonnqvist, F.; Schalling, M.; Heimburger, O.; Nordfors, L. Reduced gene expression of adiponectin in fat tissue from patients with end-stage renal disease. *Kidney Int.* **2004**, *66*, 46–50. [CrossRef] [PubMed]

71. Izadi, V.; Saraf-Bank, S.; Azadbakht, L. Dietary intakes and leptin concentrations. *ARYA Atheroscler.* **2014**, *10*, 266–272. [PubMed]

72. Gastaldelli, A.; Sironi, A.M.; Ciociaro, D.; Positano, V.; Buzzigoli, E.; Giannessi, D.; Lombardi, M.; Mari, A.; Ferrannini, E. Visceral fat and beta cell function in non-diabetic humans. *Diabetologia* **2005**, *48*, 2090–2096. [CrossRef] [PubMed]

73. Maffei, M.; Halaas, J.; Ravussin, E.; Pratley, R.E.; Lee, G.H.; Zhang, Y.; Fei, H.; Kim, S.; Lallone, R.; Ranganathan, S.; et al. Leptin levels in human and rodent: Measurement of plasma leptin and ob RNA in obese and weight-reduced subjects. *Nat. Med.* **1995**, *1*, 1155–1161. [CrossRef] [PubMed]

74. Adya, R.; Tan, B.K.; Randeva, H.S. Differential effects of leptin and adiponectin in endothelial angiogenesis. *J. Diabetes Res.* **2015**, *2015*, 648239. [CrossRef] [PubMed]

75. Martin, L.J.; Siliart, B.; Lutz, T.A.; Biourge, V.; Nguyen, P.; Dumon, H.J. Postprandial response of plasma insulin, amylin and acylated ghrelin to various test meals in lean and obese cats. *Br. J. Nutr.* **2010**, *103*, 1610–1619. [CrossRef] [PubMed]

76. Hall, M.E.; Harmancey, R.; Stec, D.E. Lean heart: Role of leptin in cardiac hypertrophy and metabolism. *World J. Cardiol.* **2015**, *7*, 511–524. [PubMed]

77. Masquio, D.C.; de Piano, A.; Sanches, P.L.; Corgosinho, F.C.; Campos, R.M.; Carnier, J.; da Silva, P.L.; Caranti, D.A.; Tock, L.; Oyama, L.M.; et al. The effect of weight loss magnitude on pro-/anti-inflammatory adipokines and carotid intima-media thickness in obese adolescents engaged in interdisciplinary weight loss therapy. *Clin. Endocrinol.* **2013**, *79*, 55–64. [CrossRef] [PubMed]

78. La Cava, A.; Matarese, G. The weight of leptin in immunity. *Nat. Rev. Immunol.* **2004**, *4*, 371–379. [CrossRef] [PubMed]

79. Cumin, F.; Baum, H.P.; de Gasparo, M.; Levens, N. Removal of endogenous leptin from the circulation by the kidney. *Int. J. Obes. Relat. Metab. Disord.* **1997**, *21*, 495–504. [CrossRef] [PubMed]

80. Stenvinkel, P.; Lindholm, B.; Lonnqvist, F.; Katzarski, K.; Heimburger, O. Increases in serum leptin levels during peritoneal dialysis are associated with inflammation and a decrease in lean body mass. *J. Am. Soc. Nephrol.* **2000**, *11*, 1303–1309. [PubMed]

81. Polyzos, S.A.; Aronis, K.N.; Kountouras, J.; Raptis, D.D.; Vasiloglou, M.F.; Mantzoros, C.S. Circulating leptin in non-alcoholic fatty liver disease: A systematic review and meta-analysis. *Diabetologia* **2016**, *59*, 30–43. [CrossRef] [PubMed]

82. Mak, R.H.; Cheung, W.; Cone, R.D.; Marks, D.L. Leptin and inflammation-associated cachexia in chronic kidney disease. *Kidney Int.* **2006**, *69*, 794–797. [CrossRef] [PubMed]

83. Carrero, J.J.; Nakashima, A.; Qureshi, A.R.; Lindholm, B.; Heimburger, O.; Barany, P.; Stenvinkel, P. Protein-energy wasting modifies the association of ghrelin with inflammation, leptin, and mortality in hemodialysis patients. *Kidney Int.* **2011**, *79*, 749–756. [CrossRef] [PubMed]

84. Gastaldelli, A.; Cusi, K.; Pettiti, M.; Hardies, J.; Miyazaki, Y.; Berria, R.; Buzzigoli, E.; Sironi, A.M.; Cersosimo, E.; Ferrannini, E.; et al. Relationship between hepatic/visceral fat and hepatic insulin resistance in nondiabetic and type 2 diabetic subjects. *Gastroenterology* **2007**, *133*, 496–506. [CrossRef] [PubMed]

85. Gastaldelli, A.; Baldi, S.; Pettiti, M.; Toschi, E.; Camastra, S.; Natali, A.; Landau, B.R.; Ferrannini, E. Influence of obesity and type 2 diabetes on gluconeogenesis and glucose output in humans: A quantitative study. *Diabetes* **2000**, *49*, 1367–1373. [CrossRef] [PubMed]

86. Khodabandehloo, H.; Gorgani-Firuzjaee, S.; Panahi, G.; Meshkani, R. Molecular and cellular mechanisms linking inflammation to insulin resistance and β-cell dysfunction. *Transl. Res.* **2016**, *167*, 228–256. [CrossRef] [PubMed]

87. Keane, K.N.; Cruzat, V.F.; Carlessi, R.; de Bittencourt, P.I., Jr.; Newsholme, P. Molecular events linking oxidative stress and inflammation to insulin resistance and β-cell dysfunction. *Oxid. Med. Cell. Longev.* **2015**, *2015*, 181643. [CrossRef] [PubMed]

88. Chen, L.; Chen, R. Mechanisms linking inflammation to insulin resistance. *Int. J. Endocrinol.* **2015**, *2015*, 508409. [CrossRef] [PubMed]

89. Lindgren, O.; Pacini, G.; Tura, A.; Holst, J.J.; Deacon, C.F.; Ahren, B. Incretin effect after oral amino acid ingestion in humans. *J. Clin. Endocrinol. Metab.* **2015**, *100*, 1172–1176. [CrossRef] [PubMed]

90. Dobbins, R.L.; Szczepaniak, L.S.; Myhill, J.; Tamura, Y.; Uchino, H.; Giacca, A.; McGarry, J.D. The composition of dietary fat directly influences glucose-stimulated insulin secretion in rats. *Diabetes* **2002**, *51*, 1825–1833. [CrossRef] [PubMed]

91. Kashyap, S.; Belfort, R.; Gastaldelli, A.; Pratipanawatr, T.; Berria, R.; Pratipanawatr, W.; Bajaj, M.; Mandarino, L.; DeFronzo, R.; Cusi, K. A sustained increase in plasma free fatty acids impairs insulin secretion in nondiabetic subjects genetically predisposed to develop type 2 diabetes. *Diabetes* **2003**, *52*, 2461–2474. [CrossRef] [PubMed]

92. Hyotylainen, T.; Jerby, L.; Petaja, E.M.; Mattila, I.; Jantti, S.; Auvinen, P.; Gastaldelli, A.; Yki-Jarvinen, H.; Ruppin, E.; Oresic, M. Genome-scale study reveals reduced metabolic adaptability in patients with non-alcoholic fatty liver disease. *Nat. Commun.* **2016**, *7*, 8994. [CrossRef] [PubMed]

93. Donnelly, K.L.; Smith, C.I.; Schwarzenberg, S.J.; Jessurun, J.; Boldt, M.D.; Parks, E.J. Sources of fatty acids stored in liver and secreted via lipoproteins in patients with nonalcoholic fatty liver disease. *J. Clin. Investig.* **2005**, *115*, 1343–1351. [CrossRef] [PubMed]

94. Paradis, V.; Perlemuter, G.; Bonvoust, F.; Dargere, D.; Parfait, B.; Vidaud, M.; Conti, M.; Huet, S.; Ba, N.; Buffet, C.; et al. High glucose and hyperinsulinemia stimulate connective tissue growth factor expression: A potential mechanism involved in progression to fibrosis in nonalcoholic steatohepatitis. *Hepatology* **2001**, *34*, 738–744. [CrossRef] [PubMed]

95. Svegliati-Baroni, G.; Ridolfi, F.; Di Sario, A.; Casini, A.; Marucci, L.; Gaggiotti, G.; Orlandoni, P.; Macarri, G.; Perego, L.; Benedetti, A.; et al. Insulin and insulin-like growth factor-1 stimulate proliferation and type I collagen accumulation by human hepatic stellate cells: Differential effects on signal transduction pathways. *Hepatology* **1999**, *29*, 1743–1751. [CrossRef] [PubMed]

96. Coggan, A.R.; Raguso, C.A.; Gastaldelli, A.; Williams, B.D.; Wolfe, R.R. Regulation of glucose production during exercise at 80% of VO_2 peak in untrained humans. *Am. J. Physiol.* **1997**, *273*, E348–E354. [PubMed]

97. Cabrera, O.; Berman, D.M.; Kenyon, N.S.; Ricordi, C.; Berggren, P.O.; Caicedo, A. The unique cytoarchitecture of human pancreatic islets has implications for islet cell function. *Proc. Natl. Acad. Sci. USA* **2006**, *103*, 2334–2339. [CrossRef] [PubMed]

98. Wewer Albrechtsen, N.J.; Kuhre, R.E.; Pedersen, J.; Knop, F.K.; Holst, J.J. The biology of glucagon and the consequences of hyperglucagonemia. *Biomark. Med.* **2016**, *10*, 1141–1151. [CrossRef] [PubMed]

99. Unger, R.H. Glucagon physiology and pathophysiology in the light of new advances. *Diabetologia* **1985**, *28*, 574–578. [CrossRef] [PubMed]

100. Gromada, J.; Franklin, I.; Wollheim, C.B. α-Cells of the endocrine pancreas: 35 years of research but the enigma remains. *Endocr. Rev.* **2007**, *28*, 84–116. [CrossRef] [PubMed]

101. Mitrakou, A.; Ryan, C.; Veneman, T.; Mokan, M.; Jenssen, T.; Kiss, I.; Durrant, J.; Cryer, P.; Gerich, J. Hierarchy of glycemic thresholds for counterregulatory hormone secretion, symptoms, and cerebral dysfunction. *Am. J. Physiol.* **1991**, *260*, E67–E74. [PubMed]

102. Bagger, J.I.; Knop, F.K.; Lund, A.; Holst, J.J.; Vilsboll, T. Glucagon responses to increasing oral loads of glucose and corresponding isoglycaemic intravenous glucose infusions in patients with type 2 diabetes and healthy individuals. *Diabetologia* **2014**, *57*, 1720–1725. [CrossRef] [PubMed]

103. Rocha, D.M.; Faloona, G.R.; Unger, R.H. Glucagon stimulating activity of 20 amino acids in dogs. *J. Clin. Investig.* **1972**, *51*, 2346–2351. [CrossRef] [PubMed]

104. Palmer, J.P.; Benson, J.W.; Walter, R.M.; Ensinck, J.W. Arginine-stimulated acute phase of insulin and glucagon secretion in diabetic subjects. *J. Clin. Investig.* **1976**, *58*, 565–570. [CrossRef] [PubMed]

105. Radulescu, A.; Gannon, M.C.; Nuttall, F.Q. The effect on glucagon, glucagon-like peptide-1, total and acyl-ghrelin of dietary fats ingested with and without potato. *J. Clin. Endocrinol. Metab.* **2010**, *95*, 3385–3391. [CrossRef] [PubMed]

106. Hippen, A.R. Glucagon as a potential therapy for ketosis and fatty liver. *Vet. Clin. N. Am. Food Anim. Pract.* **2000**, *16*, 267–282. [CrossRef]

107. Jiang, G.; Zhang, B.B. Glucagon and regulation of glucose metabolism. *Am. J. Physiol. Endocrinol. Metab.* **2003**, *284*, E671–E678. [CrossRef] [PubMed]

108. Conarello, S.L.; Jiang, G.; Mu, J.; Li, Z.; Woods, J.; Zycband, E.; Ronan, J.; Liu, F.; Roy, R.S.; Zhu, L.; et al. Glucagon receptor knockout mice are resistant to diet-induced obesity and streptozotocin-mediated beta cell loss and hyperglycaemia. *Diabetologia* **2007**, *50*, 142–150. [CrossRef] [PubMed]

109. Junker, A.E.; Gluud, L.; Holst, J.J.; Knop, F.K.; Vilsboll, T. Diabetic and nondiabetic patients with nonalcoholic fatty liver disease have an impaired incretin effect and fasting hyperglucagonaemia. *J. Intern. Med.* **2016**, *279*, 485–493. [CrossRef] [PubMed]

110. Liang, Y.; Osborne, M.C.; Monia, B.P.; Bhanot, S.; Gaarde, W.A.; Reed, C.; She, P.; Jetton, T.L.; Demarest, K.T. Reduction in glucagon receptor expression by an antisense oligonucleotide ameliorates diabetic syndrome in *db/db* mice. *Diabetes* **2004**, *53*, 410–417. [CrossRef] [PubMed]

111. Ortega, F.J.; Moreno-Navarrete, J.M.; Sabater, M.; Ricart, W.; Fruhbeck, G.; Fernandez-Real, J.M. Circulating glucagon is associated with inflammatory mediators in metabolically compromised subjects. *Eur. J. Endocrinol.* **2011**, *165*, 639–645. [CrossRef] [PubMed]

112. Dandona, P.; Ghanim, H.; Abuaysheh, S.; Green, K.; Batra, M.; Dhindsa, S.; Makdissi, A.; Patel, R.; Chaudhuri, A. Decreased insulin secretion and incretin concentrations and increased glucagon concentrations after a high-fat meal when compared with a high-fruit and -fiber meal. *Am. J. Physiol. Endocrinol. Metab.* **2015**, *308*, E185–E191. [CrossRef] [PubMed]

113. Pedersen, B.K.; Steensberg, A.; Schjerling, P. Exercise and interleukin-6. *Curr. Opin. Hematol.* **2001**, *8*, 137–141. [CrossRef] [PubMed]

114. Bastard, J.P.; Maachi, M.; Van Nhieu, J.T.; Jardel, C.; Bruckert, E.; Grimaldi, A.; Robert, J.J.; Capeau, J.; Hainque, B. Adipose tissue IL-6 content correlates with resistance to insulin activation of glucose uptake both in vivo and in vitro. *J. Clin. Endocrinol. Metab.* **2002**, *87*, 2084–2089. [CrossRef] [PubMed]

115. Hirano, T. Interleukin 6 in autoimmune and inflammatory diseases: A personal memoir. *Proc. Jpn. Acad. Ser. B Phys. Biol. Sci.* **2010**, *86*, 717–730. [CrossRef] [PubMed]

116. Tweedell, A.; Mulligan, K.X.; Martel, J.E.; Chueh, F.Y.; Santomango, T.; McGuinness, O.P. Metabolic response to endotoxin in vivo in the conscious mouse: Role of interleukin-6. *Metabolism* **2011**, *60*, 92–98. [CrossRef] [PubMed]

117. Campbell, J.E.; Drucker, D.J. Pharmacology, physiology, and mechanisms of incretin hormone action. *Cell Metab.* **2013**, *17*, 819–837. [CrossRef] [PubMed]

118. Holst, J.J. Enteroendocrine secretion of gut hormones in diabetes, obesity and after bariatric surgery. *Curr. Opin. Pharmacol.* **2013**, *13*, 983–988. [CrossRef] [PubMed]

119. Fava, S. Glucagon-like peptide 1 and the cardiovascular system. *Curr. Diabetes Rev.* **2014**, *10*, 302–310. [CrossRef] [PubMed]

120. Unger, R.H.; Ohneda, A.; Valverde, I.; Eisentraut, A.M.; Exton, J. Characterization of the responses of circulating glucagon-like immunoreactivity to intraduodenal and intravenous administration of glucose. *J. Clin. Investig.* **1968**, *47*, 48–65. [CrossRef] [PubMed]

121. McAlpine, C.S.; Bowes, A.J.; Werstuck, G.H. Diabetes, hyperglycemia and accelerated atherosclerosis: Evidence supporting a role for endoplasmic reticulum (ER) stress signaling. *Cardiovasc. Hematol. Disord. Drug Targets* **2010**, *10*, 151–157. [CrossRef] [PubMed]

122. Lee, S.S.; Yoo, J.H.; So, Y.S. Effect of the low- versus high-intensity exercise training on endoplasmic reticulum stress and GLP-1 in adolescents with type 2 diabetes mellitus. *J. Phys. Ther. Sci.* **2015**, *27*, 3063–3068. [CrossRef] [PubMed]

123. Kodera, R.; Shikata, K.; Kataoka, H.U.; Takatsuka, T.; Miyamoto, S.; Sasaki, M.; Kajitani, N.; Nishishita, S.; Sarai, K.; Hirota, D.; et al. Glucagon-like peptide-1 receptor agonist ameliorates renal injury through its anti-inflammatory action without lowering blood glucose level in a rat model of type 1 diabetes. *Diabetologia* **2011**, *54*, 965–978. [CrossRef] [PubMed]

124. Arakawa, M.; Mita, T.; Azuma, K.; Ebato, C.; Goto, H.; Nomiyama, T.; Fujitani, Y.; Hirose, T.; Kawamori, R.; Watada, H. Inhibition of monocyte adhesion to endothelial cells and attenuation of atherosclerotic lesion by a glucagon-like peptide-1 receptor agonist, exendin-4. *Diabetes* **2010**, *59*, 1030–1037. [CrossRef] [PubMed]

125. Varanasi, A.; Patel, P.; Makdissi, A.; Dhindsa, S.; Chaudhuri, A.; Dandona, P. Clinical use of liraglutide in type 2 diabetes and its effects on cardiovascular risk factors. *Endocr. Pract.* **2012**, *18*, 140–145. [CrossRef] [PubMed]

126. Lehrskov-Schmidt, L.; Lehrskov-Schmidt, L.; Nielsen, S.T.; Holst, J.J.; Moller, K.; Solomon, T.P. The effects of TNF-α on GLP-1-stimulated plasma glucose kinetics. *J. Clin. Endocrinol. Metab.* **2015**, *100*, E616–E622. [CrossRef] [PubMed]

127. Gupta, N.A.; Mells, J.; Dunham, R.M.; Grakoui, A.; Handy, J.; Saxena, N.K.; Anania, F.A. Glucagon-like peptide-1 receptor is present on human hepatocytes and has a direct role in decreasing hepatic steatosis in vitro by modulating elements of the insulin signaling pathway. *Hepatology* **2010**, *51*, 1584–1592. [CrossRef] [PubMed]
128. Svegliati-Baroni, G.; Saccomanno, S.; Rychlicki, C.; Agostinelli, L.; de Minicis, S.; Candelaresi, C.; Faraci, G.; Pacetti, D.; Vivarelli, M.; Nicolini, D.; et al. Glucagon-like peptide-1 receptor activation stimulates hepatic lipid oxidation and restores hepatic signalling alteration induced by a high-fat diet in nonalcoholic steatohepatitis. *Liver Int.* **2011**, *31*, 1285–1297. [CrossRef] [PubMed]
129. Klonoff, D.C.; Buse, J.B.; Nielsen, L.L.; Guan, X.; Bowlus, C.L.; Holcombe, J.H.; Wintle, M.E.; Maggs, D.G. Exenatide effects on diabetes, obesity, cardiovascular risk factors and hepatic biomarkers in patients with type 2 diabetes treated for at least 3 years. *Curr. Med. Res. Opin.* **2008**, *24*, 275–286. [CrossRef] [PubMed]
130. Cuthbertson, D.J.; Irwin, A.; Gardner, C.J.; Daousi, C.; Purewal, T.; Furlong, N.; Goenka, N.; Thomas, E.L.; Adams, V.L.; Pushpakom, S.P.; et al. Improved glycaemia correlates with liver fat reduction in obese, type 2 diabetes, patients given glucagon-like peptide-1 (GLP-1) receptor agonists. *PLoS ONE* **2012**, *7*, e50117. [CrossRef] [PubMed]
131. Kenny, P.R.; Brady, D.E.; Torres, D.M.; Ragozzino, L.; Chalasani, N.; Harrison, S.A. Exenatide in the treatment of diabetic patients with non-alcoholic steatohepatitis: A case series. *Am. J. Gastroenterol.* **2010**, *105*, 2707–2709. [CrossRef] [PubMed]
132. Armstrong, M.J.; Gaunt, P.; Aithal, G.P.; Barton, D.; Hull, D.; Parker, R.; Hazlehurst, J.M.; Guo, K.; LEAN trial team; Abouda, G.; et al. Liraglutide safety and efficacy in patients with non-alcoholic steatohepatitis (LEAN): A multicentre, double-blind, randomised, placebo-controlled phase 2 study. *Lancet* **2015**, *387*, 679–690. [CrossRef]
133. Gastaldelli, A.; Marchesini, G. Time for Glucagon like peptide-1 receptor agonists treatment for patients with NAFLD? *J. Hepatol.* **2016**, *64*, 262–264. [CrossRef] [PubMed]
134. Jendle, J.; Nauck, M.A.; Matthews, D.R.; Frid, A.; Hermansen, K.; During, M.; Zdravkovic, M.; Strauss, B.J.; Garber, A.J.; LEAD-2 and LEAD-3 Study Groups. Weight loss with liraglutide, a once-daily human glucagon-like peptide-1 analogue for type 2 diabetes treatment as monotherapy or added to metformin, is primarily as a result of a reduction in fat tissue. *Diabetes Obes. Metab.* **2009**, *11*, 1163–1172. [CrossRef] [PubMed]
135. Muller, T.D.; Nogueiras, R.; Andermann, M.L.; Andrews, Z.B.; Anker, S.D.; Argente, J.; Batterham, R.L.; Benoit, S.C.; Bowers, C.Y.; Broglio, F.; et al. Ghrelin. *Mol. Metab.* **2015**, *4*, 437–460. [CrossRef] [PubMed]
136. Buscher, A.K.; Buscher, R.; Hauffa, B.P.; Hoyer, P.F. Alterations in appetite-regulating hormones influence protein-energy wasting in pediatric patients with chronic kidney disease. *Pediatr. Nephrol.* **2010**, *25*, 2295–2301. [CrossRef] [PubMed]
137. Zhang, S.R.; Fan, X.M. Ghrelin-ghrelin *O*-acyltransferase system in the pathogenesis of nonalcoholic fatty liver disease. *World J. Gastroenterol.* **2015**, *21*, 3214–3222. [PubMed]
138. Al Massadi, O.; Tschop, M.H.; Tong, J. Ghrelin acylation and metabolic control. *Peptides* **2011**, *32*, 2301–2308. [CrossRef] [PubMed]
139. Cummings, D.E.; Frayo, R.S.; Marmonier, C.; Aubert, R.; Chapelot, D. Plasma ghrelin levels and hunger scores in humans initiating meals voluntarily without time- and food related cues. *Am. J. Physiol. Endocrinol. Metab.* **2004**, *287*, E297–E304. [CrossRef] [PubMed]
140. Rodriguez, A. Novel molecular aspects of ghrelin and leptin in the control of adipobiology and the cardiovascular system. *Obes. Facts* **2014**, *7*, 82–95. [CrossRef] [PubMed]
141. Foster-Schubert, K.E.; Overduin, J.; Prudom, C.E.; Liu, J.; Callahan, H.S.; Gaylinn, B.D.; Thorner, M.O.; Cummings, D.E. Acyl and total ghrelin are suppressed strongly by ingested proteins, weakly by lipids, and biphasically by carbohydrates. *J. Clin. Endocrinol. Metab.* **2008**, *93*, 1971–1979. [CrossRef] [PubMed]
142. Van Name, M.; Giannini, C.; Santoro, N.; Jastreboff, A.M.; Kubat, J.; Li, F.; Kursawe, R.; Savoye, M.; Duran, E.; Dziura, J.; et al. Blunted suppression of acyl-ghrelin in response to fructose ingestion in obese adolescents: The role of insulin resistance. *Obesity* **2015**, *23*, 653–661. [CrossRef] [PubMed]
143. Muller, T.D.; Tschop, M.H.; Jarick, I.; Ehrlich, S.; Scherag, S.; Herpertz-Dahlmann, B.; Zipfel, S.; Herzog, W.; de Zwaan, M.; Burghardt, R.; et al. Genetic variation of the ghrelin activator gene ghrelin *O*-acyltransferase (GOAT) is associated with anorexia nervosa. *J. Psychiatr. Res.* **2011**, *45*, 706–711. [CrossRef] [PubMed]
144. Burns, S.F.; Broom, D.R.; Miyashita, M.; Mundy, C.; Stensel, D.J. A single session of treadmill running has no effect on plasma total ghrelin concentrations. *J. Sports Sci.* **2007**, *25*, 635–642. [CrossRef] [PubMed]

145. Schmidt, A.; Maier, C.; Schaller, G.; Nowotny, P.; Bayerle-Eder, M.; Buranyi, B.; Luger, A.; Wolzt, M. Acute exercise has no effect on ghrelin plasma concentrations. *Horm. Metab. Res.* **2004**, *36*, 174–177. [PubMed]

146. Mackelvie, K.J.; Meneilly, G.S.; Elahi, D.; Wong, A.C.; Barr, S.I.; Chanoine, J.P. Regulation of appetite in lean and obese adolescents after exercise: Role of acylated and desacyl ghrelin. *J. Clin. Endocrinol. Metab.* **2007**, *92*, 648–654. [CrossRef] [PubMed]

147. Athinarayanan, S.; Wei, R.; Zhang, M.; Bai, S.; Traber, M.G.; Yates, K.; Cummings, O.W.; Molleston, J.; Liu, W.; Chalasani, N. Genetic polymorphism of cytochrome P450 4F2, vitamin E level and histological response in adults and children with nonalcoholic fatty liver disease who participated in PIVENS and TONIC clinical trials. *PLoS ONE* **2014**, *9*, e95366. [CrossRef] [PubMed]

148. Prodam, F.; Filigheddu, N. Ghrelin gene products in acute and chronic inflammation. *Arch. Immunol. Ther. Exp.* **2014**, *62*, 369–384. [CrossRef] [PubMed]

149. Delhanty, P.J.; Huisman, M.; Baldeon-Rojas, L.Y.; van den Berge, I.; Grefhorst, A.; Abribat, T.; Leenen, P.J.; Themmen, A.P.; van der Lely, A.J. Des-acyl ghrelin analogs prevent high-fat-diet-induced dysregulation of glucose homeostasis. *FASEB J.* **2013**, *27*, 1690–1700. [CrossRef] [PubMed]

150. Tokudome, T.; Kishimoto, I.; Miyazato, M.; Kangawa, K. Ghrelin and the cardiovascular system. *Front. Horm. Res.* **2014**, *43*, 125–133. [PubMed]

151. Marchesini, G.; Pagotto, U.; Bugianesi, E.; de Iasio, R.; Manini, R.; Vanni, E.; Pasquali, R.; Melchionda, N.; Rizzetto, M. Low ghrelin concentrations in nonalcoholic fatty liver disease are related to insulin resistance. *J. Clin. Endocrinol. Metab.* **2003**, *88*, 5674–5679. [CrossRef] [PubMed]

152. Mykhalchyshyn, G.; Kobyliak, N.; Bodnar, P. Diagnostic accuracy of acyl-ghrelin and it association with non-alcoholic fatty liver disease in type 2 diabetic patients. *J. Diabetes Metab. Disord.* **2015**, *14*, 44. [CrossRef] [PubMed]

153. Gunta, S.S.; Mak, R.H. Ghrelin and leptin pathophysiology in chronic kidney disease. *Pediatr. Nephrol.* **2013**, *28*, 611–616. [CrossRef] [PubMed]

154. Suneja, M.; Murry, D.J.; Stokes, J.B.; Lim, V.S. Hormonal regulation of energy-protein homeostasis in hemodialysis patients: An anorexigenic profile that may predispose to adverse cardiovascular outcomes. *Am. J. Physiol. Endocrinol. Metab.* **2011**, *300*, E55–E64. [CrossRef] [PubMed]

155. Raschke, S.; Eckel, J. Adipo-myokines: Two sides of the same coin—Mediators of inflammation and mediators of exercise. *Mediat. Inflamm.* **2013**, *2013*, 320724. [CrossRef] [PubMed]

156. Arias-Loste, M.T.; Ranchal, I.; Romero-Gomez, M.; Crespo, J. Irisin, a link among fatty liver disease, physical inactivity and insulin resistance. *Int. J. Mol. Sci.* **2014**, *15*, 23163–23178. [CrossRef] [PubMed]

157. Anastasilakis, A.D.; Polyzos, S.A.; Saridakis, Z.G.; Kynigopoulos, G.; Skouvaklidou, E.C.; Molyvas, D.; Vasiloglou, M.F.; Apostolou, A.; Karagiozoglou-Lampoudi, T.; Siopi, A.; et al. Circulating irisin in healthy, young individuals: Day-night rhythm, effects of food intake and exercise, and associations with gender, physical activity, diet, and body composition. *J. Clin. Endocrinol. Metab.* **2014**, *99*, 3247–3255. [CrossRef] [PubMed]

158. Ko, B.J.; Park, K.H.; Shin, S.; Zaichenko, L.; Davis, C.R.; Crowell, J.A.; Joung, H.; Mantzoros, C.S. Diet quality and diet patterns in relation to circulating cardiometabolic biomarkers. *Clin. Nutr.* **2016**, *35*, 484–490. [CrossRef] [PubMed]

159. Schlogl, M.; Piaggi, P.; Votruba, S.B.; Walter, M.; Krakoff, J.; Thearle, M.S. Increased 24-hour ad libitum food intake is associated with lower plasma irisin concentrations the following morning in adult humans. *Appetite* **2015**, *90*, 154–159. [CrossRef] [PubMed]

160. Qiu, S.; Cai, X.; Sun, Z.; Schumann, U.; Zugel, M.; Steinacker, J.M. Chronic exercise training and circulating irisin in adults: A meta-analysis. *Sports Med.* **2015**, *45*, 1577–1588. [CrossRef] [PubMed]

161. Zhang, H.J.; Zhang, X.F.; Ma, Z.M.; Pan, L.L.; Chen, Z.; Han, H.W.; Han, C.K.; Zhuang, X.J.; Lu, Y.; Li, X.J.; et al. Irisin is inversely associated with intrahepatic triglyceride contents in obese adults. *J. Hepatol.* **2013**, *59*, 557–562. [CrossRef] [PubMed]

162. Polyzos, S.A.; Kountouras, J.; Anastasilakis, A.D.; Geladari, E.V.; Mantzoros, C.S. Irisin in patients with nonalcoholic fatty liver disease. *Metabolism* **2014**, *63*, 207–217. [CrossRef] [PubMed]

163. Zurlo, F.; Larson, K.; Bogardus, C.; Ravussin, E. Skeletal muscle metabolism is a major determinant of resting energy expenditure. *J. Clin. Investig.* **1990**, *86*, 1423–1427. [CrossRef] [PubMed]

164. Panesar, A.; Agarwal, R. Resting energy expenditure in chronic kidney disease: Relationship with glomerular filtration rate. *Clin. Nephrol.* **2003**, *59*, 360–366. [CrossRef] [PubMed]

165. Lee, M.J.; Lee, S.A.; Nam, B.Y.; Park, S.; Lee, S.H.; Ryu, H.J.; Kwon, Y.E.; Kim, Y.L.; Park, K.S.; Oh, H.J.; et al. Irisin, a novel myokine is an independent predictor for sarcopenia and carotid atherosclerosis in dialysis patients. *Atherosclerosis* **2015**, *242*, 476–482. [CrossRef] [PubMed]

166. Wen, M.S.; Wang, C.Y.; Lin, S.L.; Hung, K.C. Decrease in irisin in patients with chronic kidney disease. *PLoS ONE* **2013**, *8*, e64025. [CrossRef] [PubMed]

167. Ebert, T.; Focke, D.; Petroff, D.; Wurst, U.; Richter, J.; Bachmann, A.; Lossner, U.; Kralisch, S.; Kratzsch, J.; Beige, J.; et al. Serum levels of the myokine irisin in relation to metabolic and renal function. *Eur. J. Endocrinol.* **2014**, *170*, 501–506. [CrossRef] [PubMed]

168. Burk, R.F.; Hill, K.E. Selenoprotein P: An extracellular protein with unique physical characteristics and a role in selenium homeostasis. *Annu. Rev. Nutr.* **2005**, *25*, 215–235. [CrossRef] [PubMed]

169. Carlson, B.A.; Novoselov, S.V.; Kumaraswamy, E.; Lee, B.J.; Anver, M.R.; Gladyshev, V.N.; Hatfield, D.L. Specific excision of the selenocysteine tRNA[Ser]Sec (*Trsp*) gene in mouse liver demonstrates an essential role of selenoproteins in liver function. *J. Biol. Chem.* **2004**, *279*, 8011–8017. [CrossRef] [PubMed]

170. Hill, K.E.; Zhou, J.; McMahan, W.J.; Motley, A.K.; Atkins, J.F.; Gesteland, R.F.; Burk, R.F. Deletion of selenoprotein P alters distribution of selenium in the mouse. *J. Biol. Chem.* **2003**, *278*, 13640–13646. [CrossRef] [PubMed]

171. Schomburg, L.; Schweizer, U.; Holtmann, B.; Flohe, L.; Sendtner, M.; Kohrle, J. Gene disruption discloses role of selenoprotein P in selenium delivery to target tissues. *Biochem. J.* **2003**, *370*, 397–402. [CrossRef] [PubMed]

172. Misu, H.; Takamura, T.; Takayama, H.; Hayashi, H.; Matsuzawa-Nagata, N.; Kurita, S.; Ishikura, K.; Ando, H.; Takeshita, Y.; Ota, T.; et al. A liver-derived secretory protein, selenoprotein P, causes insulin resistance. *Cell Metab.* **2010**, *12*, 483–495. [CrossRef] [PubMed]

173. Misu, H.; Ishikura, K.; Kurita, S.; Takeshita, Y.; Ota, T.; Saito, Y.; Takahashi, K.; Kaneko, S.; Takamura, T. Inverse correlation between serum levels of selenoprotein P and adiponectin in patients with type 2 diabetes. *PLoS ONE* **2012**, *7*, e34952. [CrossRef] [PubMed]

174. Yang, J.G.; Hill, K.E.; Burk, R.F. Dietary selenium intake controls rat plasma selenoprotein P concentration. *J. Nutr.* **1989**, *119*, 1010–1012. [PubMed]

175. Falnoga, I.; Kobal, A.B.; Stibilj, V.; Horvat, M. Selenoprotein P in subjects exposed to mercury and other stress situations such as physical load or metal chelation treatment. *Biol. Trace Elem. Res.* **2002**, *89*, 25–33. [CrossRef]

176. Huang, Z.; Rose, A.H.; Hoffmann, P.R. The role of selenium in inflammation and immunity: From molecular mechanisms to therapeutic opportunities. *Antioxid. Redox Signal.* **2012**, *16*, 705–743. [CrossRef] [PubMed]

177. Mattmiller, S.A.; Carlson, B.A.; Sordillo, L.M. Regulation of inflammation by selenium and selenoproteins: Impact on eicosanoid biosynthesis. *J. Nutr. Sci.* **2013**, *2*, e28. [PubMed]

178. Nichol, C.; Herdman, J.; Sattar, N.; O'Dwyer, P.J.; St, J.O.R.D.; Littlejohn, D.; Fell, G. Changes in the concentrations of plasma selenium and selenoproteins after minor elective surgery: Further evidence for a negative acute phase response? *Clin. Chem.* **1998**, *44*, 1764–1766. [PubMed]

179. Hesse-Bahr, K.; Dreher, I.; Kohrle, J. The influence of the cytokines Il-1beta and INFgamma on the expression of selenoproteins in the human hepatocarcinoma cell line HepG2. *Biofactors* **2000**, *11*, 83–85. [CrossRef] [PubMed]

180. Dreher, I.; Jakobs, T.C.; Kohrle, J. Cloning and characterization of the human selenoprotein P promoter. Response of selenoprotein P expression to cytokines in liver cells. *J. Biol. Chem.* **1997**, *272*, 29364–29371 [CrossRef] [PubMed]

181. Rayman, M.P. Selenium and human health. *Lancet* **2012**, *379*, 1256–1268. [CrossRef]

182. Yang, S.J.; Hwang, S.Y.; Choi, H.Y.; Yoo, H.J.; Seo, J.A.; Kim, S.G.; Kim, N.H.; Baik, S.H.; Choi, D.S.; Choi, K.M. Serum selenoprotein P levels in patients with type 2 diabetes and prediabetes: Implications for insulin resistance, inflammation, and atherosclerosis. *J. Clin. Endocrinol. Metab.* **2011**, *96*, E1325–E1329. [CrossRef] [PubMed]

183. Rose, A.H.; Hoffmann, P.R. Selenoproteins and cardiovascular stress. *Thromb. Haemost.* **2015**, *113*, 494–504. [CrossRef] [PubMed]

184. Choi, H.Y.; Hwang, S.Y.; Lee, C.H.; Hong, H.C.; Yang, S.J.; Yoo, H.J.; Seo, J.A.; Kim, S.G.; Kim, N.H.; Baik, S.H.; et al. Increased selenoprotein p levels in subjects with visceral obesity and nonalcoholic Fatty liver disease. *Diabetes Metab. J.* **2013**, *37*, 63–71. [CrossRef] [PubMed]

185. Takayama, H.; Misu, H.; Iwama, H.; Chikamoto, K.; Saito, Y.; Murao, K.; Teraguchi, A.; Lan, F.; Kikuchi, A.; Saito, R.; et al. Metformin suppresses expression of the selenoprotein P gene via an AMP-activated kinase (AMPK)/FoxO3a pathway in H4IIEC3 hepatocytes. *J. Biol. Chem.* **2014**, *289*, 335–345. [CrossRef] [PubMed]

186. Burk, R.F.; Hill, K.E. Regulation of selenium metabolism and transport. *Annu. Rev. Nutr.* **2015**, *35*, 109–134. [CrossRef] [PubMed]

187. Reinhardt, W.; Dolff, S.; Benson, S.; Broecker-Preuss, M.; Behrendt, S.; Hog, A.; Fuhrer, D.; Schomburg, L.; Kohrle, J. Chronic kidney disease distinctly affects relationship between selenoprotein P status and serum thyroid hormone parameters. *Thyroid* **2015**, *25*, 1091–1096. [CrossRef] [PubMed]

188. Meyer, T.W.; Hostetter, T.H. Uremia. *N. Engl. J. Med.* **2007**, *357*, 1316–1325. [CrossRef] [PubMed]

189. Denecke, B.; Graber, S.; Schafer, C.; Heiss, A.; Woltje, M.; Jahnen-Dechent, W. Tissue distribution and activity testing suggest a similar but not identical function of fetuin-B and fetuin-A. *Biochem. J.* **2003**, *376*, 135–145. [CrossRef] [PubMed]

190. Mathews, S.T.; Chellam, N.; Srinivas, P.R.; Cintron, V.J.; Leon, M.A.; Goustin, A.S.; Grunberger, G. α2-HSG, a specific inhibitor of insulin receptor autophosphorylation, interacts with the insulin receptor. *Mol. Cell. Endocrinol.* **2000**, *164*, 87–98. [CrossRef]

191. Stefan, N.; Hennige, A.M.; Staiger, H.; Machann, J.; Schick, F.; Krober, S.M.; Machicao, F.; Fritsche, A.; Haring, H.U. α2-Heremans-Schmid glycoprotein/fetuin-A is associated with insulin resistance and fat accumulation in the liver in humans. *Diabetes Care* **2006**, *29*, 853–857. [CrossRef] [PubMed]

192. Mathews, S.T.; Singh, G.P.; Ranalletta, M.; Cintron, V.J.; Qiang, X.; Goustin, A.S.; Jen, K.L.; Charron, M.J.; Jahnen-Dechent, W.; Grunberger, G. Improved insulin sensitivity and resistance to weight gain in mice null for the Ahsg gene. *Diabetes* **2002**, *51*, 2450–2458. [CrossRef] [PubMed]

193. Siddiq, A.; Lepretre, F.; Hercberg, S.; Froguel, P.; Gibson, F. A synonymous coding polymorphism in the α2-Heremans-schmid glycoprotein gene is associated with type 2 diabetes in French Caucasians. *Diabetes* **2005**, *54*, 2477–2481. [CrossRef] [PubMed]

194. Dahlman, I.; Eriksson, P.; Kaaman, M.; Jiao, H.; Lindgren, C.M.; Kere, J.; Arner, P. α2-Heremans-Schmid glycoprotein gene polymorphisms are associated with adipocyte insulin action. *Diabetologia* **2004**, *47*, 1974–1979. [CrossRef] [PubMed]

195. Nimptsch, K.; Janke, J.; Pischon, T.; Linseisen, J. Association between dietary factors and plasma fetuin-A concentrations in the general population. *Br. J. Nutr.* **2015**, *114*, 1278–1285. [CrossRef] [PubMed]

196. Seyithanoglu, M.; Oner-Iyidogan, Y.; Dogru-Abbasoglu, S.; Tanrikulu-Kucuk, S.; Kocak, H.; Beyhan-Ozdas, S.; Kocak-Toker, N. The effect of dietary curcumin and capsaicin on hepatic fetuin-A expression and fat accumulation in rats fed on a high-fat diet. *Arch. Physiol. Biochem.* **2016**, *122*, 94–102. [CrossRef] [PubMed]

197. Malin, S.K.; Mulya, A.; Fealy, C.E.; Haus, J.M.; Pagadala, M.R.; Scelsi, A.R.; Huang, H.; Flask, C.A.; McCullough, A.J.; Kirwan, J.P. Fetuin-A is linked to improved glucose tolerance after short-term exercise training in nonalcoholic fatty liver disease. *J. Appl. Physiol.* **2013**, *115*, 988–994. [CrossRef] [PubMed]

198. Yang, S.J.; Hong, H.C.; Choi, H.Y.; Yoo, H.J.; Cho, G.J.; Hwang, T.G.; Baik, S.H.; Choi, D.S.; Kim, S.M.; Choi, K.M. Effects of a three-month combined exercise programme on fibroblast growth factor 21 and fetuin-A levels and arterial stiffness in obese women. *Clin. Endocrinol.* **2011**, *75*, 464–469. [CrossRef] [PubMed]

199. Rametta, R.; Ruscica, M.; Dongiovanni, P.; Macchi, C.; Fracanzani, A.L.; Steffani, L.; Fargion, S.; Magni, P.; Valenti, L. Hepatic steatosis and PNPLA3 I148M variant are associated with serum Fetuin-A independently of insulin resistance. *Eur. J. Clin. Investig.* **2014**, *44*, 627–633. [CrossRef] [PubMed]

200. Yilmaz, Y.; Yonal, O.; Kurt, R.; Ari, F.; Oral, A.Y.; Celikel, C.A.; Korkmaz, S.; Ulukaya, E.; Ozdogan, O.; Imeryuz, N.; et al. Serum fetuin A/α2HS-glycoprotein levels in patients with non-alcoholic fatty liver disease: Relation with liver fibrosis. *Ann. Clin. Biochem.* **2010**, *47*, 549–553. [CrossRef] [PubMed]

201. Ou, H.Y.; Yang, Y.C.; Wu, H.T.; Wu, J.S.; Lu, F.H.; Chang, C.J. Increased fetuin-A concentrations in impaired glucose tolerance with or without nonalcoholic fatty liver disease, but not impaired fasting glucose. *J. Clin. Endocrinol. Metab.* **2012**, *97*, 4717–4723. [CrossRef] [PubMed]

202. Cottone, S.; Palermo, A.; Arsena, R.; Riccobene, R.; Guarneri, M.; Mule, G.; Tornese, F.; Altieri, C.; Vaccaro, F.; Previti, A.; et al. Relationship of fetuin-A with glomerular filtration rate and endothelial dysfunction in moderate-severe chronic kidney disease. *J. Nephrol.* **2010**, *23*, 62–69. [PubMed]

9

Type 2 Diabetes in Non-Alcoholic Fatty Liver Disease and Hepatitis C Virus Infection—Liver: The *"Musketeer"* in the Spotlight

Stefano Ballestri [1], Fabio Nascimbeni [2,3], Dante Romagnoli [2], Enrica Baldelli [3], Giovanni Targher [4] and Amedeo Lonardo [2,*]

[1] Operating Unit Internal Medicine, Pavullo General Hospital, Azienda USL Modena, ViaSuore di San Giuseppe Benedetto Cottolengo, 5, Pavullo, 41026 Modena, Italy; stefanoballestri@tiscali.it

[2] Outpatient Liver Clinic and Operating Unit Internal Medicine, NOCSAE, Azienda USL Modena, Via P. Giardini, 1355, 41126 Modena, Italy; fabio.nascimbeni@libero.it (F.N.); danter1@alice.it (D.R.)

[3] Department of Biomedical, Metabolic and Neural Sciences, University of Modena and Reggio Emilia, Via P. Giardini, 1355, 41126 Modena, Italy; enrica.baldelli@unimore.it

[4] Section of Endocrinology, Diabetes and Metabolism, Department of Medicine, University and Azienda Ospedaliera Universitaria Integrata of Verona, Piazzale Stefani, 1, 37126 Verona, Italy; giovanni.targher@univr.it

* Correspondence: a.lonardo@libero.it

Academic Editor: Giovanni Tarantino

Abstract: The pathogenesis of type 2 diabetes (T2D) involves chronic hyperinsulinemia due to systemic and hepatic insulin resistance (IR), which if uncorrected, will lead to progressive pancreatic beta cell failure in predisposed individuals. Non-alcoholic fatty liver disease (NAFLD) encompasses a spectrum of fatty (simple steatosis and steatohepatitis) and non-fatty liver changes (NASH-cirrhosis with or without hepatocellular carcinoma (HCC)) that are commonly observed among individuals with multiple metabolic derangements, notably including visceral obesity, IR and T2D. Hepatitis C virus (HCV) infection is also often associated with both hepatic steatosis and features of a specific HCV-associated dysmetabolic syndrome. In recent years, the key role of the steatotic liver in the development of IR and T2D has been increasingly recognized. Thus, in this comprehensive review we summarize the rapidly expanding body of evidence that links T2D with NAFLD and HCV infection. For each of these two liver diseases with systemic manifestations, we discuss the epidemiological burden, the pathophysiologic mechanisms and the clinical implications. To date, substantial evidence suggests that NAFLD and HCV play a key role in T2D development and that the interaction of T2D with liver disease may result in a "vicious circle", eventually leading to an increased risk of all-cause mortality and liver-related and cardiovascular complications. Preliminary evidence also suggests that improvement of NAFLD is associated with a decreased incidence of T2D. Similarly, the prevention of T2D following HCV eradication in the era of direct-acting antiviral agents is a biologically plausible result. However, additional studies are required for further clarification of mechanisms involved.

Keywords: epidemiology; cirrhosis; clinical implications; direct acting antivirals; fibrosis; insulin resistance; hepatocellular carcinoma; NASH; pathophysiology

1. Introduction

1.1. Definitions

Type 2 diabetes (T2D) identifies the more prevalent category of diabetes mellitus and is due to a progressive insulin secretory defect in the background of insulin resistance (IR) [1]. T2D is typically found in obese and overweight middle-aged individuals though the age of its initial manifestation has now been observed shifting towards adolescents and even children [2].

Non-alcoholic fatty liver disease (NAFLD) describes a cluster of hepatic disorders predominantly (though not exclusively) characterized by fatty changes with or without ballooning degeneration and fibrosis (*i.e.*, simple steatosis, steatohepatitis (NASH) and advanced fibrosis), which may evolve into cirrhosis (NASH-cirrhosis will typically lose fatty changes) and hepatocellular carcinoma (HCC); NAFLD is commonly observed in insulin-resistant, dysmetabolic individuals without excessive alcohol consumption and other competing etiologies of liver disease [3,4]. There is now compelling evidence that NAFLD is a multisystem disease associated with a wide range of extra-hepatic manifestations, notably including, among others, IR, dysglycemia and premature atherosclerosis [5,6].

Hepatitis C virus (HCV) is a small enveloped RNA virus belonging to the genus Flaviviridae, of which six different genotypes are recognized and which is transmitted via the parenteral route [7]. In several countries there have been two major HCV epidemics. The first one (mostly sustained by genotype 1 HCV) took place in the 1960s as a result of HCV being transmitted via medical procedures. The second one (predominantly due to genotype 3 HCV) occurred in the 1980s owing to needle-sharing practices among intravenous illicit drug users [7].

The natural course of HCV infection is variable and modulated by the interaction of host and viral factors. Of concern, the chronicity rate following acute infection approximates 85%, giving way to dreadful *sequelae*, such as chronic hepatitis, cirrhosis, end-stage liver failure and HCC [7]. Similarly to NAFLD, HCV infection is increasingly identified as a systemic disease which may be conducive to metabolic disorders (including IR and T2D) and premature atherosclerosis [8].

1.2. Epidemiology and Burden of Type 2 Diabetes

The world prevalence of T2D was estimated to be 6.4% in 2010 and is projected to rise to 7.7% in 2030 [9]. Recent estimates of T2D prevalence in the main five European countries (France, Germany, Italy, Spain and UK) ranged from 4.8% in Italy to 8.9% in Germany, with rates increasing steadily over the past two decades in all these countries. Of concern, in these European countries the total direct medical costs of T2D in 2010 were estimated to range from 5.45 billion euros in Spain to 43.2 billion euros in Germany, with hospitalizations due to T2D-related complications accounting for the greatest proportion of these costs [10]. In the USA, T2D now affects up to 8%–10% of adults in the general population in whom it increases up to four-fold the risk of major cardiovascular events and is the leading cause of blindness, chronic kidney failure and non-traumatic lower extremity amputations [11]. In 2007, T2D posed on society a cost as high as 174 billion dollars in the USA [12]. Of concern, this already alarming prevalence of T2D is predicted to be increasing in all age groups, making it urgent for clinicians, researchers and health authorities to gain a better understanding of the pathophysiology of T2D aimed at preventing the further spread of its disastrous pandemic [13].

1.3. Liver and Type 2 Diabetes: Historical Overview

In the past, clinicians and pathologists viewed the hepatic fatty changes as a histological correlate of the coexistence of T2D and obesity (the so-called *"diabesity"*) [14], a conclusion which has been fully supported by contemporary studies [15]. Stated otherwise, the liver was essentially regarded as a target organ affected by either concurrent or pre-existent *"diabesity"*.

More recently, however, this perspective has been fully overturned. Several studies have now exhaustively proven that hepatic steatosis precedes the development of T2D and Metabolic Syndrome (MetS) in a large proportion of cases [16–18]. *In tandem*, epidemiological evidence has also suggested that HCV infection almost doubles the risk of incident T2D compared to both HBV infection and virus-free individuals [19]. This is of outstanding interest given that HCV infection is a systemic disease [20] that often exhibits hepatic histological changes of variable severity, including hepatic steatosis, which makes it conceptually similar to NAFLD [7,21]. Excitingly, a cure for HCV has recently become available with direct acting antivirals [22–24].

Collectively, all the above findings support the notion that there is a causal, bi-directional link between NAFLD and T2D [25]; that HCV infection is a diabetogenic condition [19]; and that T2D is potentially preventable by curing NAFLD [26] and HCV infection [27].

1.4. Aim of the Review and Evidence Acquisition

The liver, the skeletal muscle and the pancreas are the anatomic basis of IR and they have collectively been alluded as the *"three musketeers"* [28]. Along with these three organs, the adipose tissue is the *"fourth musketeer"* which is implicated in the pathogenesis of IR (Figure 1) [29]. Over the last decade, the liver has been put in the spotlight of research and our group has been gaining particular interest in the association between the steatotic liver and risk of incident T2D. Accordingly, the main purpose of this article was to review data linking T2D with either NAFLD or HCV infection. For each of these two liver diseases, we will discuss systematically the epidemiological burden, the pathophysiologic mechanisms and the clinical implications.

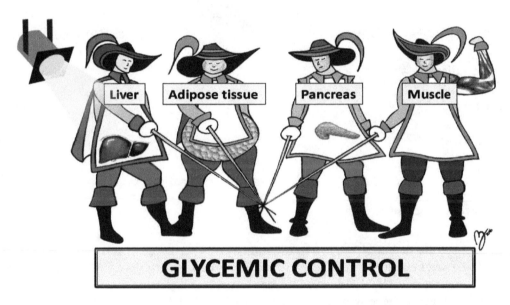

Figure 1. The *"four musketeers"* fighting for maintaining glucose homeostasis. Under normal conditions, muscle and pancreas improve glycemic control. However, an expanded adipose tissue will usually lead to dysglycemia. Similarly, fatty changes occurring in the liver will result in the development of insulin resistance. Hence, this review article puts the liver in the spotlight.

In order to retrieve pertinent articles, the PubMed database was extensively searched for reports published through 31 January 2016. To this end, we used the following keywords "nonalcoholic fatty liver disease" or "NAFLD" combined with "insulin resistance", "type 2 diabetes" or "diabetes". The same keywords were used to identify those articles in which "insulin resistance", "type 2 diabetes" or "diabetes" were combined with either "HCV" or "hepatitis C virus".

The selection of articles was performed based on agreement among the authors. Cross-references were taken in consideration based on the authors' judgment.

2. NAFLD and Type 2 Diabetes

2.1. Epidemiology

The wide spectrum of the extra-hepatic manifestations and correlates of NAFLD includes cardiovascular diseases (CVD), chronic kidney disease, colorectal cancer, obstructive sleep apnea syndrome, psoriasis, endocrine disorders, notably including IR/T2D, thyroid dysfunction, polycystic ovarian syndrome and osteoporosis (Figure 2) [5,6,30–36]. Epidemiological data fully support a bi-directional relationship between NAFLD and T2D [25]. Stated otherwise, NAFLD is associated with established T2D in cross-sectional studies and precedes the development of T2D in follow-up studies [3,16,18].

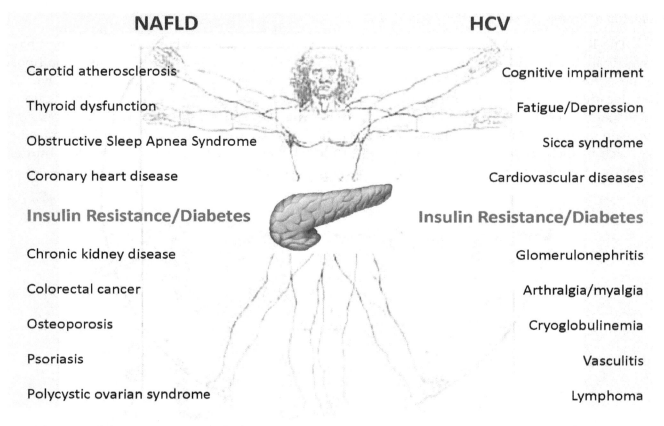

Figure 2. The spectrum of extra-hepatic manifestations and correlates of both non-alcoholic fatty liver disease (NAFLD) and hepatitis C virus (HCV) infection: type 2 diabetes is a shared feature. This figure illustrates the concept that NAFLD and HCV infection are two systemic diseases whose spectrum of clinical manifestations tends to overlap significantly. Type 2 diabetes is a feature shared among the various pathologic conditions included in the NAFLD clinical spectrum [5,6,30–36] as well as in the clinical spectrum of chronic HCV infection [8,37,38].

2.1.1. NAFLD as a "Manifestation" of Type 2 Diabetes

A consistent body of epidemiological evidence supports the conclusion that NAFLD is strongly associated with T2D and that T2D is a major modifier of the epidemiological features of NAFLD [3,39]. For example, the prevalence of NAFLD (assessed by ultrasonography) is approximately 25%–30% in the general adult population, and men outnumber women by 20% to 40%. In patients with T2D, the prevalence of NAFLD is considerably higher (occurring in up to 75% of these patients), and, remarkably, T2D abrogates sex differences among patients with NAFLD [3,39]. The prevalence of NAFLD in patients with T2D ranges widely from 45% to 75% in large hospital-based studies and from 30% to 70% in population-based studies; this wide inter-study variability is largely due to differences in the ethnicity, population characteristics and criteria adopted for the diagnosis of diabetes [39]. The prevalence of histologically diagnosed NASH, *i.e.*, the more rapidly progressive form of NAFLD [40], is estimated to occur in 2%–3% of the general adult population [6]; conversely, it ranges from 56% to 76% in hospital-based studies [41,42] and from 22% to 83% in outpatient cohort-based studies among individuals with T2D [15,43,44]. Notably, a recent study reported a high prevalence of NAFLD (76%) and NASH (56%) in obese T2D patients with normal serum aminotransferase levels [42]. The finding that many T2D patients with NAFLD have fairly normal serum transaminase concentrations is not reassuring given that NASH, advanced fibrosis and even cirrhosis may occur in such patients with "normal" serum aminotransferases [39,45,46]. Taken together, these studies suggest that the "normal" range of serum liver enzymes needs to be lowered to capture more NAFLD cases.

2.1.2. NAFLD as a Precursor of Type 2 Diabetes

Accumulating data from observational prospective studies indicate that NAFLD (as diagnosed by serum liver enzymes or imaging) is strongly associated with an increased incidence of both T2D and MetS [3,45]. Two large meta-analytic studies have provided further evidence for a strong association between NAFLD and increased risk of incident T2D [17,18]. The first of such meta-analyses, published by Musso et al., [17] found an approximately two-fold increased risk of incident T2D among patients with NAFLD. The second one, recently published by our group, confirmed that NAFLD was associated with an almost two-fold increased risk of developing both T2D and MetS over a median period of five years. Worryingly, our meta-analysis is first in suggesting that the risk of developing MetS was much higher in those in whom NAFLD was identified by ultrasonography compared to those in whom NAFLD was identified based on abnormal liver enzymes [18]. In agreement with these findings, a retrospective cohort study by Sung et al. [47] showed that individuals in whom ultrasonography-assessed NAFLD developed or worsened over five years had a marked increase in T2D risk, suggesting that more severe NAFLD is associated with a higher risk of incident T2D [47]. Conversely, individuals in whom NAFLD resolved over five years did not show an increased T2D risk [47]. Similarly, a recent retrospective study reported a strong and independent association between NAFLD improvement and reduced incidence of T2D [48]. Moreover, another recent study has shown that non-overweight individuals with NAFLD had a substantially increased risk of incident T2D compared with both overweight and non-overweight NAFLD-free individuals [49]. Finally, the Multi-Ethnic Study of Atherosclerosis [50] has shown that NAFLD, assessed by computed tomography, was associated with an increased risk of incident T2D independent of common risk factors of T2D.

To date, there is a paucity of published data regarding the association between biopsy proven-NAFLD and the risk of incident T2D or MetS. In a retrospective cohort of 129 Swedish adults with histologically confirmed NAFLD and elevated liver enzymes, the baseline prevalence of T2D was 8.5% and approximately 80% of cases developed T2D (58%) or pre-diabetes (20%) at the end of a 14-year follow-up period [51].

In conclusion, a large body of epidemiological evidence supports the notion that the prevalence of NAFLD is remarkably increased in patients with T2D and that NAFLD is closely associated with an increased risk of incident T2D and MetS.

2.2. Pathophysiology

The pathogenic mechanisms linking NAFLD and T2D encompass a complex cross-talk among different organ systems, notably including the gut and the nervous system further to the previously alluded "four musketeers": the adipose tissue, the skeletal muscle, the liver and the pancreas.

2.2.1. Remodeling of White Adipose Tissue

Excess visceral adiposity is a key factor in connecting NAFLD and T2D. The expansion of white adipose tissue (WAT) is associated with hypoxia and adipocytes necrosis [52–55]. The former causes the release of hypoxia inducible factor 1α (HIF1α), while adipocytes necrosis induces infiltration and M1-polarization of macrophages, thus producing WAT dysfunction, inflammation and fibrosis [53,55–62]. Such a WAT remodeling causes a dysregulation of multiple endocrine and lipid storage functions [54,62]. Dysfunctional WAT, in its turn, is associated with an imbalanced cytokine release, i.e., over-production of multiple pro-inflammatory adipocytokines, such as tumor necrosis factor (TNF)-α and monocyte chemoattractant protein-1/C-C chemokine receptor-2 (MCP-1/CCR-2), and reduction of adiponectin, which contribute to worsen local and systemic metabolic derangements [62–72]. Increased interstitial fibrosis in WAT limits adipose tissue expandability [52,53,62]. Reduction in lipid storage capacity also contributes to ectopic lipid accumulation in the liver, skeletal muscles and pancreas where lipotoxicity triggers multiple pathways that hinder insulin signaling [53,62,73,74]. All of these mechanisms may contribute to the development of IR in the adipose tissue with its inherent failure to suppress adipose lipolysis that results in an overflow of free fatty acids (FFAs) to the liver [74].

2.2.2. Role of Skeletal Muscle and Brown Adipose Tissue

Muscle IR, due to intra-myocellular lipid accumulation, occurs early in the course of T2D. It has been suggested that intra-myocellular diacylglycerol (DAG) accumulation activates protein kinase C-θ (PKCθ), which impairs insulin signaling, impeding muscle glucose uptake and leading to increased delivery of glucose to the liver, where it becomes substrate for hepatic *de-novo* lipogenesis (DNL) [74–77]. Accordingly, it has recently been shown that skeletal muscle steatosis is associated with NAFLD [78].

The myokines, *i.e.*, cytokines produced by the skeletal muscle, have been recently identified as another piece in the interplay linking NAFLD to T2D. Irisin is produced by the skeletal muscle in response to physical exercise and exerts beneficial metabolic effects by recruiting brown adipose tissue (BAT) and triggering thermogenesis [79,80]. Evidence has recently shown that BAT is recruitable post-natally within either WAT or skeletal muscle [81–85]. BAT, through the expression of uncoupling C protein-1 (UCP-1), generates heat and regulates energy expenditure, lipid and glucose metabolism [81,86,87]. For these reasons, both irisin and BAT could be potential targets for the treatment of obesity-related complications. Interestingly, low levels of irisin have been associated with NAFLD and T2D in humans, thus confirming the important role of this myokine in the regulation of energy homeostasis and preservation of a healthy metabolism [88–90].

2.2.3. Intrahepatic Fat Accumulation, Hepatic Insulin Resistance and Hepatokines

In NAFLD, steatogenesis results mainly from increased hepatic esterification of FFAs originating from dysfunctional/inflamed WAT (60%), DNL (25%) and diet (15%) [91,92]. Increased lipolysis drives hepatic lipid synthesis through esterification of FFAs and stimulates hepatic gluconeogenesis [92–94], thus promoting hepatic IR [74,95]. Muscle IR increases glucose delivery to the liver, thus enhancing DNL. Moreover, dietary monosaccharides, particularly fructose, directly promotes hepatic lipogenesis by increasing sterol regulatory element binding protein 1c (SREBP1c), carbohydrate-responsive element-binding protein (chREBP), peroxisome proliferator-activated receptor (PPAR)-γ coactivator 1-β, and liver X receptor expression [74,96–101].

The resulting intrahepatic ectopic storage of lipids has been specifically associated with hepatic IR [74,102]. However, hepatic triglyceride accumulation *per se* is not always harmful. Experimentally, the inhibition of diacylglycerol acyltransferase 2 (DGAT2), an enzyme devoted to hepatocyte triglyceride biosynthesis, decreases hepatic steatosis, but increases markers of lipid peroxidation/oxidant stress, hepatic lobular necro-inflammation and fibrosis [103]. Several lines of evidence support that intrahepatic diacylglycerol (DAG), via activation of PKCε, and ceramides, by impairing Akt2 action and inducing endoplasmic-reticulum stress and mitochondrial dysfunction, are the two major lipid mediators of hepatic IR [74,102,104–114]. Also intracellular localization of lipids in the liver matters [102]. A common single-nucleotide polymorphism of patatin-like phospholipase domain-containing protein 3 (PNPLA3), a lipid droplet protein with triglyceride lipase activity, has been strongly associated with NAFLD, but not with IR [114–120]. This dissociation between hepatic steatosis and IR is likely due to the accumulation of metabolically inert polyunsaturated triacylglycerols in lipid droplets caused by the PNPLA3 I148M variant [114,121,122]. Other underlying mechanisms clearly implicated in the development of hepatic IR and in the progression of NAFLD are low-grade chronic inflammation, elevated production of reactive oxygen species, activation of unfolded protein response and endoplasmic-reticulum stress, activation of Jun N-terminal kinase (JNK)-1, increased hepatocyte apoptosis and lipo-autophagy [25,92,102,123–127].

Finally, the liver releases several endocrine mediators, the so-called hepatokines, able to impact glucose metabolism, insulin action and secretion. Fetuin-A, which is abundantly secreted by steatotic hepatocytes, mediates IR by inhibiting the insulin receptor, reducing adiponectin expression, and enhancing WAT inflammation and dysfunction, and is independently associated with T2D development [128–132]. More recently, also fetuin-B has emerged as a potentially major player in T2D pathogenesis. Indeed, in their seminal study, Meex *et al.* [133], have shown that 32 hepatokines are differently secreted in steatotic *versus* non-steatotic hepatocytes. By inducing inflammation and IR in macrophages and skeletal muscles, these changes in the secretory products may contribute to the development of metabolic dysfunction in other cell types. These authors have identified higher levels of fetuin-B in the altered hepatokine secretory profile of steatotic livers in obese patients, and have also experimentally demonstrated that fetuin-B impairs insulin sensitivity in myotubes and hepatocytes and causes glucose intolerance in mice [133]. Fibroblast growth factor (FGF)-21 acts as a potent activator of glucose uptake and inhibitor of WAT lipolysis, recruits BAT and is associated with obesity, NAFLD and T2D [134–140]. Finally, serpinB1 increases pancreatic β-cell proliferation and its deficiency leads to maladaptive β-cell proliferation in IR [141,142].

2.2.4. Gut-Liver Axis

Compelling evidence links gut microbiota, intestinal barrier integrity and NAFLD. Dysbiosis and impaired gut permeability favor the occurrence of endotoxemia and toll like receptor (TLR) 4-mediated inflammation, thereby contributing to the development of IR and other metabolic complications in obese individuals [143–145]. Other interactions between the gut and the liver may occur through the production of multiple gut hormones and the entero-hepatic circulation of bile acids that activate farnesoid X receptor in the liver [26].

Although further research is needed, these findings underline the importance of NAFLD as a precursor for the development of hepatic and systemic IR. However, the presence of long-standing IR *per se* is not sufficient to lead to the development of T2D. Gluco-lipotoxicity and genetic factors are additional requirements, which induce T2D through the development of pancreatic β-cell failure [25,74,146].

2.3. Clinical Implications

2.3.1. NASH and Fibrosis

Several studies have shown that T2D patients with NAFLD are at a high risk of NASH and cirrhosis [39,147–149]. Data from cross sectional studies [15,150–153] and longitudinal retrospective studies with sequential liver biopsies [154–156] clearly indicate that T2D strongly predicts fibrosis severity and progression in NAFLD patients. Consistently, two studies have demonstrated that poor glycemic control was associated with an increased risk of fibrosis in NASH [157,158].

Interestingly, one study showed that T2D and IR were strongly associated with NASH and severe fibrosis in patients with normal serum liver enzymes [159]. This finding provides further evidence to the clinical wisdom that "normal" serum liver enzyme levels are not a sufficient reason for excluding from liver biopsy those "high-risk" patients in whom advanced liver disease is strongly suggested by non-invasive evaluation. To this end, transient elastography and semi-quantitative ultrasound or non-invasive clinical scores (such as the US-FLI, the NAFLD fibrosis or the Fib4 scores) may be used in most patients with T2D [39,45,160,161].

2.3.2. Cirrhosis and Hepatocellular Carcinoma

Many studies have reported T2D as an established risk factor for cirrhosis [162,163] and HCC [164–166]. Worryingly, a significant proportion of NAFLD patients with HCC have no evidence of cirrhosis [164], implying that they have escaped the normal surveillance strategies implemented in patients with cirrhosis of viral or alcoholic origin, and thus are diagnosed too late to receive radical treatment [167,168].

The presence of NAFLD among patients with T2D is also an important risk factor of increased all-cause and cause-specific mortality. Patients with T2D have an increased mortality risk from cirrhosis of any aetiology [39]. Accordingly, a recent cohort study showed that, compared to the age- and sex-matched general population, patients with T2D had a two- to three-fold higher risk of dying of non-viral and non-alcoholic chronic liver disease, largely attributable to NAFLD [169]. Consistently, a recent Scottish national retrospective cohort study reported that T2D was associated with an increased risk of hospital admissions or deaths for all common chronic liver diseases and, among them, NAFLD had the strongest association with T2D [170]. In agreement, a retrospective USA cohort study on 132 NAFLD patients found that T2D patients with NAFLD were at risk for the development of poor clinical outcomes, such as increased all-cause and liver-related mortality or morbidity after adjusting for potential confounding factors [162]. Finally, NAFLD was associated with a two-fold increased risk of all-cause mortality (mainly due to malignancy (33%), liver-related complications (19%) or ischemic heart disease (19%)) in a cohort study of 337 T2D patients followed-up for a mean period of 11 years [171].

2.3.3. Atherosclerosis

Accumulating evidence indicates that NAFLD is strongly associated not only with liver-related morbidity or mortality, but also with an excess risk of CVD, which is the most common cause of death in T2D [39]. Several studies have reported a strong association between NAFLD and early subclinical or advanced atherosclerosis among patients with and without T2D [172]. These findings have been further confirmed by multiple prospective studies that showed an increased risk of fatal and non-fatal CVD events in patients with and without T2D, independently of several cardiometabolic risk factors [39,172–174]. The association between NAFLD and risk of CVD mortality has been further supported by a milestone meta-analysis [17], although some recent follow-up studies are conflicting [172,175].

Emerging evidence also indicates that NAFLD is independently associated with the development of microvascular diabetic complications, *i.e.*, chronic kidney disease and advanced diabetic retinopathy [5].

Collectively, the above-mentioned studies convincingly show that T2D is strongly associated with an increased risk of progressive NAFLD and an excess risk of overall and cause-specific mortality, including not only liver-related but also CVD-related mortality. These findings fully support careful monitoring and screening for NAFLD and/or advanced fibrosis among patients with T2D.

3. HCV and Type 2 Diabetes

3.1. Epidemiology

3.1.1. HCV and Diabetes: A Non-chance Association

The notion that cirrhosis is a potentially diabetogenic condition dates back to as early as 1906 [176]. More recently, such a view was confirmed in the pre-HBV and pre-HCV age [177]. It was more than 20 years ago that Allison *et al.*, [178] by comparing the rates of T2D among cirrhotic patients undergoing evaluation for liver transplantation, showed that T2D prevalence was 50% in patients with HCV-related *versus* 9% in those with non-HCV-related cirrhosis. Since that pioneering report, this topic has developed into a major line of research and, at the time of this writing, more than 1340 articles can be retrieved [179].

3.1.2. The Burden

Licensing of oral direct acting antivirals (DAA), which deliver sustained virological response (SVR) rates >90%, has led to the revolutionary expectation that HCV infection will possibly be the first chronic viral infection totally eradicated [22]. However, such an inference is premature and, for the time being, HCV still infects from 150,000,000 to 185,000,000 people worldwide, namely up to 2.8% of the world population [180,181]. Moreover, in developing countries, the case-finding and management have not improved *in tandem*, suggesting that continued refinement of epidemiology, cost-utility models and targeted diagnostic strategies remain an unmet need [182]. Worldwide, chronic HCV infection remains a significant public health burden, given that it can lead to cirrhosis in approximately 15% to 20% of those infected within 20 years, resulting in end-stage liver disease and HCC [182]. In Europe, although the iatrogenic HCV transmission was enormously reduced over the last 20 years, transmission related to intravenous recreational drug use is on the increase, especially in Eastern Europe, and the high HCV prevalence in the migrant populations is a challenge [183]. Moreover, HCV-related morbidity and mortality are projected to increase in Europe until 2030 [183]. In the USA, up to 35% of patients on the liver-transplant waiting list are infected with HCV, and global HCV-associated mortality estimates approximate 500,000 deaths per year [184,185].

3.1.3. Extra-Hepatic Manifestations of HCV Infection: Type 2 Diabetes

The clinical spectrum of chronic HCV infection is not limited to liver disease but also includes major extra-hepatic conditions, affecting eyes, salivary glands, skin, kidneys, genital tract, endocrine, neurologic, cardiovascular and immune systems (Figure 2) [8,37,38].

Among the extra-hepatic manifestations of HCV, a mutual and bi-directional relationship connects T2D with HCV infection. HCV infection is more common in patients with T2D than in those without T2D and, conversely, T2D abounds among patients with chronic HCV infection [177]. That said, however, the usual clinical scenario depicts a vignette in which, in predisposed individuals, HCV infection precedes and accelerates the development of new-onset T2D by approximately 10 years [38,186]. This finding suggests that HCV infection observed in T2D patients does not result from the risk of HCV infection associated with medical procedures in the highly medicalized T2D population but is the primary event which may adversely affect the subsequent development of T2D [187].

3.1.4. Heterogeneity in the Distribution of HCV and Type 2 Diabetes and Differential Features of Hepatitis C-Associated Dysmetabolic Syndrome and MetS

There are 170,000,000 individuals with T2D worldwide, namely the same number of individuals with HCV infection [177]. However, HCV infection has undergone epidemiological diffusion in certain age groups and geographical areas as a result of specific lifestyle risk behaviors or transmission via medical practices, whereas T2D reaches its zenith among 45-to-64 year old individuals, particularly in obese and sedentary individuals [177]. Stated otherwise, the epidemiological distribution of HCV infection and T2D does not identify the same geographical areas and groups of individuals. Accordingly, screening campaigns to identify either HCV infection among T2D patients or T2D among those with HCV infection are not justifiable at this time and more accurate strategies are needed in screening selected cohorts of individuals [188].

Finally, it should be pointed out that while T2D is a prominent feature of the MetS which is bi-directionally associated with NAFLD [3], HCV infection is also associated with a specific hepatitis C-associated dysmetabolic syndrome (HCADS), which was first described by Lonardo *et al.* [189]. Table 1 schematically compares the main features of the MetS with those of the HCADS [3,7,168,190–193].

Table 1. Metabolic Syndrome *versus* Hepatitis C-Associated Dysmetabolic Syndrome (HCADS)—A comparison at a glance.

Criteria	Metabolic Syndrome	HCADS	Reference(s)
T2D	Yes	Yes	[3]
Hypertension	Yes	Yes	[3]
Visceral Obesity	Yes	Preliminary evidence suggests that HCV patients have abdominal fat distribution	[3]
Atherogenic dyslipidemia	Yes	Acquired, reversible hypocholesterolemia	[6]
Hepatic steatosis	Not included among diagnostic criteria but often found as a concurrent or precursor finding	In chronic HCV patients, steatosis is two- to three-fold more prevalent than in chronic hepatitides of other etiologies. HCV genotype 3 is associated with a higher prevalence and more severe steatosis	[3,6]
Hyperuricemia	Not included in diagnostic criteria but often associated on pathophysiological grounds	Strongly associated with severity of steatosis	[3,190]
Accelerated atherogenesis	Whether the full-blown MetS adds to the risk of its individual components, particularly T2D, is controversial	Individuals with HCV infection (particularly those with T2D and hypertension) have an excess of cardiovascular morbidity and mortality	[3,191]
HCC risk	Both the MetS and T2D increase the risk of HCC. This likely results via NAFLD/NASH even in non-cirrhotic livers	Concurrent T2D and chronic HCV infection lead to increased risk of HCC. Steatosis and overweight/obesity possibly play a role	[168,192,193]

3.2. Pathophysiology

3.2.1. HCV Increases T2D Risk via Insulin Resistance

Consistent with the development of new-onset T2D observed in the setting of NAFLD, HCV promotes a state of IR that leads, over time, to pancreatic beta-cell dysfunction, eventually culminating in the irreversible damage of such cells and the development of overt T2D [177].

3.2.2. IR Associated with HCV: Antigens, Sites and Determinants

HCV antigens, such as the core protein, play a key role in determining post-receptor defects causing IR by interfering with the AKT signaling pathway via cytokines (such as TNF-α and interleukin-6) and the suppressors of cytokine signaling [194–197]. Strong evidence suggests that the site of IR is not only hepatic but also extra-hepatic [198], predominantly in the skeletal muscle, correlates with subcutaneous, rather than visceral adiposity, and is independent of liver fat content [199]. These findings conflict with the notion that HCV predominantly infects hepatocytes and suggest that either HCV-infected hepatocytes release a soluble mediator capable of inducing IR in skeletal muscles [38] or, alternatively, that HCV directly infects myocytes. This latter hypothesis appears to be conceptually sustainable based on the findings of a recent case-control study, which provided evidence for a significant association between inclusion body myositis and HCV infection [200].

3.2.3. T2D in the Setting of the HCADS

T2D is not the only metabolic disease observed in the setting of HCV infection. Over time, several features of what is now alluded to as the HCADS have been increasingly identified. For example, hepatic steatosis, which is one of such features, was first identified as a distinct disease entity [7,21,201]. Data comparing hepatic steatosis due to varying viral (HIV-related) and non-viral (NAFLD) steatogenic disorders suggest that IR is a prominent feature specifically associated with HCV infection [202].

Over time, several features have been added to the initial description of the HCADS [203–205], which, presently, is deemed to characterize hyperuricemia, reversible hypocholesterolemia, IR, hypertension and visceral obesity [189]. Collectively, these dysmetabolic disorders may best be interpreted as a Darwinian survival strategy favoring the survival of HCV at the expenses of the host's metabolism [189]. The finding of expanded visceral adipose tissue in patients with HCV infection is consistent with the hepatic and extra-hepatic origin of IR discussed above and prompts further research as to the potential ability of HCV infection to localize directly within adipocytes [206,207].

3.3. Clinical Implications

3.3.1. Risk of Fibrosis

A consistent body of evidence supports the notion that T2D is closely associated with fibrosis in the setting of chronic HCV infection [188]. More recently, a large study conducted in USA in approximately 10,000 patients with hepatitis C found that age, sex, race, HCV genotype, HIV co-infection, alcohol abuse, antiviral therapy and T2D were independently associated with the risk of cirrhosis [208]. Moreover, a recent meta-analysis of 14 studies, involving 3659 participants with HCV infection, reported a significant association between IR and advanced hepatic fibrosis among patients with HCV genotype 1 infection but not among those with HCV genotype 3 [209]. These findings are consistent with those of previous studies reporting that IR was strongly associated with HCV genotypes 1 and 4 [210,211].

3.3.2. Risk of Hepatocellular Carcinoma

Population-based studies fully support T2D being as an emerging risk factor for HCC [192]. In a recent meta-analysis, Dyal *et al.*, [193] have reported that concurrent T2D is strongly associated with an increased risk of HCC among chronic HCV patients. It may be argued, however, that, in these patients, T2D may either be a proxy of more advanced metabolic derangement which leads to excess fibrosis via NASH or that T2D *per se* exposes these individuals to higher risk of developing HCC via increased oxidative stress and hormonal changes (*e.g.*, IR, increased IGF-1 and activation of the renin-angiotensin-aldosterone system) [193,212,213].

An Italian study conducted in 163 consecutive HCV-positive patients with cirrhosis followed-up for a median period of 10.7 years found that HCV genotype 1b was strongly associated with a higher risk of developing HCC [214].

Further studies are needed to control accurately for all viral and host's confounders, such as genotype, obesity and ethnicity, given that an improved understanding of HCC risk factors may provide specific areas of targeted interventions to reduce HCC risk in chronic HCV patients [193].

3.3.3. Risk of Atherosclerosis

The strong association between HCV infection and T2D development is one of the most important mechanisms that may lead to accelerated atherogenesis in chronic HCV patients [215]. Three studies showed that HCV infection is a strong risk factor for carotid subclinical atherosclerosis [216–218]. Consistent with the notion that HCV infection is a systemic disease, the risk of major CVD events is higher in patients with HCV infection than in HCV-negative controls, independently of traditional CVD risk factors and other potential confounding variables [219,220]. In a recent meta-analysis conducted on 22 studies, Petta *et al.* [191] showed that patients with chronic HCV infection had an increased risk of CVD-related morbidity and mortality, especially those with T2D and hypertension. On these grounds, all chronic HCV patients should be non-invasively screened for atherosclerosis [215].

4. Conclusions

Among the *"four musketeers"* fighting for controlling glucose homeostasis, the liver is now in the spotlight of basic, epidemiological and clinical investigations (Figure 1). Indeed, by reviewing the role of HCV and NAFLD in the development of T2D, we found that there is a substantial body of evidence indicating that the liver plays a pathogenic role in T2D development and that the close inter-connections connecting T2D with liver disease may result in a *"vicious circle"* eventually leading to an excess risk of liver-related and CVD complications (Figure 3).

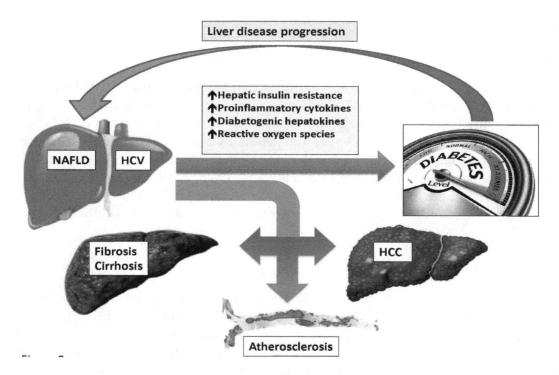

Figure 3. Non-alcoholic fatty liver disease, hepatitis C virus infection and type 2 diabetes: the *"vicious circle"*. The liver plays a pathogenic role in the development of type 2 diabetes both in the context of non-alcoholic fatty liver disease and hepatitis C virus infection through the development of systemic and hepatic insulin resistance, partly mediated by the release of multiple pro-inflammatory cytokines, diabetogenic hepatokines and reactive oxygen species. If left uncorrected, insulin resistance will eventually lead to progressive pancreatic beta cell failure in predisposed individuals. Moreover, the strong interconnection between type 2 diabetes and liver disease may result into a "vicious circle" [25] eventually leading to liver disease progression with an excess risk of liver-related, *i.e.*, cirrhosis and hepatocellular carcinoma (HCC), and cardiovascular complications, *i.e.*, atherosclerosis.

NAFLD and HCV infection are two multisystem diseases whose spectrum of clinical manifestations, seemingly as a result of their sharing hepatic steatosis and IR as prominent features (Figure 2) [205], tends to overlap more and more. Basic research is very active in the arena of NAFLD pathophysiology and extrapolation of notions from the NAFLD to the HCV research field appears to be justified and potentially fruitful [21].

However, several questions remain largely unanswered. For instance: is NAFLD treatment able to reduce the development of T2D and its major complications? Based on preliminary evidence [47,48] one may be tempted to answer affirmatively, though this remains to be fully proven by studies *ad hoc*. Does T2D impair SVR in the era of new direct-acting antivirals? While T2D was associated with a lower SVR rate following interferon-based therapy [7], regimens based on new direct-acting antiviral agents do not appear to be affected by coexisting T2D [221]. Moreover, whether HCV eradication may also have an impact on the future morbidity and mortality due to T2D is a clinically relevant and biologically plausible outcome. However, further studies with new direct-acting antivirals are needed to ultimately settle this issue [27].

In the meantime, it is important to underline that lifestyle changes are the mainstay of treatment for all patients with NAFLD and T2D [173,222]. It has been reported that a combination of educational, behavioral and motivational strategies may help patients with NAFLD in achieving lifestyle changes [223–225]. Preliminary evidence also suggests that body weight reduction may improve liver histology in those patients in whom HCV infection is associated with hepatic steatosis [226]. However, future studies are required to better define effective weight loss strategies in these patients.

Acknowledgments: Giovanni Targher is supported in part by grants from the University School of Medicine of Verona. We are indebted to Ms. Elisa Gibertini for her helping us as a graphic artist.

Author Contributions: Amedeo Lonardo conceived the idea of this article, wrote the first draft of Chapters 1 and 4, the Table and, with Dante Romagnoli, Chapter 3; Amedeo Lonardo also drew the figures in collaboration with Giovanni Targher and Fabio Nascimbeni; Stefano Ballestri and Fabio Nascimbeni wrote the first draft of Abstract and Chapter 2; Giovanni Targher and Enrica Baldelli contributed to the discussion and reviewed the manuscript. All the Authors took part in the bibliographic research, discussed, edited and approved the final version of the article.

Abbreviations

The following abbreviations are used in this manuscript:

CCR-2	C-C chemokine receptor-2
CHD	coronary heart disease
chREBP	carbohydrate-responsive element-binding protein
CVD	cardiovascular disease
DAA	direct acting antivirals
DAG	diacylglycerol
DGAT2	diacylglycerolacyltransferase 2
DNL	de-novo lipogenesis
FA	fatty acids
FGF-21	fibroblast growth factor 21
FXR	farnesoid X receptor
HCC	hepatocellular carcinoma
HIF1α	hypoxia inducible factor 1α
HCV	hepatitis C virus
IR	insulin resistance
MCP-1	monocyte chemoattractant protein-1
MetS	metabolic syndrome
PNPLA3	patatin-like phospholipase domain-containing protein 3
PPAR-γ	peroxisome proliferator–activated receptor
ROS	reactive oxygen species
SREBP1c	sterol regulatory element binding protein 1c
T2D	type 2 diabetes
TLR-4	toll-like receptor 4
TNFα	tumor necrosis factor α
UCP-1	uncoupling protein-1
WAT	white adipose tissue

References

1. Inzucchi, S.E. Clinical practice. Diagnosis of diabetes. *N. Engl. J. Med.* **2012**, *367*, 542–550. [CrossRef] [PubMed]
2. Cameron, F.J.; Wherrett, D.K. Care of diabetes in children and adolescents: Controversies, changes, and consensus. *Lancet* **2015**, *385*, 2096–2106. [CrossRef]
3. Lonardo, A.; Ballestri, S.; Marchesini, G.; Angulo, P.; Loria, P. Nonalcoholic fatty liver disease: Aprecursor of the metabolic syndrome. *Dig. Liver Dis.* **2015**, *47*, 181–190. [CrossRef] [PubMed]
4. Nascimbeni, F.; Pais, R.; Bellentani, S.; Day, C.P.; Ratziu, V.; Loria, P.; Lonardo, A. From NAFLD in clinical practice to answers from guidelines. *J. Hepatol.* **2013**, *59*, 859–871. [CrossRef] [PubMed]
5. Byrne, C.D.; Targher, G. NAFLD: A multisystem disease. *J. Hepatol.* **2015**, *62*, S47–S64. [CrossRef] [PubMed]
6. Petta, S.; Valenti, L.; Bugianesi, E.; Targher, G.; Bellentani, S.; Bonino, F.; Special Interest Group on Personalised Hepatology of the Italian Association for the Study of the Liver (AISF). A "systems medicine" approach to the study of non-alcoholic fatty liver disease. *Dig. Liver Dis.* **2016**, *48*, 333–342. [CrossRef] [PubMed]
7. Lonardo, A.; Loria, P.; Adinolfi, L.E.; Carulli, N.; Ruggiero, G. Hepatitis C and steatosis: A reappraisal. *J. Viral Hepat.* **2006**, *13*, 73–80. [CrossRef] [PubMed]

8.   Negro, F.; Forton, D.; Craxi, A.; Sulkowski, M.S.; Feld, J.J.; Manns, M.P. Extrahepatic morbidity and mortality of chronic hepatitis C. *Gastroenterology* **2015**, *149*, 1345–1360. [CrossRef] [PubMed]

9.   Shaw, J.E.; Sicree, R.A.; Zimmet, P.Z. Global estimates of the prevalence of diabetes for 2010 and 2030. *Diabetes Res. Clin. Pract.* **2010**, *87*, 4–14. [CrossRef] [PubMed]

10.   Kanavos, P.; van den Aardweg, S.; Schurer, W. Diabetes Expenditure, Burden of Disease and Management in 5 EU Countries. Available online: http://www.lse.ac.uk/LSEHealthAndSocialCare/research/LSEHealth/MTRG/LSEDiabetesReport26Jan2012.pdf (accessed on 8 February 2016).

11.   Centers for Disease Control and Prevention. *National Diabetes Fact Sheet: National Estimates and General Information on Diabetes and Prediabetes in the United States*; U.S. Department of Health and Human Services, Centers for Disease Control and Prevention: Atlanta, GA, USA, 2011.

12.   American Diabetes Association. Economic costs of diabetes in the U.S. in 2007. *Diabetes Care* **2008**, *31*, 596–615.

13.   Sherwin, R.; Jastreboff, A.M. Year in diabetes 2012: The diabetes tsunami. *J. Clin. Endocrinol. Metab.* **2012**, *97*, 4293–4301. [CrossRef] [PubMed]

14.   Zimmerman, H.J.; Mac, M.F.; Rappaport, H.; Alpert, L.K. Studies on the liver in diabetes mellitus. II. The significance of fatty metamorphosis and its correlation with insulin sensitivity. *J. Lab. Clin. Med.* **1950**, *36*, 922–928. [PubMed]

15.   Ballestri, S.; Nascimbeni, F.; Romagnoli, D.; Lonardo, A. The independent predictors of NASH and its individual histological features. Insulin resistance, serum uric acid, metabolic syndrome, alt and serum total cholesterol are a clue to pathogenesis and candidate targets for treatment. *Hepatol. Res.* **2016**. [CrossRef] [PubMed]

16.   Zhang, Y.; Zhang, T.; Zhang, C.; Tang, F.; Zhong, N.; Li, H.; Song, X.; Lin, H.; Liu, Y.; Xue, F. Identification of reciprocal causality between non-alcoholic fatty liver disease and metabolic syndrome by a simplified bayesian network in a chinese population. *BMJ Open* **2015**, *5*, e008204. [CrossRef] [PubMed]

17.   Musso, G.; Gambino, R.; Cassader, M.; Pagano, G. Meta-analysis: Natural history of non-alcoholic fatty liver disease (NAFLD) and diagnostic accuracy of non-invasive tests for liver disease severity. *Ann. Med.* **2011**, *43*, 617–649. [CrossRef] [PubMed]

18.   Ballestri, S.; Zona, S.; Targher, G.; Romagnoli, D.; Baldelli, E.; Nascimbeni, F.; Roverato, A.; Guaraldi, G.; Lonardo, A. Nonalcoholic fatty liver disease is associated with an almost two-fold increased risk of incident type 2 diabetes and metabolic syndrome. Evidence from a systematic review and meta-analysis. *J. Gastroenterol. Hepatol.* **2015**. [CrossRef] [PubMed]

19.   White, D.L.; Ratziu, V.; El-Serag, H.B. Hepatitis Cinfection and risk of diabetes: A systematic review and meta-analysis. *J. Hepatol.* **2008**, *49*, 831–844. [CrossRef] [PubMed]

20.   Cacoub, P.; Gragnani, L.; Comarmond, C.; Zignego, A.L. Extrahepatic manifestations of chronic hepatitis Cvirus infection. *Dig. Liver Dis.* **2014**, *46*, S165–S173. [CrossRef] [PubMed]

21.   Lonardo, A.; Adinolfi, L.E.; Loria, P.; Carulli, N.; Ruggiero, G.; Day, C.P. Steatosis and hepatitis Cvirus: Mechanisms and significance for hepatic and extrahepatic disease. *Gastroenterology* **2004**, *126*, 586–597. [CrossRef] [PubMed]

22.   Asselah, T.; Boyer, N.; Saadoun, D.; Martinot-Peignoux, M.; Marcellin, P. Direct-acting antivirals for the treatment of hepatitis Cvirus infection: Optimizing current IFN-free treatment and future perspectives. *Liver Int.* **2016**, *36*, 47–57. [CrossRef] [PubMed]

23.   Ilyas, J.A.; Vierling, J.M. An overview of emerging therapies for the treatment of chronic hepatitis C. *Med. Clin. N. Am.* **2014**, *98*, 17–38. [CrossRef] [PubMed]

24.   Welsch, C.; Jesudian, A.; Zeuzem, S.; Jacobson, I. New direct-acting antiviral agents for the treatment of hepatitis Cvirus infection and perspectives. *Gut* **2012**, *61*, i36–i46. [CrossRef] [PubMed]

25.   Loria, P.; Lonardo, A.; Anania, F. Liver and diabetes. A vicious circle. *Hepatol. Res.* **2013**, *43*, 51–64. [CrossRef] [PubMed]

26.   Ballestri, S.; Nascimbeni, F.; Romagnoli, D.; Baldelli, E.; Lonardo, A. The role of nuclear receptors in the pathophysiology, natural course, and drug treatment of NAFLDin humans. *Adv. Ther.* **2016**. [CrossRef] [PubMed]

27.   Vanni, E.; Bugianesi, E.; Saracco, G. Treatment of type 2 diabetes mellitus by viral eradication in chronic hepatitis C: Myth or reality? *Dig. Liver Dis.* **2016**, *48*, 105–111. [CrossRef] [PubMed]

28. Klip, A.; Vranic, M. Muscle, liver, and pancreas: Three musketeers fighting to control glycemia. *Am. J. Physiol. Endocrinol. Metab.* **2006**, *291*, E1141–E1143. [CrossRef] [PubMed]

29. Reaven, G.M. The fourth musketeer—From Alexandre Dumas to Claude Bernard. *Diabetologia* **1995**, *38*, 3–13. [CrossRef] [PubMed]

30. Armstrong, M.J.; Adams, L.A.; Canbay, A.; Syn, W.K. Extrahepatic complications of nonalcoholic fatty liver disease. *Hepatology* **2014**, *59*, 1174–1197. [CrossRef] [PubMed]

31. Carulli, L.; Ballestri, S.; Lonardo, A.; Lami, F.; Violi, E.; Losi, L.; Bonilauri, L.; Verrone, A.M.; Odoardi, M.R.; Scaglioni, F.; *et al*. Is nonalcoholic steatohepatitis associated with a high-though-normal thyroid stimulating hormone level and lower cholesterol levels? *Intern. Emerg. Med.* **2013**, *8*, 297–305. [CrossRef] [PubMed]

32. Nascimbeni, F.; Ballestri, S.; Di Tommaso, L.; Piccoli, M.; Lonardo, A. Inflammatory hepatocellular adenomatosis, metabolic syndrome, polycystic ovary syndrome and non-alcoholic steatohepatitis: Chance tetrad or association by necessity? *Dig. Liver Dis.* **2014**, *46*, 288–289. [CrossRef] [PubMed]

33. Loria, P.; Carulli, L.; Bertolotti, M.; Lonardo, A. Endocrine and liver interaction: The role of endocrine pathways in NASH. *Nat.Rev. Gastroenterol. Hepatol.* **2009**, *6*, 236–247. [CrossRef] [PubMed]

34. Targher, G.; Rossini, M.; Lonardo, A. Evidence that non-alcoholic fatty liver disease and polycystic ovary syndrome are associated by necessity rather than chance: Anovel hepato-ovarian axis? *Endocrine* **2016**, *51*, 211–221. [CrossRef] [PubMed]

35. Targher, G.; Lonardo, A.; Rossini, M. Nonalcoholic fatty liver disease and decreased bone mineral density: Is there a link? *J. Endocrinol. Investig.* **2015**, *38*, 817–825. [CrossRef] [PubMed]

36. Mantovani, A.; Gisondi, P.; Lonardo, A.; Targher, G. Relationship between non-alcoholic fatty liver disease and psoriasis: A novel hepato-dermal axis? *Int. J. Mol. Sci.* **2016**, *17*, 217. [CrossRef] [PubMed]

37. Vigano, M.; Colombo, M. Extrahepatic manifestations of hepatitis C virus. *Gastroenterol. Clin. N. Am.* **2015**, *44*, 775–791. [CrossRef] [PubMed]

38. Negro, F. Facts and fictions of HCV and comorbidities: Steatosis, diabetes mellitus, and cardiovascular diseases. *J. Hepatol.* **2014**, *61*, S69–S78. [CrossRef] [PubMed]

39. Lonardo, A.; Bellentani, S.; Argo, C.K.; Ballestri, S.; Byrne, C.D.; Caldwell, S.H.; Cortez-Pinto, H.; Grieco, A.; Machado, M.V.; *et al*. Epidemiological modifiers of non-alcoholic fatty liver disease: Focus on high-risk groups. *Dig Liver Dis.* **2015**, *47*, 997–1006.

40. Singh, S.; Allen, A.M.; Wang, Z.; Prokop, L.J.; Murad, M.H.; Loomba, R. Fibrosis progression in nonalcoholic fatty liver vs nonalcoholic steatohepatitis: Asystematic review and meta-analysis of paired-biopsy studies. *Clin. Gastroenterol. Hepatol.* **2015**, *13*, 643–654. [CrossRef] [PubMed]

41. Leite, N.C.; Villela-Nogueira, C.A.; Pannain, V.L.; Bottino, A.C.; Rezende, G.F.; Cardoso, C.R.; Salles, G.F. Histopathological stages of nonalcoholic fatty liver disease in type 2 diabetes: Prevalences and correlated factors. *Liver Int.* **2011**, *31*, 700–706. [CrossRef] [PubMed]

42. Portillo Sanchez, P.; Bril, F.; Maximos, M.; Lomonaco, R.; Biernacki, D.; Orsak, B.; Subbarayan, S.; Webb, A.; Hecht, J.; Cusi, K. High prevalence of nonalcoholic fatty liver disease in patients with type 2 diabetes mellitus and normal plasma aminotransferase levels. *J. Clin. Endocrinol. Metab.* **2015**, *100*, 2231–2238. [CrossRef] [PubMed]

43. Williams, C.D.; Stengel, J.; Asike, M.I.; Torres, D.M.; Shaw, J.; Contreras, M.; Landt, C.L.; Harrison, S.A. Prevalence of nonalcoholic fatty liver disease and nonalcoholic steatohepatitis among a largely middle-aged population utilizing ultrasound and liver biopsy: Aprospective study. *Gastroenterology* **2011**, *140*, 124–131. [CrossRef] [PubMed]

44. Kwok, R.; Choi, K.C.; Wong, G.L.; Zhang, Y.; Chan, H.L.; Luk, A.O.; Shu, S.S.; Chan, A.W.; Yeung, M.W.; Chan, J.C.; *et al*. Screening diabetic patients for non-alcoholic fatty liver disease with controlled attenuation parameter and liver stiffness measurements: Aprospective cohort study. *Gut* **2015**. [CrossRef] [PubMed]

45. Anstee, Q.M.; Targher, G.; Day, C.P. Progression of NAFLD to diabetes mellitus, cardiovascular disease or cirrhosis. *Nat.Rev. Gastroenterol. Hepatol.* **2013**, *10*, 330–344. [CrossRef] [PubMed]

46. Maximos, M.; Bril, F.; Portillo Sanchez, P.; Lomonaco, R.; Orsak, B.; Biernacki, D.; Suman, A.; Weber, M.; Cusi, K. The role of liver fat and insulin resistance as determinants of plasma aminotransferase elevation in nonalcoholic fatty liver disease. *Hepatology* **2015**, *61*, 153–160. [CrossRef] [PubMed]

47. Sung, K.C.; Wild, S.H.; Byrne, C.D. Resolution of fatty liver and risk of incident diabetes. *J. Clin. Endocrinol. Metab.* **2013**, *98*, 3637–3643. [CrossRef] [PubMed]

48. Yamazaki, H.; Tsuboya, T.; Tsuji, K.; Dohke, M.; Maguchi, H. Independent association between improvement of nonalcoholic fatty liver disease and reduced incidence of type 2 diabetes. *Diabetes Care* **2015**, *38*, 1673–1679. [CrossRef] [PubMed]

49. Fukuda, T.; Hamaguchi, M.; Kojima, T.; Hashimoto, Y.; Ohbora, A.; Kato, T.; Nakamura, N.; Fukui, M. The impact of non-alcoholic fatty liver disease on incident type 2 diabetes mellitus in non-overweight individuals. *Liver Int.* **2016**, *36*, 275–283. [CrossRef] [PubMed]

50. Shah, R.V.; Allison, M.A.; Lima, J.A.; Bluemke, D.A.; Abbasi, S.A.; Ouyang, P.; Jerosch-Herold, M.; Ding, J.; Budoff, M.J.; Murthy, V.L. Liver fat, statin use, and incident diabetes: The multi-ethnic study of atherosclerosis. *Atherosclerosis* **2015**, *242*, 211–217. [CrossRef] [PubMed]

51. Ekstedt, M.; Franzen, L.E.; Mathiesen, U.L.; Thorelius, L.; Holmqvist, M.; Bodemar, G.; Kechagias, S. Long-term follow-up of patients with NAFLD and elevated liver enzymes. *Hepatology* **2006**, *44*, 865–873. [CrossRef] [PubMed]

52. Buechler, C.; Krautbauer, S.; Eisinger, K. Adipose tissue fibrosis. *World J. Diabetes* **2015**, *6*, 548–553. [PubMed]

53. Sun, K.; Tordjman, J.; Clement, K.; Scherer, P.E. Fibrosis and adipose tissue dysfunction. *Cell Metab.* **2013**, *18*, 470–477. [CrossRef] [PubMed]

54. Sun, K.; Kusminski, C.M.; Scherer, P.E. Adipose tissue remodeling and obesity. *J. Clin. Investig.* **2011**, *121*, 2094–2101. [CrossRef] [PubMed]

55. Cinti, S.; Mitchell, G.; Barbatelli, G.; Murano, I.; Ceresi, E.; Faloia, E.; Wang, S.; Fortier, M.; Greenberg, A.S.; Obin, M.S. Adipocyte death defines macrophage localization and function in adipose tissue of obese mice and humans. *J. Lipid Res.* **2005**, *46*, 2347–2355. [CrossRef] [PubMed]

56. Cancello, R.; Henegar, C.; Viguerie, N.; Taleb, S.; Poitou, C.; Rouault, C.; Coupaye, M.; Pelloux, V.; Hugol, D.; Bouillot, J.L.; *et al.* Reduction of macrophage infiltration and chemoattractant gene expression changes in white adipose tissue of morbidly obese subjects after surgery-induced weight loss. *Diabetes* **2005**, *54*, 2277–2286. [CrossRef] [PubMed]

57. Halberg, N.; Khan, T.; Trujillo, M.E.; Wernstedt-Asterholm, I.; Attie, A.D.; Sherwani, S.; Wang, Z.V.; Landskroner-Eiger, S.; Dineen, S.; Magalang, U.J.; *et al.* Hypoxia-inducible factor 1alpha induces fibrosis and insulin resistance in white adipose tissue. *Mol. Cell. Biol.* **2009**, *29*, 4467–4483. [CrossRef] [PubMed]

58. Jiang, C.; Qu, A.; Matsubara, T.; Chanturiya, T.; Jou, W.; Gavrilova, O.; Shah, Y.M.; Gonzalez, F.J. Disruption of hypoxia-inducible factor 1 in adipocytes improves insulin sensitivity and decreases adiposity in high-fat diet-fed mice. *Diabetes* **2011**, *60*, 2484–2495. [CrossRef] [PubMed]

59. Sun, K.; Halberg, N.; Khan, M.; Magalang, U.J.; Scherer, P.E. Selective inhibition of hypoxia-inducible factor 1alpha ameliorates adipose tissue dysfunction. *Mol. Cell. Biol.* **2013**, *33*, 904–917. [CrossRef] [PubMed]

60. Lumeng, C.N.; Bodzin, J.L.; Saltiel, A.R. Obesity induces a phenotypic switch in adipose tissue macrophage polarization. *J. Clin. Investig.* **2007**, *117*, 175–184. [CrossRef] [PubMed]

61. Lumeng, C.N.; DelProposto, J.B.; Westcott, D.J.; Saltiel, A.R. Phenotypic switching of adipose tissue macrophages with obesity is generated by spatiotemporal differences in macrophage subtypes. *Diabetes* **2008**, *57*, 3239–3246. [CrossRef] [PubMed]

62. Suganami, T.; Tanaka, M.; Ogawa, Y. Adipose tissue inflammation and ectopic lipid accumulation. *Endocr. J.* **2012**, *59*, 849–857. [CrossRef] [PubMed]

63. Berg, A.H.; Scherer, P.E. Adipose tissue, inflammation, and cardiovascular disease. *Circ. Res.* **2005**, *96*, 939–949. [CrossRef] [PubMed]

64. Rocha, V.Z.; Libby, P. Obesity, inflammation, and atherosclerosis. *Nat. Rev. Cardiol.* **2009**, *6*, 399–409. [CrossRef] [PubMed]

65. Hotamisligil, G.S.; Shargill, N.S.; Spiegelman, B.M. Adipose expression of tumor necrosis factor-α: Direct role in obesity-linked insulin resistance. *Science* **1993**, *259*, 87–91. [CrossRef] [PubMed]

66. Uysal, K.T.; Wiesbrock, S.M.; Marino, M.W.; Hotamisligil, G.S. Protection from obesity-induced insulin resistance in mice lacking TNF-alpha function. *Nature* **1997**, *389*, 610–614. [PubMed]

67. Kanda, H.; Tateya, S.; Tamori, Y.; Kotani, K.; Hiasa, K.; Kitazawa, R.; Kitazawa, S.; Miyachi, H.; Maeda, S.; Egashira, K.; *et al.* Mcp-1 contributes to macrophage infiltration into adipose tissue, insulin resistance, and hepatic steatosis in obesity. *J. Clin. Investig.* **2006**, *116*, 1494–1505. [CrossRef] [PubMed]

68. Kamei, N.; Tobe, K.; Suzuki, R.; Ohsugi, M.; Watanabe, T.; Kubota, N.; Ohtsuka-Kowatari, N.; Kumagai, K.; Sakamoto, K.; Kobayashi, M.; *et al.* Overexpression of monocyte chemoattractant protein-1 in adipose tissues

causes macrophage recruitment and insulin resistance. *J. Biol. Chem.* **2006**, *281*, 26602–26614. [CrossRef] [PubMed]

69. Weisberg, S.P.; Hunter, D.; Huber, R.; Lemieux, J.; Slaymaker, S.; Vaddi, K.; Charo, I.; Leibel, R.L.; Ferrante, A.W., Jr. CCR2 modulates inflammatory and metabolic effects of high-fat feeding. *J. Clin. Investig.* **2006**, *116*, 115–124. [CrossRef] [PubMed]

70. Yamauchi, T.; Kamon, J.; Waki, H.; Terauchi, Y.; Kubota, N.; Hara, K.; Mori, Y.; Ide, T.; Murakami, K.; Tsuboyama-Kasaoka, N.; *et al.* The fat-derived hormone adiponectin reverses insulin resistance associated with both lipoatrophy and obesity. *Nat. Med.* **2001**, *7*, 941–946. [CrossRef] [PubMed]

71. Maeda, N.; Shimomura, I.; Kishida, K.; Nishizawa, H.; Matsuda, M.; Nagaretani, H.; Furuyama, N.; Kondo, H.; Takahashi, M.; Arita, Y.; *et al.* Diet-induced insulin resistance in mice lacking adiponectin/ACRP 30. *Nat. Med.* **2002**, *8*, 731–737. [CrossRef] [PubMed]

72. Wernstedt Asterholm, I.; Tao, C.; Morley, T.S.; Wang, Q.A.; Delgado-Lopez, F.; Wang, Z.V.; Scherer, P.E. Adipocyte inflammation is essential for healthy adipose tissue expansion and remodeling. *Cell Metab.* **2014**, *20*, 103–118. [CrossRef] [PubMed]

73. Divoux, A.; Tordjman, J.; Lacasa, D.; Veyrie, N.; Hugol, D.; Aissat, A.; Basdevant, A.; Guerre-Millo, M.; Poitou, C.; Zucker, J.D.; *et al.* Fibrosis in human adipose tissue: Composition, distribution, and link with lipid metabolism and fat mass loss. *Diabetes* **2010**, *59*, 2817–2825. [CrossRef] [PubMed]

74. Samuel, V.T.; Shulman, G.I. The pathogenesis of insulin resistance: Integrating signaling pathways and substrate flux. *J. Clin. Investig.* **2016**, *126*, 12–22. [CrossRef] [PubMed]

75. Yu, C.; Chen, Y.; Cline, G.W.; Zhang, D.; Zong, H.; Wang, Y.; Bergeron, R.; Kim, J.K.; Cushman, S.W.; Cooney, G.J.; *et al.* Mechanism by which fatty acids inhibit insulin activation of insulin receptor substrate-1 (IRS-1)-associated phosphatidylinositol 3-kinase activity in muscle. *J. Biol. Chem.* **2002**, *277*, 50230–50236. [CrossRef] [PubMed]

76. Griffin, M.E.; Marcucci, M.J.; Cline, G.W.; Bell, K.; Barucci, N.; Lee, D.; Goodyear, L.J.; Kraegen, E.W.; White, M.F.; Shulman, G.I. Free fatty acid-induced insulin resistance is associated with activation of protein kinase Ctheta and alterations in the insulin signaling cascade. *Diabetes* **1999**, *48*, 1270–1274. [CrossRef] [PubMed]

77. Szendroedi, J.; Yoshimura, T.; Phielix, E.; Koliaki, C.; Marcucci, M.; Zhang, D.; Jelenik, T.; Muller, J.; Herder, C.; Nowotny, P.; *et al.* Role of diacylglycerol activation of PKCθ in lipid-induced muscle insulin resistance in humans. *Proc. Natl. Acad. Sci. USA* **2014**, *111*, 9597–9602. [CrossRef] [PubMed]

78. Kitajima, Y.; Hyogo, H.; Sumida, Y.; Eguchi, Y.; Ono, N.; Kuwashiro, T.; Tanaka, K.; Takahashi, H.; Mizuta, T.; Ozaki, I.; *et al.* Severity of non-alcoholic steatohepatitis is associated with substitution of adipose tissue in skeletal muscle. *J. Gastroenterol. Hepatol.* **2013**, *28*, 1507–1514. [CrossRef] [PubMed]

79. Arias-Loste, M.T.; Ranchal, I.; Romero-Gomez, M.; Crespo, J. Irisin, a link among fatty liver disease, physical inactivity and insulin resistance. *Int. J. Mol. Sci.* **2014**, *15*, 23163–23178. [CrossRef] [PubMed]

80. Bostrom, P.; Wu, J.; Jedrychowski, M.P.; Korde, A.; Ye, L.; Lo, J.C.; Rasbach, K.A.; Bostrom, E.A.; Choi, J.H.; Long, J.Z.; *et al.* A PGC 1-α-dependent myokine that drives brown-fat-like development of white fat and thermogenesis. *Nature* **2012**, *481*, 463–468. [CrossRef] [PubMed]

81. Schulz, T.J.; Tseng, Y.H. Brown adipose tissue: Development, metabolism and beyond. *Biochem. J.* **2013**, *453*, 167–178. [CrossRef] [PubMed]

82. Seale, P.; Bjork, B.; Yang, W.; Kajimura, S.; Chin, S.; Kuang, S.; Scime, A.; Devarakonda, S.; Conroe, H.M.; Erdjument-Bromage, H.; *et al.* PRDM16 controls a brown fat/skeletal muscle switch. *Nature* **2008**, *454*, 961–967. [CrossRef] [PubMed]

83. Ishibashi, J.; Seale, P. Medicine. Beige can be slimming. *Science* **2010**, *328*, 1113–1114. [CrossRef] [PubMed]

84. Enerback, S. The origins of brown adipose tissue. *N. Engl. J. Med.* **2009**, *360*, 2021–2023. [CrossRef] [PubMed]

85. Scheja, L.; Heeren, J. Metabolic interplay between white, beige, brown adipocytes and the liver. *J. Hepatol.* **2016**. [CrossRef] [PubMed]

86. Guerra, C.; Navarro, P.; Valverde, A.M.; Arribas, M.; Bruning, J.; Kozak, L.P.; Kahn, C.R.; Benito, M. Brown adipose tissue-specific insulin receptor knockout shows diabetic phenotype without insulin resistance. *J. Clin. Investig.* **2001**, *108*, 1205–1213. [CrossRef] [PubMed]

87. Bartelt, A.; Bruns, O.T.; Reimer, R.; Hohenberg, H.; Ittrich, H.; Peldschus, K.; Kaul, M.G.; Tromsdorf, U.I.; Weller, H.; Waurisch, C.; *et al.* Brown adipose tissue activity controls triglyceride clearance. *Nat. Med.* **2011**, *17*, 200–205. [CrossRef] [PubMed]

88.   Assyov, Y.; Gateva, A.; Tsakova, A.; Kamenov, Z. Irisin in the glucose continuum. *Exp. Clin. Endocrinol. Diabetes* **2016**, *124*, 22–27. [CrossRef] [PubMed]

89.   Liu, J.J.; Wong, M.D.; Toy, W.C.; Tan, C.S.; Liu, S.; Ng, X.W.; Tavintharan, S.; Sum, C.F.; Lim, S.C. Lower circulating irisin is associated with type 2 diabetes mellitus. *J. Diabetes Complicat.* **2013**, *27*, 365–369. [CrossRef] [PubMed]

90.   Zhang, H.J.; Zhang, X.F.; Ma, Z.M.; Pan, L.L.; Chen, Z.; Han, H.W.; Han, C.K.; Zhuang, X.J.; Lu, Y.; Li, X.J.; et al. Irisin is inversely associated with intrahepatic triglyceride contents in obese adults. *J. Hepatol.* **2013**, *59*, 557–562. [CrossRef] [PubMed]

91.   Donnelly, K.L.; Smith, C.I.; Schwarzenberg, S.J.; Jessurun, J.; Boldt, M.D.; Parks, E.J. Sources of fatty acids stored in liver and secreted via lipoproteins in patients with nonalcoholic fatty liver disease. *J. Clin. Investig.* **2005**, *115*, 1343–1351. [CrossRef] [PubMed]

92.   Haas, J.T.; Francque, S.; Staels, B. Pathophysiology and mechanisms of nonalcoholic fatty liver disease. *Ann. Rev. Physiol.* **2016**, *78*, 181–205. [CrossRef] [PubMed]

93.   Seppala-Lindroos, A.; Vehkavaara, S.; Hakkinen, A.M.; Goto, T.; Westerbacka, J.; Sovijarvi, A.; Halavaara, J.; Yki-Jarvinen, H. Fat accumulation in the liver is associated with defects in insulin suppression of glucose production and serum free fatty acids independent of obesity in normal men. *J. Clin. Endocrinol. Metab.* **2002**, *87*, 3023–3028. [CrossRef] [PubMed]

94.   Bugianesi, E.; Gastaldelli, A.; Vanni, E.; Gambino, R.; Cassader, M.; Baldi, S.; Ponti, V.; Pagano, G.; Ferrannini, E.; Rizzetto, M. Insulin resistance in non-diabetic patients with non-alcoholic fatty liver disease: Sites and mechanisms. *Diabetologia* **2005**, *48*, 634–642. [CrossRef] [PubMed]

95.   Vatner, D.F.; Majumdar, S.K.; Kumashiro, N.; Petersen, M.C.; Rahimi, Y.; Gattu, A.K.; Bears, M.; Camporez, J.P.; Cline, G.W.; Jurczak, M.J.; et al. Insulin-independent regulation of hepatic triglyceride synthesis by fatty acids. *Proc. Natl. Acad. Sci. USA* **2015**, *112*, 1143–1148. [CrossRef] [PubMed]

96.   Matsuzaka, T.; Shimano, H.; Yahagi, N.; Amemiya-Kudo, M.; Okazaki, H.; Tamura, Y.; Iizuka, Y.; Ohashi, K.; Tomita, S.; Sekiya, M.; et al. Insulin-independent induction of sterol regulatory element-binding protein-1c expression in the livers of streptozotocin-treated mice. *Diabetes* **2004**, *53*, 560–569. [CrossRef] [PubMed]

97.   Stanhope, K.L.; Schwarz, J.M.; Keim, N.L.; Griffen, S.C.; Bremer, A.A.; Graham, J.L.; Hatcher, B.; Cox, C.L.; Dyachenko, A.; Zhang, W.; et al. Consuming fructose-sweetened, not glucose-sweetened, beverages increases visceral adiposity and lipids and decreases insulin sensitivity in overweight/obese humans. *J. Clin. Investig.* **2009**, *119*, 1322–1334. [CrossRef] [PubMed]

98.   Uyeda, K.; Repa, J.J. Carbohydrate response element binding protein, chrebp, a transcription factor coupling hepatic glucose utilization and lipid synthesis. *Cell Metab.* **2006**, *4*, 107–110. [CrossRef] [PubMed]

99.   Erion, D.M.; Popov, V.; Hsiao, J.J.; Vatner, D.; Mitchell, K.; Yonemitsu, S.; Nagai, Y.; Kahn, M.; Gillum, M.P.; Dong, J.; et al. The role of the carbohydrate response element-binding protein in male fructose-fed rats. *Endocrinology* **2013**, *154*, 36–44. [CrossRef] [PubMed]

100. Nagai, Y.; Yonemitsu, S.; Erion, D.M.; Iwasaki, T.; Stark, R.; Weismann, D.; Dong, J.; Zhang, D.; Jurczak, M.J.; Loffler, M.G.; et al. The role of peroxisome proliferator-activated receptor gamma coactivator-1 β in the pathogenesis of fructose-induced insulin resistance. *Cell Metab.* **2009**, *9*, 252–264. [CrossRef] [PubMed]

101. Bindesboll, C.; Fan, Q.; Norgaard, R.C.; MacPherson, L.; Ruan, H.B.; Wu, J.; Pedersen, T.A.; Steffensen, K.R.; Yang, X.; Matthews, J.; et al. Liver Xreceptor regulates hepatic nuclear O-GlcNAc signaling and carbohydrate responsive element-binding protein activity. *J. Lipid Res.* **2015**, *56*, 771–785. [CrossRef] [PubMed]

102. Samuel, V.T.; Shulman, G.I. Mechanisms for insulin resistance: Common threads and missing links. *Cell* **2012**, *148*, 852–871. [CrossRef] [PubMed]

103. Yamaguchi, K.; Yang, L.; McCall, S.; Huang, J.; Yu, X.X.; Pandey, S.K.; Bhanot, S.; Monia, B.P.; Li, Y.X.; Diehl, A.M. Inhibiting triglyceride synthesis improves hepatic steatosis but exacerbates liver damage and fibrosis in obese mice with nonalcoholic steatohepatitis. *Hepatology* **2007**, *45*, 1366–1374. [CrossRef] [PubMed]

104. Samuel, V.T.; Liu, Z.X.; Wang, A.; Beddow, S.A.; Geisler, J.G.; Kahn, M.; Zhang, X.M.; Monia, B.P.; Bhanot, S.; Shulman, G.I. Inhibition of protein kinase cepsilon prevents hepatic insulin resistance in nonalcoholic fatty liver disease. *J. Clin. Investig.* **2007**, *117*, 739–745. [CrossRef] [PubMed]

105. Qu, X.; Seale, J.P.; Donnelly, R. Tissue and isoform-selective activation of protein kinase Cin insulin-resistant obese zucker rats—Effects of feeding. *J. Endocrinol.* **1999**, *162*, 207–214. [CrossRef] [PubMed]

106. Kumashiro, N.; Erion, D.M.; Zhang, D.; Kahn, M.; Beddow, S.A.; Chu, X.; Still, C.D.; Gerhard, G.S.; Han, X.; Dziura, J.; et al. Cellular mechanism of insulin resistance in nonalcoholic fatty liver disease. *Proc. Natl. Acad. Sci. USA* **2011**, *108*, 16381–16385. [CrossRef] [PubMed]

107. Magkos, F.; Su, X.; Bradley, D.; Fabbrini, E.; Conte, C.; Eagon, J.C.; Varela, J.E.; Brunt, E.M.; Patterson, B.W.; Klein, S. Intrahepatic diacylglycerol content is associated with hepatic insulin resistance in obese subjects. *Gastroenterology* **2012**, *142*, 1444–1446. [CrossRef] [PubMed]

108. Schmitz-Peiffer, C.; Craig, D.L.; Biden, T.J. Ceramide generation is sufficient to account for the inhibition of the insulin-stimulated PKBpathway in C2C12 skeletal muscle cells pretreated with palmitate. *J. Biol. Chem.* **1999**, *274*, 24202–24210. [CrossRef] [PubMed]

109. Stratford, S.; Hoehn, K.L.; Liu, F.; Summers, S.A. Regulation of insulin action by ceramide: Dual mechanisms linking ceramide accumulation to the inhibition of AKT/protein kinase B. *J. Biol. Chem.* **2004**, *279*, 36608–36615. [CrossRef] [PubMed]

110. Turinsky, J.; O'Sullivan, D.M.; Bayly, B.P. 1,2-Diacylglycerol and ceramide levels in insulin-resistant tissues of the rat *in vivo*. *J. Biol. Chem.* **1990**, *265*, 16880–16885. [PubMed]

111. Chavez, J.A.; Summers, S.A. A ceramide-centric view of insulin resistance. *Cell Metab.* **2012**, *15*, 585–594. [CrossRef] [PubMed]

112. Hla, T.; Kolesnick, R. C16:0-ceramide signals insulin resistance. *Cell Metab.* **2014**, *20*, 703–705. [CrossRef] [PubMed]

113. Turpin, S.M.; Nicholls, H.T.; Willmes, D.M.; Mourier, A.; Brodesser, S.; Wunderlich, C.M.; Mauer, J.; Xu, E.; Hammerschmidt, P.; Bronneke, H.S.; et al. Obesity-induced CERS6-dependent C16:0 ceramide production promotes weight gain and glucose intolerance. *Cell Metab.* **2014**, *20*, 678–686. [CrossRef] [PubMed]

114. Luukkonen, P.K.; Zhou, Y.; Sadevirta, S.; Leivonen, M.; Arola, J.; Oresic, M.; Hyotylainen, T.; Yki-Jarvinen, H. Ceramides dissociate steatosis and insulin resistance in the human liver in non-alcoholic fatty liver disease. *J. Hepatol.* **2016**. [CrossRef] [PubMed]

115. Jenkins, C.M.; Mancuso, D.J.; Yan, W.; Sims, H.F.; Gibson, B.; Gross, R.W. Identification, cloning, expression, and purification of three novel human calcium-independent phospholipase A2 family members possessing triacylglycerol lipase and acylglycerol transacylase activities. *J. Biol. Chem.* **2004**, *279*, 48968–48975. [CrossRef] [PubMed]

116. Romeo, S.; Kozlitina, J.; Xing, C.; Pertsemlidis, A.; Cox, D.; Pennacchio, L.A.; Boerwinkle, E.; Cohen, J.C.; Hobbs, H.H. Genetic variation in PNPLA3 confers susceptibility to nonalcoholic fatty liver disease. *Nat. Genet.* **2008**, *40*, 1461–1465. [CrossRef] [PubMed]

117. Kantartzis, K.; Peter, A.; Machicao, F.; Machann, J.; Wagner, S.; Konigsrainer, I.; Konigsrainer, A.; Schick, F.; Fritsche, A.; Haring, H.U.; et al. Dissociation between fatty liver and insulin resistance in humans carrying a variant of the patatin-like phospholipase 3 gene. *Diabetes* **2009**, *58*, 2616–2623. [CrossRef] [PubMed]

118. Kotronen, A.; Johansson, L.E.; Johansson, L.M.; Roos, C.; Westerbacka, J.; Hamsten, A.; Bergholm, R.; Arkkila, P.; Arola, J.; Kiviluoto, T.; et al. A common variant in PNPLA3, which encodes adiponutrin, is associated with liver fat content in humans. *Diabetologia* **2009**, *52*, 1056–1060. [CrossRef] [PubMed]

119. Speliotes, E.K.; Butler, J.L.; Palmer, C.D.; Voight, B.F.; Consortium, G.; Consortium, M.I.; Nash, C.R.N.; Hirschhorn, J.N. PNPLA3 variants specifically confer increased risk for histologic nonalcoholic fatty liver disease but not metabolic disease. *Hepatology* **2010**, *52*, 904–912. [CrossRef] [PubMed]

120. Kumari, M.; Schoiswohl, G.; Chitraju, C.; Paar, M.; Cornaciu, I.; Rangrez, A.Y.; Wongsiriroj, N.; Nagy, H.M.; Ivanova, P.T.; Scott, S.A.; et al. Adiponutrin functions as a nutritionally regulated lysophosphatidic acid acyltransferase. *Cell Metab.* **2012**, *15*, 691–702. [CrossRef] [PubMed]

121. Smagris, E.; BasuRay, S.; Li, J.; Huang, Y.; Lai, K.M.; Gromada, J.; Cohen, J.C.; Hobbs, H.H. PNPLA3I148Mknockin mice accumulate PNPLA3 on lipid droplets and develop hepatic steatosis. *Hepatology* **2015**, *61*, 108–118. [CrossRef] [PubMed]

122. Wu, J.W.; Yang, H.; Mitchell, G.A. Potential mechanism underlying the PNPLA3^{I148M}-hepatic steatosis connection. *Hepatology* **2016**, *63*, 676–677. [CrossRef] [PubMed]

123. Puri, P.; Mirshahi, F.; Cheung, O.; Natarajan, R.; Maher, J.W.; Kellum, J.M.; Sanyal, A.J. Activation and dysregulation of the unfolded protein response in nonalcoholic fatty liver disease. *Gastroenterology* **2008**, *134*, 568–576. [CrossRef] [PubMed]

124. Malhi, H.; Gores, G.J. Molecular mechanisms of lipotoxicity in nonalcoholic fatty liver disease. *Semin. Liver Dis.* **2008**, *28*, 360–369. [CrossRef] [PubMed]

125. Singh, R.; Kaushik, S.; Wang, Y.; Xiang, Y.; Novak, I.; Komatsu, M.; Tanaka, K.; Cuervo, A.M.; Czaja, M.J. Autophagy regulates lipid metabolism. *Nature* **2009**, *458*, 1131–1135. [CrossRef] [PubMed]

126. Wang, Y.; Singh, R.; Xiang, Y.; Czaja, M.J. Macroautophagy and chaperone-mediated autophagy are required for hepatocyte resistance to oxidant stress. *Hepatology* **2010**, *52*, 266–277. [CrossRef] [PubMed]

127. Czaja, M.J. Autophagy in health and disease. 2. Regulation of lipid metabolism and storage by autophagy: Pathophysiological implications. *Am. J. Physiol. Cell Physiol.* **2010**, *298*, C973–C978. [CrossRef] [PubMed]

128. Pal, D.; Dasgupta, S.; Kundu, R.; Maitra, S.; Das, G.; Mukhopadhyay, S.; Ray, S.; Majumdar, S.S.; Bhattacharya, S. Fetuin-Aacts as an endogenous ligand of TLR4 to promote lipid-induced insulin resistance. *Nat. Med.* **2012**, *18*, 1279–1285. [CrossRef] [PubMed]

129. Chatterjee, P.; Seal, S.; Mukherjee, S.; Kundu, R.; Mukherjee, S.; Ray, S.; Mukhopadhyay, S.; Majumdar, S.S.; Bhattacharya, S. Adipocyte fetuin-Acontributes to macrophage migration into adipose tissue and polarization of macrophages. *J. Biol. Chem.* **2013**, *288*, 28324–28330. [CrossRef] [PubMed]

130. Ix, J.H.; Shlipak, M.G.; Brandenburg, V.M.; Ali, S.; Ketteler, M.; Whooley, M.A. Association between human fetuin-Aand the metabolic syndrome: Data from the heart and soul study. *Circulation* **2006**, *113*, 1760–1767. [CrossRef] [PubMed]

131. Ix, J.H.; Wassel, C.L.; Kanaya, A.M.; Vittinghoff, E.; Johnson, K.C.; Koster, A.; Cauley, J.A.; Harris, T.B.; Cummings, S.R.; Shlipak, M.G.; *et al.* Fetuin-Aand incident diabetes mellitus in older persons. *JAMA* **2008**, *300*, 182–188. [CrossRef] [PubMed]

132. Stefan, N.; Hennige, A.M.; Staiger, H.; Machann, J.; Schick, F.; Krober, S.M.; Machicao, F.; Fritsche, A.; Haring, H.U. Alpha2-heremans-schmid glycoprotein/fetuin-Ais associated with insulin resistance and fat accumulation in the liver in humans. *Diabetes Care* **2006**, *29*, 853–857. [CrossRef] [PubMed]

133. Meex, R.C.; Hoy, A.J.; Morris, A.; Brown, R.D.; Lo, J.C.; Burke, M.; Goode, R.J.; Kingwell, B.A.; Kraakman, M.J.; Febbraio, M.A.; *et al.* Fetuin Bis a secreted hepatocyte factor linking steatosis to impaired glucose metabolism. *Cell Metab.* **2015**, *22*, 1078–1089. [CrossRef] [PubMed]

134. Kharitonenkov, A.; Shiyanova, T.L.; Koester, A.; Ford, A.M.; Micanovic, R.; Galbreath, E.J.; Sandusky, G.E.; Hammond, L.J.; Moyers, J.S.; Owens, R.A.; *et al.* FGF-21 as a novel metabolic regulator. *J. Clin. Investig.* **2005**, *115*, 1627–1635. [CrossRef] [PubMed]

135. Zhang, X.; Yeung, D.C.; Karpisek, M.; Stejskal, D.; Zhou, Z.G.; Liu, F.; Wong, R.L.; Chow, W.S.; Tso, A.W.; Lam, K.S.; *et al.* Serum FGF21 levels are increased in obesity and are independently associated with the metabolic syndrome in humans. *Diabetes* **2008**, *57*, 1246–1253. [CrossRef] [PubMed]

136. Itoh, N. FGF21 as a hepatokine, adipokine, and myokine in metabolism and diseases. *Front. Endocrinol. (Lausanne)* **2014**, *5*, 107. [CrossRef] [PubMed]

137. Chavez, A.O.; Molina-Carrion, M.; Abdul-Ghani, M.A.; Folli, F.; Defronzo, R.A.; Tripathy, D. Circulating fibroblast growth factor-21 is elevated in impaired glucose tolerance and type 2 diabetes and correlates with muscle and hepatic insulin resistance. *Diabetes Care* **2009**, *32*, 1542–1546. [CrossRef] [PubMed]

138. Dushay, J.; Chui, P.C.; Gopalakrishnan, G.S.; Varela-Rey, M.; Crawley, M.; Fisher, F.M.; Badman, M.K.; Martinez-Chantar, M.L.; Maratos-Flier, E. Increased fibroblast growth factor 21 in obesity and nonalcoholic fatty liver disease. *Gastroenterology* **2010**, *139*, 456–463. [CrossRef] [PubMed]

139. Li, H.; Dong, K.; Fang, Q.; Hou, X.; Zhou, M.; Bao, Y.; Xiang, K.; Xu, A.; Jia, W. High serum level of fibroblast growth factor 21 is an independent predictor of non-alcoholic fatty liver disease: A3-year prospective study in china. *J. Hepatol.* **2013**, *58*, 557–563. [CrossRef] [PubMed]

140. Li, H.; Fang, Q.; Gao, F.; Fan, J.; Zhou, J.; Wang, X.; Zhang, H.; Pan, X.; Bao, Y.; Xiang, K.; *et al.* Fibroblast growth factor 21 levels are increased in nonalcoholic fatty liver disease patients and are correlated with hepatic triglyceride. *J. Hepatol.* **2010**, *53*, 934–940. [CrossRef] [PubMed]

141. El Ouaamari, A.; Dirice, E.; Gedeon, N.; Hu, J.; Zhou, J.Y.; Shirakawa, J.; Hou, L.; Goodman, J.; Karampelias, C.; Qiang, G.; *et al.* SerpinB1 promotes pancreatic beta cell proliferation. *Cell Metab.* **2016**, *23*, 194–205. [CrossRef] [PubMed]

142. Tarasov, A.I.; Rorsman, P. Dramatis personae in beta-cell mass regulation: Enter serpinB1. *Cell Metab.* **2016**, *23*, 8–10. [CrossRef] [PubMed]

143. Boursier, J.; Mueller, O.; Barret, M.; Machado, M.; Fizanne, L.; Araujo-Perez, F.; Guy, C.D.; Seed, P.C.; Rawls, J.F.; David, L.A.; *et al.* The severity of NAFLD is associated with gut dysbiosis and shift in the metabolic function of the gut microbiota. *Hepatology* **2016**, *63*, 764–775. [CrossRef] [PubMed]

144. Le Roy, T.; Llopis, M.; Lepage, P.; Bruneau, A.; Rabot, S.; Bevilacqua, C.; Martin, P.; Philippe, C.; Walker, F.; Bado, A.; *et al.* Intestinal microbiota determines development of non-alcoholic fatty liver disease in mice. *Gut* **2013**, *62*, 1787–1794. [CrossRef] [PubMed]

145. Musso, G.; Gambino, R.; Cassader, M. Gut microbiota as a regulator of energy homeostasis and ectopic fat deposition: Mechanisms and implications for metabolic disorders. *Curr. Opin. Lipidol.* **2010**, *21*, 76–83. [CrossRef] [PubMed]

146. Nolan, C.J.; Damm, P.; Prentki, M. Type 2 diabetes across generations: From pathophysiology to prevention and management. *Lancet* **2011**, *378*, 169–181. [CrossRef]

147. Shima, T.; Uto, H.; Ueki, K.; Takamura, T.; Kohgo, Y.; Kawata, S.; Yasui, K.; Park, H.; Nakamura, N.; Nakatou, T.; *et al.* Clinicopathological features of liver injury in patients with type 2 diabetes mellitus and comparative study of histologically proven nonalcoholic fatty liver diseases with or without type 2 diabetes mellitus. *J.Gastroenterol.* **2013**, *48*, 515–525. [CrossRef] [PubMed]

148. Goh, G.B.; Pagadala, M.R.; Dasarathy, J.; Unalp-Arida, A.; Sargent, R.; Hawkins, C.; Sourianarayanane, A.; Khiyami, A.; Yerian, L.; Pai, R.K.; *et al.* Clinical spectrum of non-alcoholic fatty liver disease in diabetic and non-diabetic patients. *BBA Clin.* **2015**, *3*, 141–145. [CrossRef] [PubMed]

149. Nascimbeni, F.; Aron-Wisniewsky, J.; Pais, R.; Tordjman, J.; Poitou, C.; Charlotte, F.; Bedossa, P.; Poynard, T.; Clement, K.; Ratziu, V. Statins, antidiabetic medications and liver histology in diabetic patients with non-alcoholic fatty liver disease. *BMJ Open Gastroenterol.* **2016**. in press.

150. Angulo, P.; Keach, J.C.; Batts, K.P.; Lindor, K.D. Independent predictors of liver fibrosis in patients with nonalcoholic steatohepatitis. *Hepatology* **1999**, *30*, 1356–1362. [CrossRef] [PubMed]

151. De Ledinghen, V.; Ratziu, V.; Causse, X.; Le Bail, B.; Capron, D.; Renou, C.; Pilette, C.; Oules, V.; Gelsi, E.; Oberti, F.; *et al.* Diagnostic and predictive factors of significant liver fibrosis and minimal lesions in patients with persistent unexplained elevated transaminases. A prospective multicenter study. *J. Hepatol.* **2006**, *45*, 592–599. [CrossRef] [PubMed]

152. Hossain, N.; Afendy, A.; Stepanova, M.; Nader, F.; Srishord, M.; Rafiq, N.; Goodman, Z.; Younossi, Z. Independent predictors of fibrosis in patients with nonalcoholic fatty liver disease. *Clin. Gastroenterol. Hepatol.* **2009**, *7*, 1224–1229. [CrossRef] [PubMed]

153. Nakahara, T.; Hyogo, H.; Yoneda, M.; Sumida, Y.; Eguchi, Y.; Fujii, H.; Ono, M.; Kawaguchi, T.; Imajo, K.; Aikata, H.; *et al.* Type 2 diabetes mellitus is associated with the fibrosis severity in patients with nonalcoholic fatty liver disease in a large retrospective cohort of Japanese patients. *J. Gastroenterol.* **2014**, *49*, 1477–1484. [CrossRef] [PubMed]

154. McPherson, S.; Hardy, T.; Henderson, E.; Burt, A.D.; Day, C.P.; Anstee, Q.M. Evidence of NAFLDprogression from steatosis to fibrosing-steatohepatitis using paired biopsies: Implications for prognosis and clinical management. *J. Hepatol.* **2015**, *62*, 1148–1155. [CrossRef] [PubMed]

155. Pais, R.; Charlotte, F.; Fedchuk, L.; Bedossa, P.; Lebray, P.; Poynard, T.; Ratziu, V.; Group, L.S. A systematic review of follow-up biopsies reveals disease progression in patients with non-alcoholic fatty liver. *J. Hepatol.* **2013**, *59*, 550–556. [CrossRef] [PubMed]

156. Adams, L.A.; Sanderson, S.; Lindor, K.D.; Angulo, P. The histological course of nonalcoholic fatty liver disease: A longitudinal study of 103 patients with sequential liver biopsies. *J. Hepatol.* **2005**, *42*, 132–138. [CrossRef] [PubMed]

157. Hamaguchi, E.; Takamura, T.; Sakurai, M.; Mizukoshi, E.; Zen, Y.; Takeshita, Y.; Kurita, S.; Arai, K.; Yamashita, T.; Sasaki, M.; *et al.* Histological course of nonalcoholic fatty liver disease in Japanese patients: Tight glycemic control, rather than weight reduction, ameliorates liver fibrosis. *Diabetes Care* **2010**, *33*, 284–286. [CrossRef] [PubMed]

158. Hashiba, M.; Ono, M.; Hyogo, H.; Ikeda, Y.; Masuda, K.; Yoshioka, R.; Ishikawa, Y.; Nagata, Y.; Munekage, K.; Ochi, T.; *et al.* Glycemic variability is an independent predictive factor for development of hepatic fibrosis in nonalcoholic fatty liver disease. *PLoS ONE* **2013**, *8*, e76161. [CrossRef] [PubMed]

159. Fracanzani, A.L.; Valenti, L.; Bugianesi, E.; Andreoletti, M.; Colli, A.; Vanni, E.; Bertelli, C.; Fatta, E.; Bignamini, D.; Marchesini, G.; *et al.* Risk of severe liver disease in nonalcoholic fatty liver disease with normal aminotransferase levels: Arole for insulin resistance and diabetes. *Hepatology* **2008**, *48*, 792–798. [CrossRef] [PubMed]

160. Ballestri, S.; Romagnoli, D.; Nascimbeni, F.; Francica, G.; Lonardo, A. Role of ultrasound in the diagnosis and treatment of nonalcoholic fatty liver disease and its complications. *Expert Rev. Gastroenterol. Hepatol.* **2015**, *9*, 603–627. [CrossRef] [PubMed]

161. Nascimbeni, F.; Loria, P.; Ratziu, V. Non-alcoholic fatty liver disease: Diagnosis and investigation. *Dig. Dis.* **2014**, *32*, 586–596. [CrossRef] [PubMed]

162. Younossi, Z.M.; Gramlich, T.; Matteoni, C.A.; Boparai, N.; McCullough, A.J. Nonalcoholic fatty liver disease in patients with type 2 diabetes. *Clin. Gastroenterol. Hepatol.* **2004**, *2*, 262–265. [CrossRef]

163. Hessheimer, A.J.; Forner, A.; Varela, M.; Bruix, J. Metabolic risk factors are a major comorbidity in patients with cirrhosis independent of the presence of hepatocellular carcinoma. *Eur. J. Gastroenterol. Hepatol.* **2010**, *22*, 1239–1244. [CrossRef] [PubMed]

164. Ertle, J.; Dechene, A.; Sowa, J.P.; Penndorf, V.; Herzer, K.; Kaiser, G.; Schlaak, J.F.; Gerken, G.; Syn, W.K.; Canbay, A. Non-alcoholic fatty liver disease progresses to hepatocellular carcinoma in the absence of apparent cirrhosis. *Int. J.Cancer* **2011**, *128*, 2436–2443. [CrossRef] [PubMed]

165. Yasui, K.; Hashimoto, E.; Komorizono, Y.; Koike, K.; Arii, S.; Imai, Y.; Shima, T.; Kanbara, Y.; Saibara, T.; Mori, T.; *et al.* Characteristics of patients with nonalcoholic steatohepatitis who develop hepatocellular carcinoma. *Clin. Gastroenterol. Hepatol.* **2011**, *9*, 428–433. [CrossRef] [PubMed]

166. Raff, E.J.; Kakati, D.; Bloomer, J.R.; Shoreibah, M.; Rasheed, K.; Singal, A.K. Diabetes mellitus predicts occurrence of cirrhosis and hepatocellular cancer in alcoholic liver and non-alcoholic fatty liver diseases. *J. Clin. Transl. Hepatol.* **2015**, *3*, 9–16. [CrossRef] [PubMed]

167. Giannini, E.G.; Marabotto, E.; Savarino, V.; Trevisani, F.; di Nolfo, M.A.; Del Poggio, P.; Benvegnu, L.; Farinati, F.; Zoli, M.; Borzio, F.; *et al.* Hepatocellular carcinoma in patients with cryptogenic cirrhosis. *Clin. Gastroenterol. Hepatol.* **2009**, *7*, 580–585. [CrossRef] [PubMed]

168. Piscaglia, F.; Svegliati-Baroni, G.; Barchetti, A.; Pecorelli, A.; Marinelli, S.; Tiribelli, C.; Bellentani, S. HCC-NAFLD Italian Study Group. Clinical patterns of hepatocellular carcinoma (HCC) in nonalcoholic fatty liver disease (NAFLD): Amulticenter prospective study. *Hepatology* **2016**, *63*, 827–838. [CrossRef] [PubMed]

169. Zoppini, G.; Fedeli, U.; Gennaro, N.; Saugo, M.; Targher, G.; Bonora, E. Mortality from chronic liver diseases in diabetes. *Am. J. Gastroenterol.* **2014**, *109*, 1020–1025. [CrossRef] [PubMed]

170. Wild, S.H.; Morling, J.R.; McAllister, D.A.; Kerssens, J.; Fischbacher, C.; Parkes, J.; Roderick, P.J.; Sattar, N.; Byrne, C.D. Scottish and Southampton Diabetes and Liver Disease Group and the Scottish Diabetes Research Network Epidemiology Group. Type 2 diabetes, chronic liver disease and hepatocellular cancer: A national retrospective cohort study using linked routine data. *J. Hepatol.* **2016**. [CrossRef] [PubMed]

171. Adams, L.A.; Harmsen, S.; St Sauver, J.L.; Charatcharoenwitthaya, P.; Enders, F.B.; Therneau, T.; Angulo, P. Nonalcoholic fatty liver disease increases risk of death among patients with diabetes: A community-based cohort study. *Am. J. Gastroenterol.* **2010**, *105*, 1567–1573. [CrossRef] [PubMed]

172. Ballestri, S.; Lonardo, A.; Bonapace, S.; Byrne, C.D.; Loria, P.; Targher, G. Risk of cardiovascular, cardiac and arrhythmic complications in patients with non-alcoholic fatty liver disease. *World J. Gastroenterol.* **2014**, *20*, 1724–1745. [CrossRef] [PubMed]

173. Lonardo, A.; Ballestri, S.; Targher, G.; Loria, P. Diagnosis and management of cardiovascular risk in nonalcoholic fatty liver disease. *Expert Rev. Gastroenterol. Hepatol.* **2015**, *9*, 629–650. [CrossRef] [PubMed]

174. Targher, G.; Bertolini, L.; Rodella, S.; Tessari, R.; Zenari, L.; Lippi, G.; Arcaro, G. Nonalcoholic fatty liver disease is independently associated with an increased incidence of cardiovascular events in type 2 diabetic patients. *Diabetes Care* **2007**, *30*, 2119–2121. [CrossRef] [PubMed]

175. Mantovani, A.; Ballestri, S.; Lonardo, A.; Targher, G. Cardiovascular disease and myocardial abnormalities in nonalcoholic fatty liver disease. *Dig. Dis. Sci.* **2016**. [CrossRef] [PubMed]

176. Naunyn, B. *Der Diabetes Melitis*; A Holder: Wienna, Austria, 1898.

177. Lonardo, A.; Adinolfi, L.E.; Petta, S.; Craxi, A.; Loria, P. Hepatitis C and diabetes: The inevitable coincidence? *Expert Rev. Anti. Infect. Ther.* **2009**, *7*, 293–308. [CrossRef] [PubMed]

178. Allison, M.E.; Wreghitt, T.; Palmer, C.R.; Alexander, G.J. Evidence for a link between hepatitis Cvirus infection and diabetes mellitus in a cirrhotic population. *J. Hepatol.* **1994**, *21*, 1135–1139. [CrossRef]

179. Searched on PubMed, Keywords: "HCV and diabetes". Available online: http://www.ncbi.nlm.nih.gov/pubmed/?term=HCV+and+diabetes (accessed on 24 January 2016).

180. Kohli, A.; Shaffer, A.; Sherman, A.; Kottilil, S. Treatment of hepatitis C: Asystematic review. *JAMA* **2014**, *312*, 631–640. [CrossRef] [PubMed]

181. Hajarizadeh, B.; Grebely, J.; Dore, G.J. Epidemiology and natural history of HCVinfection. *Nat. Rev. Gastroenterol. Hepatol.* **2013**, *10*, 553–562. [CrossRef] [PubMed]

182. Shire, N.J.; Sherman, K.E. Epidemiology of hepatitis Cvirus: Abattle on new frontiers. *Gastroenterol. Clin. N. Am.* **2015**, *44*, 699–716. [CrossRef] [PubMed]

183. Dultz, G.; Zeuzem, S. Hepatitis Cvirus: An European perspective. *Gastroenterol. Clin. N. Am.* **2015**, *44*, 807–824. [CrossRef] [PubMed]

184. Lozano, R.; Naghavi, M.; Foreman, K.; Lim, S.; Shibuya, K.; Aboyans, V.; Abraham, J.; Adair, T.; Aggarwal, R.; Ahn, S.Y.; *et al.* Global and regional mortality from 235 causes of death for 20 age groups in 1990 and 2010: Asystematic analysis for the global burden of disease study 2010. *Lancet* **2012**, *380*, 2095–2128. [CrossRef]

185. Wong, R.J.; Aguilar, M.; Cheung, R.; Perumpail, R.B.; Harrison, S.A.; Younossi, Z.M.; Ahmed, A. Nonalcoholic steatohepatitis is the second leading etiology of liver disease among adults awaiting liver transplantation in the united states. *Gastroenterology* **2015**, *148*, 547–555. [CrossRef] [PubMed]

186. Mehta, S.H.; Brancati, F.L.; Strathdee, S.A.; Pankow, J.S.; Netski, D.; Coresh, J.; Szklo, M.; Thomas, D.L. Hepatitis Cvirus infection and incident type 2 diabetes. *Hepatology* **2003**, *38*, 50–56. [CrossRef] [PubMed]

187. Rudoni, S.; Petit, J.M.; Bour, J.B.; Aho, L.S.; Castaneda, A.; Vaillant, G.; Verges, B.; Brun, J.M. HCV infection and diabetes mellitus: Influence of the use of finger stick devices on nosocomial transmission. *Diabetes Metab.* **1999**, *25*, 502–505. [PubMed]

188. Lonardo, A.; Carulli, N.; Loria, P. HCV and diabetes. A two-question-based reappraisal. *Dig. Liver Dis.* **2007**, *39*, 753–761. [CrossRef] [PubMed]

189. Lonardo, A.; Adinolfi, L.E.; Restivo, L.; Ballestri, S.; Romagnoli, D.; Baldelli, E.; Nascimbeni, F.; Loria, P. Pathogenesis and significance of hepatitis C virus steatosis: An update on survival strategy of a successful pathogen. *World J. Gastroenterol.* **2014**, *20*, 7089–7103. [CrossRef] [PubMed]

190. Petta, S.; Macaluso, F.S.; Camma, C.; Marco, V.D.; Cabibi, D.; Craxi, A. Hyperuricaemia: Another metabolic feature affecting the severity of chronic hepatitis because of HCV infection. *Liver Int.* **2012**, *32*, 1443–1450. [CrossRef] [PubMed]

191. Petta, S.; Maida, M.; Macaluso, F.S.; Barbara, M.; Licata, A.; Craxi, A.; Camma, C. Hepatitis C virus infection is associated with increased cardiovascular mortality: Ameta-analysis of observational studies. *Gastroenterology* **2016**, *150*, 145–155. [CrossRef] [PubMed]

192. Singal, A.G.; El-Serag, H.B. Hepatocellular carcinoma from epidemiology to prevention: Translating knowledge into practice. *Clin. Gastroenterol. Hepatol.* **2015**, *13*, 2140–2151. [CrossRef] [PubMed]

193. Dyal, H.K.; Aguilar, M.; Bartos, G.; Holt, E.W.; Bhuket, T.; Liu, B.; Cheung, R.; Wong, R.J. Diabetes mellitus increases risk of hepatocellular carcinoma in chronic hepatitis C virus patients: Asystematic review. *Dig. Dis. Sci.* **2016**, *61*, 636–645. [CrossRef] [PubMed]

194. Lecube, A.; Hernandez, C.; Genesca, J.; Simo, R. Proinflammatory cytokines, insulin resistance, and insulin secretion in chronic hepatitis C patients: A case-control study. *Diabetes Care* **2006**, *29*, 1096–1101. [CrossRef] [PubMed]

195. Knobler, H.; Zhornicky, T.; Sandler, A.; Haran, N.; Ashur, Y.; Schattner, A. Tumor necrosis factor-alpha-induced insulin resistance may mediate the hepatitis C virus diabetes association. *Am. J. Gastroenterol.* **2003**, *98*, 2751–2756. [CrossRef] [PubMed]

196. Zheng, Y.Y.; Wang, L.F.; Fan, X.H.; Wu, C.H.; Huo, N.; Lu, H.Y.; Xu, X.Y.; Wei, L. Association of suppressor of cytokine signalling 3 polymorphisms with insulin resistance in patients with chronic hepatitis C. *J. Viral Hepat.* **2013**, *20*, 273–280. [CrossRef] [PubMed]

197. Pazienza, V.; Vinciguerra, M.; Andriulli, A.; Mangia, A. Hepatitis C virus core protein genotype 3a increases SOCS-7 expression through PPAR-{gamma} in Huh-7 cells. *J. Gen. Virol.* **2010**, *91*, 1678–1686. [CrossRef] [PubMed]

198. Vanni, E.; Abate, M.L.; Gentilcore, E.; Hickman, I.; Gambino, R.; Cassader, M.; Smedile, A.; Ferrannini, E.; Rizzetto, M.; Marchesini, G.; *et al.* Sites and mechanisms of insulin resistance in nonobese, nondiabetic patients with chronic hepatitis C. *Hepatology* **2009**, *50*, 697–706. [CrossRef] [PubMed]

199. Milner, K.L.; van der Poorten, D.; Trenell, M.; Jenkins, A.B.; Xu, A.; Smythe, G.; Dore, G.J.; Zekry, A.; Weltman, M.; Fragomeli, V.; *et al.* Chronic hepatitis C is associated with peripheral rather than hepatic insulin resistance. *Gastroenterology* **2010**, *138*, 932–941. [CrossRef] [PubMed]

200. Uruha, A.; Noguchi, S.; Hayashi, Y.K.; Tsuburaya, R.S.; Yonekawa, T.; Nonaka, I.; Nishino, I. Hepatitis C virus infection in inclusion body myositis: A case-control study. *Neurology* **2016**, *86*, 211–217. [CrossRef] [PubMed]

201. Adinolfi, L.E.; Gambardella, M.; Andreana, A.; Tripodi, M.F.; Utili, R.; Ruggiero, G. Steatosis accelerates the progression of liver damage of chronic hepatitis C patients and correlates with specific HCV genotype and visceral obesity. *Hepatology* **2001**, *33*, 1358–1364. [CrossRef] [PubMed]

202. Guaraldi, G.; Lonardo, A.; Ballestri, S.; Zona, S.; Stentarelli, C.; Orlando, G.; Carli, F.; Carulli, L.; Roverato, A.; Loria, P. Human immunodeficiency virus is the major determinant of steatosis and hepatitis C virus of insulin resistance in virus-associated fatty liver disease. *Arch. Med. Res.* **2011**, *42*, 690–697. [CrossRef] [PubMed]

203. Lonardo, A.; Loria, P.; Carulli, N. Dysmetabolic changes associated with HCV: Adistinct syndrome? *Intern. Emerg. Med.* **2008**, *3*, 99–108. [CrossRef] [PubMed]

204. Adinolfi, L.E.; Restivo, L.; Zampino, R.; Lonardo, A.; Loria, P. Metabolic alterations and chronic hepatitis C: Treatment strategies. *Expert Opin. Pharmacother.* **2011**, *12*, 2215–2234. [CrossRef] [PubMed]

205. Loria, P.; Marchesini, G.; Nascimbeni, F.; Ballestri, S.; Maurantonio, M.; Carubbi, F.; Ratziu, V.; Lonardo, A. Cardiovascular risk, lipidemic phenotype and steatosis. A comparative analysis of cirrhotic and non-cirrhotic liver disease due to varying etiology. *Atherosclerosis* **2014**, *232*, 99–109. [CrossRef] [PubMed]

206. Mostafa, A.; Mohamed, M.K.; Saeed, M.; Hasan, A.; Fontanet, A.; Godsland, I.; Coady, E.; Esmat, G.; El-Hoseiny, M.; Abdul-Hamid, M.; *et al.* Hepatitis Cinfection and clearance: Impact on atherosclerosis and cardiometabolic risk factors. *Gut* **2010**, *59*, 1135–1140. [CrossRef] [PubMed]

207. Zampino, R.; Coppola, N.; Cirillo, G.; Boemio, A.; Pisaturo, M.; Marrone, A.; Macera, M.; Sagnelli, E.; Perrone, L.; Adinolfi, L.E.; *et al.* Abdominal fat interacts with PNPLA3 I148M, but not with the APOC3 variant in the pathogenesis of liver steatosis in chronic hepatitis C. *J. Viral Hepat.* **2013**, *20*, 517–523. [CrossRef] [PubMed]

208. Gordon, S.C.; Lamerato, L.E.; Rupp, L.B.; Holmberg, S.D.; Moorman, A.C.; Spradling, P.R.; Teshale, E.; Xu, F.; Boscarino, J.A.; Vijayadeva, V.; *et al.* Prevalence of cirrhosis in hepatitis Cpatients in the chronic hepatitis cohort study (CHeCS): A retrospective and prospective observational study. *Am. J. Gastroenterol.* **2015**, *110*, 1169–1177. [CrossRef] [PubMed]

209. Patel, S.; Jinjuvadia, R.; Patel, R.; Liangpunsakul, S. Insulin resistance is associated with significant liver fibrosis in chronic hepatitis C patients: Asystemic review and meta-analysis. *J. Clin. Gastroenterol.* **2016**, *50*, 80–84. [CrossRef] [PubMed]

210. Moucari, R.; Asselah, T.; Cazals-Hatem, D.; Voitot, H.; Boyer, N.; Ripault, M.P.; Sobesky, R.; Martinot-Peignoux, M.; Maylin, S.; Nicolas-Chanoine, M.H.; *et al.* Insulin resistance in chronic hepatitis C: Association with genotypes 1 and 4, serum HCVRNA level, and liver fibrosis. *Gastroenterology* **2008**, *134*, 416–423. [CrossRef] [PubMed]

211. Serste, T.; Nkuize, M.; Moucari, R.; Van Gossum, M.; Reynders, M.; Scheen, R.; Vertongen, F.; Buset, M.; Mulkay, J.P.; Marcellin, P. Metabolic disorders associated with chronic hepatitis C: Impact of genotype and ethnicity. *Liver Int.* **2010**, *30*, 1131–1136. [CrossRef] [PubMed]

212. Wang, C.S.; Yao, W.J.; Chang, T.T.; Wang, S.T.; Chou, P. The impact of type 2 diabetes on the development of hepatocellular carcinoma in different viral hepatitis statuses. *Cancer Epidemiol. Biomarkers Prev.* **2009**, *18*, 2054–2060. [CrossRef] [PubMed]

213. Arase, Y.; Kobayashi, M.; Suzuki, F.; Suzuki, Y.; Kawamura, Y.; Akuta, N.; Kobayashi, M.; Sezaki, H.; Saito, S.; Hosaka, T.; *et al.* Effect of type 2 diabetes on risk for malignancies includes hepatocellular carcinoma in chronic hepatitis C. *Hepatology* **2013**, *57*, 964–973. [CrossRef] [PubMed]

214. Bruno, S.; Crosignani, A.; Maisonneuve, P.; Rossi, S.; Silini, E.; Mondelli, M.U. Hepatitis C virus genotype 1b as a major risk factor associated with hepatocellular carcinoma in patients with cirrhosis: Aseventeen-year prospective cohort study. *Hepatology* **2007**, *46*, 1350–1356. [CrossRef] [PubMed]

215. Adinolfi, L.E.; Zampino, R.; Restivo, L.; Lonardo, A.; Guerrera, B.; Marrone, A.; Nascimbeni, F.; Florio, A.; Loria, P. Chronic hepatitis C virus infection and atherosclerosis: Clinical impact and mechanisms. *World J. Gastroenterol.* **2014**, *20*, 3410–3417. [CrossRef] [PubMed]

216. Adinolfi, L.E.; Restivo, L.; Zampino, R.; Guerrera, B.; Lonardo, A.; Ruggiero, L.; Riello, F.; Loria, P.; Florio, A. Chronic HCV infection is a risk of atherosclerosis. Role of HCVand HCV-related steatosis. *Atherosclerosis* **2012**, *221*, 496–502. [CrossRef] [PubMed]

217. Petta, S.; Torres, D.; Fazio, G.; Camma, C.; Cabibi, D.; Di Marco, V.; Licata, A.; Marchesini, G.; Mazzola, A.; Parrinello, G.; et al. Carotid atherosclerosis and chronic hepatitis C: A prospective study of risk associations. *Hepatology* **2012**, *55*, 1317–1323. [CrossRef] [PubMed]

218. Targher, G.; Bertolini, L.; Padovani, R.; Rodella, S.; Arcaro, G.; Day, C. Differences and similarities in early atherosclerosis between patients with non-alcoholic steatohepatitis and chronic hepatitis Band C. *J. Hepatol.* **2007**, *46*, 1126–1132. [CrossRef] [PubMed]

219. Gill, K.; Ghazinian, H.; Manch, R.; Gish, R. Hepatitis C virus as a systemic disease: Reaching beyond the liver. *Hepatol. Int.* **2015**. in press. [CrossRef] [PubMed]

220. Domont, F.; Cacoub, P. Chronic hepatitis C virus infection, a new cardiovascular risk factor? *Liver Int.* **2016**. [CrossRef] [PubMed]

221. Backus, L.I.; Belperio, P.S.; Shahoumian, T.A.; Loomis, T.P.; Mole, L.A. Effectiveness of sofosbuvir-based regimens in genotype 1 and 2 hepatitis C virus infection in 4026 U.S. Veterans. *Aliment. Pharmacol. Ther.* **2015**, *42*, 559–573. [CrossRef] [PubMed]

222. Rinella, M.E. Nonalcoholic fatty liver disease: A systematic review. *JAMA* **2015**, *313*, 2263–2273. [CrossRef] [PubMed]

223. Montesi, L.; Caselli, C.; Centis, E.; Nuccitelli, C.; Moscatiello, S.; Suppini, A.; Marchesini, G. Physical activity support or weight loss counseling for nonalcoholic fatty liver disease? *World J. Gastroenterol.* **2014**, *20*, 10128–10136. [CrossRef] [PubMed]

224. Oliveira, C.P.; de Lima Sanches, P.; de Abreu-Silva, E.O.; Marcadenti, A. Nutrition and physical activity in nonalcoholic fatty liver disease. *J. Diabetes Res.* **2016**, *2016*, 4597246. [CrossRef] [PubMed]

225. Hallsworth, K.; Avery, L.; Trenell, M.I. Targeting lifestyle behavior change in adults with NAFLD during a 20-min consultation: Summary of the dietary and exercise literature. *Curr. Gastroenterol. Rep.* **2016**, *18*, 11. [CrossRef] [PubMed]

226. Hickman, I.J.; Clouston, A.D.; Macdonald, G.A.; Purdie, D.M.; Prins, J.B.; Ash, S.; Jonsson, J.R.; Powell, E.E. Effect of weight reduction on liver histology and biochemistry in patients with chronic hepatitis C. *Gut* **2002**, *51*, 89–94. [CrossRef] [PubMed]

10

NAFLD and Increased Aortic Stiffness: Parallel or Common Physiopathological Mechanisms?

Cristiane A. Villela-Nogueira, Nathalie C. Leite, Claudia R. L. Cardoso and Gil F. Salles *

Department of Internal Medicine, Medical School and University Hospital Clementino Fraga Filho, Universidade Federal do Rio de Janeiro, Rua Croton 72, Rio de Janeiro 22750-240, Brasil; crisvillelanog@gmail.com (C.A.V.-N.); nathaliecleite@gmail.com (N.C.L.); claudiacardoso@hucff.ufrj.br (C.R.L.C.)
* Correspondence: gilsalles@hucff.ufrj.br

Academic Editor: Giovanni Targher

Abstract: Non-alcoholic fatty liver disease (NAFLD) has become the leading cause of chronic liver diseases worldwide. Liver inflammation and fibrosis related to NAFLD contribute to disease progression and increasing liver-related mortality and morbidity. Increasing data suggest that NAFLD may be linked to atherosclerotic vascular disease independent of other established cardiovascular risk factors. Central arterial stiffness has been recognized as a measure of cumulative cardiovascular risk marker load, and the measure of carotid-femoral pulse wave velocity (cf-PWV) is regarded as the gold standard assessment of aortic stiffness. It has been shown that increased aortic stiffness predicts cardiovascular morbidity and mortality in several clinical settings, including type 2 diabetes mellitus, a well-known condition associated with advanced stages of NAFLD. Furthermore, recently-published studies reported a strong association between NAFLD and increased arterial stiffness, suggesting a possible link in the pathogenesis of atherosclerosis and NAFLD. We sought to review the published data on the associations between NAFLD and aortic stiffness, in order to better understand the interplay between these two conditions and identify possible common physiopathological mechanisms.

Keywords: non-alcoholic fatty liver disease; steatohepatitis; liver fibrosis; arterial stiffness; pulse wave velocity

1. Introduction

Non-alcoholic fatty liver disease (NAFLD) is currently the most prevalent chronic liver disease worldwide and the most frequent cause of abnormal liver enzymes in daily practice [1]. It is clearly related to metabolic syndrome, and its association with progressive liver fibrosis leading to cirrhosis and hepatocellular carcinoma has also been well established [2–5]. In addition to liver disease, NAFLD is also associated with extrahepatic diseases. Type 2 diabetes mellitus, an increasingly prevalent disease worldwide, is currently regarded as one of NAFLD's main risk factors, and it correlates with the severest histological aspects of NAFLD, with a growing prevalence of hepatocellular carcinoma [6–9]. Furthermore, NAFLD has also been linked to increased cardiovascular risk. A recent meta-analysis showed a 57% increase in overall mortality in patients with NAFLD, not only related to liver disease, but also due to cardiovascular disease (CVD) [10].

Regarding epidemiological aspects, NAFLD affects nearly 20% of the population worldwide, with its highest prevalence being described in South America (35%) and in Middle East (32%) [11]. In patients with associated risk factors, such as morbidly obese patients, NAFLD prevalence can achieve rates as high as 80% [12].

The spectrum of NAFLD encompasses a group of distinct liver diseases. Excluding alcohol ingestion greater than 20 g/day in women and 30 g/day in men and additional specific causes of steatosis, such as drug-induced and malnutrition among others, NAFLD ranges from simple steatosis, defined when at least 5% of hepatocytes are affected by fat; steatohepatitis (NASH), which comprises inflammation with ballooning; and ultimately, fibrosis, evolving to cirrhosis and its complications, such as hepatocellular carcinoma [13,14].

Increased arterial stiffness is an established cardiovascular risk marker in several clinical settings and had been proposed to reflect the cumulative burden of cardiovascular risk factors on the vascular wall [15,16]. Moreover, some recent studies have reported strong associations between increased aortic stiffness and NAFLD, particularly at its more advanced stages [17]. Hence, the aim of this review is to provide a comprehensive overview of previous studies assessing relationships between NAFLD and increased arterial stiffness in order to better understand the interplay between these two conditions and identify possible common physiopathological mechanisms.

2. Cardiovascular Risk and Non-Alcoholic Fatty Liver Disease (NAFLD)

Growing evidence has shown that NAFLD may be closely related to atherosclerotic vascular disease over and beyond other well-known cardiovascular risk factors [18,19]. Cardiovascular disease is the most common cause of mortality among patients with NAFLD [20,21]. Kim *et al.*, in 4023 individuals without any suspicion of liver disease or coronary artery disease, described that increased coronary artery calcification scores were associated with the presence of NAFLD, independent of traditional risk factors and of visceral adiposity, suggesting that NAFLD might be a risk factor for coronary artery disease [22]. A recent meta-analysis showed that NAFLD was associated with increased carotid-artery intima media thickness, impaired flow-mediated vasodilatation, increased arterial stiffness and increased coronary artery calcification. These associations were all independent of known risk factors and metabolic syndrome traits in a wide range of patient populations [23]. Further, the Framingham Heart study observed, among 3014 participants who performed a multidetector computed tomography (CT)-scan, that there was a significant association between NAFLD and coronary artery calcium and a trend towards a significant association between hepatic steatosis and previous clinical cardiovascular disease [24]. In a cohort of 755 healthy males who performed 18F-fluorodeoxyglucose (FDG) positron emission tomography with computed tomography, patients with NAFLD showed elevated carotid FDG uptake, besides an augmented carotid intima media thickness. These findings hinted that they might be at an increased risk of having inflammatory atherosclerotic plaques in the carotid arteries [25]. Targher *et al.* also demonstrated that patients with steatohepatitis when compared to those with simple steatosis and to controls had a greater carotid artery intima media thickness. Moreover, the same study showed that the histologic severity of nonalcoholic steatohepatitis was also related to carotid artery intima media thickness, regardless of traditional cardiovascular risk factors, insulin resistance and metabolic syndrome elements [26]. In resume, there is well-established evidence of associations between NAFLD and clinical and pre-clinical cardiovascular diseases.

Nevertheless, the physiopathological mechanisms underlying the associations between NAFLD and cardiovascular disease development are much debated, but still largely unsettled. Yoneda *et al.* showed, for the first time, elevated levels of high-sensitivity C-reactive protein (hs-CRP) in patients with biopsy-proven NASH, implying there may be a shared pathway between the severity of liver disease and the levels of hs-CRP, a well-known marker of cardiovascular risk [27]. Some studies observed that intrahepatic messenger RNA expression of C-reactive protein, interleukin-6 or plasminogen activator inhibitor 1 (PAI-1) was associated with the severest forms of NAFLD, mostly steatohepatitis [27–29]. Wieckoswska *et al.* correlated interleukin-6 liver expression with plasma levels and liver histology in patients with NASH and diabetes, hinting at a possible link between NAFLD and insulin resistance [28]. Similarly, Thuy *et al.* demonstrated an association between PAI-1, ingestion of a fructose-enriched diet and NAFLD [29]. Cigolini *et al.* also showed that increased PAI-1 was correlated with liver steatosis, implying that it might be mediated by concomitant alterations in plasma triglycerides and insulin concentrations [30]. In the same direction, Targher *et al.* reported that levels of fibrinogen and PAI-1 activity were higher in men with NASH, as well as plasma hs-CRP levels. They also had lower adiponectin levels compared to overweight men without steatosis with comparable visceral adiposity, suggesting that nonalcoholic steatohepatitis may be a factor for a more atherogenic risk profile besides its contribution to visceral adiposity [31]. In this setting, adiponectin concentrations may play a role [32–34]. Higher adiponectin levels were associated with a minor risk of myocardial infarction on a nested case control study among 18,225 male participants [33]. Low adiponectin levels are frequently observed in patients with NAFLD. We evaluated cytokine levels in 84 diabetic patients with biopsy-proven NAFLD: patients with NASH or with advanced fibrosis had equal cytokine levels to those without NASH or with absent/light fibrosis, except for lower serum adiponectin levels [34].

3. Prognostic Markers: The Role of Fibrosis

The conundrum of NAFLD is to identify patients whose disease will progress and impact survival. The natural history of NAFLD is a dynamic process that has been frequently revised. NAFLD has been considered a stable disease that seldom leads to advanced fibrosis. In a long-term follow-up study, only 1% of patients with simple steatosis presented cirrhosis, whereas among those with NASH, 11% developed cirrhosis and 7.3% died from a liver-related cause after 15.6 years of follow-up [35]. Overall liver-related survival was reduced in Swedish subjects with NAFLD and NASH, particularly in those with significant liver fibrosis, whereas bland steatosis was not associated with any increase in mortality risk, compared to the Swedish general population, followed for a median of 21 years [36]. Thus, current studies support the concept that the presence and severity of liver fibrosis on liver biopsy is the main surrogate marker of long-term prognosis. Hence, it would be important to implement accurate non-invasive markers to identify fibrosis to help to manage high risk patients.

Besides identifying early fibrosis, the recognition of patients who might be at risk for fibrosis progression is of utmost importance in order to define the best management for this specific population. Studies with paired biopsies identified clinical and biochemical aspects that helped in risk stratification regarding fibrosis progression. A recent meta-analysis [37], which included 11 cohort studies with biopsy-proven NAFLD (150 with simple steatosis and 261 with NASH), described that arterial hypertension and a low AST/ALT ratio at baseline predicted liver fibrosis progression. In this meta-analysis, two subgroups of patients were identified according to the rate of fibrosis progression: rapid and slow progressors. The first group comprised 21.1% of patients who had Stage 0 fibrosis at baseline, but in an average of 5.9 years developed fibrosis Stages 3 or 4. The majority of patients were categorized in the second group, which consisted of patients who had low fibrosis progression rate, changing their subsequent biopsies by one or two stages. Two of four studies in the systematic review observed that patients with a higher steatosis grade were more likely to develop progressive fibrosis. Remarkably, in this meta-analysis, no association was found between baseline severity of necroinflammation and risk of progressive fibrosis. This led to the concept that both patients with simple steatosis and with NASH may develop progressive liver fibrosis [37]. However, comparing patients with simple steatosis and NASH at baseline who had no fibrosis at baseline (F0), the rate of fibrosis progression was twice faster in patients with NASH (0.14 *vs.* 0.07 stages). Hence, although fibrosis progression was observed in both groups, it was slower in the simple steatosis group. Nevertheless, these findings differ from those reported in a previous meta-analysis of patients with NASH [38]. It estimated an overall fibrosis progression of 0.03 stages per year, and only age and inflammation on initial biopsy were predictors of progression to advanced fibrosis. Otherwise, in a review of 70 patients with untreated NAFLD who performed two liver biopsies with an interval of more than one year, a significant proportion of patients with NAFLD progressed towards well-defined NASH with bridging fibrosis, especially if metabolic risk factors deteriorated [39]. In this study, even mild inflammation or fibrosis could be considered as prognostic markers, increasing the risk of progression when compared to steatosis alone [39]. It is thus important to define two distinct situations in NAFLD that is simple steatosis, which seems to have a benign course with slower liver fibrosis progression, and steatosis with inflammation that could point to a progressive disease [40].

4. Aortic Stiffness and NAFLD

Arterial stiffness is the consequence of a complex interaction between stable and dynamic effects in structural and cellular components of the vascular wall. These vascular changes result from hemodynamic forces and extrinsic factors, like hormones, salt and glucose regulation. Arterial stiffness depends on the structural and geometric properties of the arterial wall and on the distending pressure. Its main determinants are aging and blood pressure [41,42]. Increased arterial stiffness occurs in a heterogeneous pattern predominantly on central segments, sparing peripheral arteries [43]. The stability, resiliency and compliancy properties of the vascular wall rely on two important scaffolding proteins: collagen and elastin. The quantity of such molecules is generally kept stable by a slow, but dynamic interplay of production and degradation. Deregulation of this balance, which may be stimulated by an inflammatory milieu, may lead to overproduction of altered collagen and reduced quantities of normal elastin, leading to increased arterial stiffness [44]. Prevalent diseases, such as arterial hypertension and diabetes mellitus in conjunction with ageing, augment these vascular alterations that worsen artery stiffening in different and synergistic ways. The evaluation of carotid-femoral pulse wave velocity (cf-PWV) can be easily obtained and is regarded as the gold standard method of assessing central aortic stiffness [40]. Further, increased aortic stiffness has been shown to predict cardiovascular morbidity and mortality in individuals with end-stage renal disease [45], hypertension [46], diabetes [47] and in general population-based samples [48,49].

Several previous studies [50–65], resumed in Table 1, have evaluated the relationships between NAFLD and arterial stiffness. All studies, except two of them [64,65], had cross-sectional designs, and all confirmed an association between increased arterial stiffness and NAFLD (mainly detected by ultrasonography), independent of other traditional cardiometabolic risk factors. Of note, one of these studies [56] demonstrated that the association between NAFLD and increased arterial stiffness was already present at adolescence. In this study, on a 17-year old population cohort from Australia, two groups were categorized according to their metabolic profile as a "high risk" and a "low risk" metabolic cluster. Central PWV was evaluated in both group, and NAFLD was diagnosed by abdominal ultrasound. Males and females with NAFLD in the presence of the metabolic cluster had greater PWV. They concluded that NAFLD was associated with increased arterial stiffness only in the presence of the "high risk" metabolic cluster, suggesting that arterial stiffness associated with NAFLD was linked to the presence of an adverse metabolic profile in adolescents [56]. However, because of their cross-sectional designs, no causal deductions could be drawn, only mere correlations. Of note, only three studies were performed in patients with NAFLD confirmed by histologic evaluation [52,57,62]. Sunbul et al. [57] evaluated in 100 biopsy-proven NAFLD patients the relation among arterial stiffness measures and the histological severity of NAFLD and epicardial fat thickness. Among the included patients matched to 50 control individuals, 33% were diabetic, and 55% fulfilled the criteria for metabolic syndrome. Measurements of arterial stiffness using cf-PWV and the augmentation index (AIx) were performed, and epicardial fat thickness was assessed by echocardiography. Patients with NAFLD showed significantly higher aortic PWV (7.0 ± 1.1 vs. 6.2 ± 0.8 m/s, $p < 0.001$) and AIx values ($22.2\% \pm 13.1\%$ vs. $17.4\% \pm 12.3\%$, $p = 0.02$) compared to controls, after adjusting for all potential confounders. Their results corroborated that NAFLD patients had an increased arterial stiffness, which was independently related to the severity of the liver fibrosis and increased epicardial fat thickness [57]. Otherwise, Ozturk et al. [62], evaluating 61 biopsy-proven NAFLD patients and 40 matched controls, found significant associations between NAFLD and aortic stiffness, independent of the presence of metabolic syndrome; but no correlation with histological liver fibrosis or inflammatory activity. Chen et al. [60] also described the association of advanced fibrosis with subclinical atherosclerosis in 2550 participants with ultrasound-diagnosed NAFLD. In this study, the NAFLD fibrosis score was calculated to assess the severity of the fibrosis of NAFLD patients. An NAFLD score >0.676

indicated the presence of advanced fibrosis in their study. The indicators of early atherosclerosis in the study were the carotid intima media thickness, carotid plaques and brachial-ankle pulse wave velocity (ba-PWV). They found that advanced fibrosis indicated by the NAFLD score was associated with carotid intima media thickness, with the presence of carotid plaques and with increased arterial stiffness, independent of usual cardiometabolic risk factors and insulin resistance [60]. There are only two longitudinal studies [64,65] evaluating the progression of arterial stiffness and the presence of NAFLD. The first one [64], with two arterial stiffness evaluations, employed brachial-ankle PWV, hence measuring principally peripheral arterial stiffness. It was accomplished in 1225 individuals on a five-year follow-up. This study concluded that individuals with NAFLD at first evaluation (diagnosed by ultrasonography) had a faster arterial stiffening than individuals without NAFLD, regardless of the concomitance of metabolic syndrome. We [65] performed serial cf-PWV measurements and evaluated liver fibrosis by transient elastography in 291 diabetic patients with NAFLD over a median follow-up of seven years. We observed that both a high aortic stiffness at the second cf-PWV examination (odds ratio (OR): 3.0; 95% confidence interval (CI): 1.3–7.2; $p = 0.011$) and a further augment in aortic stiffness (OR: 2.1; 95% CI: 1.0–4.3; $p = 0.046$) pointed to the increased likelihood of presenting advanced liver fibrosis on transient elastography examination [65]. Thus, it is possible that the chronological longitudinal associations between NAFLD and arterial stiffness may be bidirectional: NAFLD may hasten arterial stiffness progression, whilst increasing aortic stiffness may lead prior NAFLD in the direction of advanced liver fibrosis [65].

Table 1. Studies evaluating associations between non-alcoholic fatty liver disease (NAFLD) and arterial stiffness.

Author, Year	Number of Participants and Methods of Liver Investigation	Study Design	Aims	Conclusions
Shiotani et al., 2005 [50]	353 young university Japanese adults, submitted to abdominal ultrasound.	Transversal	To evaluate the validity of noninvasive ba-PWV measurements in overweight young adults.	ba-PWV was increased in males with NAFLD and might conceivably be useful to predict NAFLD.
Salvi et al., 2010 [51]	220 participants (123 women), aged between 30 and 70 years, from the Cardio-gambettola observatory liver steatosis estimation (GOOSE) study, submitted to abdominal ultrasound.	Transversal	To evaluate the relationship between metabolic syndrome, NAFLD and subclinical vascular disease, evaluated by carotid IMT and cf-PWV.	A possible independent role of NAFLD in determining arterial stiffness.
Vlachopoulos et al., 2010 [52]	23 biopsy-proven NAFLD patients and 28 matched controls.	Transversal	To investigate associations between NAFLD and functional arterial changes and early atherosclerosis.	NAFLD was associated with endothelial dysfunction and aortic stiffness (cf-PWV).
Kim et al., 2012 [53]	4467 patients submitted to abdominal ultrasound.	Transversal	To evaluate the association of NAFLD and ba-PWV in patients with and without metabolic syndrome.	NAFLD was independently associated with increased ba-PWV, irrespective of multiple covariates, only in patients without metabolic syndrome.
Huang et al., 2012 [54]	8632 Chinese from a population-based sample; NAFLD detected by ultrasound.	Transversal	To evaluate associations between NAFLD and early atherosclerosis (carotid IMT and ba-PWV).	NAFLD was associated with increased carotid IMT and ba-PWV, independent of traditional CV risk factors and metabolic syndrome.
Lee et al., 2012 [55]	1442 healthy adults; NAFLD detected by ultrasound.	Transversal	To evaluate association between NAFLD and arterial stiffness (ba-PWV).	Arterial stiffness was associated with NAFD, independent of classical CV risk factors.
Huang et al., 2013 [56]	964 adolescents (17-year-olds) from an Australian birth cohort, submitted to abdominal ultrasound.	Transversal	To examine if NAFLD was associated with aortic PWV, independent of cardiometabolic factors.	Aortic PWV was related to the presence of NAFLD that was predicated by the presence of an adverse metabolic profile in adolescents.
Sunbul et al., 2014 [57]	100 patients with biopsy-proven NAFLD and 50 age- and sex-matched controls.	Transversal	To examine the relationship between aortic PWV and AIx, the histological severity of NAFLD and epicardial fat thickness (EFT).	Patients with NAFLD have an increased arterial stiffness, which reflects both the severity of liver fibrosis and increased EFT values.
Omelchenko et al., 2014 [58]	52 NAFLD patients detected by ultrasound.	Transversal	To evaluate associations between adiponectin levels and arterial stiffness parameters (cf-PWV and AIx).	Adiponectin remained a significant predictor of PWV, even after controlling for age and gender, suggesting an active role of adiponectin in the pathophysiology of vascular disease in NAFLD patients.

Table 1. *Cont.*

Author, Year	Number of Participants and Methods of Liver Investigation	Study Design	Aims	Conclusions
Yu *et al.*, 2014 [59]	1296 non-obese, non-hypertensive, non-diabetic adults, NAFLD by ultrasound.	Transversal	To evaluate then association between NAFLD and arterial stiffness (ba-PWV).	NAFLD was associated with ba-PWV in Chinese individuals without obesity, hypertension and diabetes.
Chen *et al.*, 2015 [60]	2550 participants with ultrasound-confirmed NAFLD from a community-based sample.	Transversal	To evaluate whether advanced fibrosis assessed by NAFLD fibrosis score was associated with subclinical atherosclerosis in NAFLD patients.	Advanced fibrosis was associated with carotid intima media thickness, the presence of carotid plaques and arterial stiffness, independent of cardiometabolic risk factors and insulin resistance.
Chou *et al.*, 2015 [61]	4860 non-diabetic, pre-diabetic and newly-diagnosed T2DM individuals, evaluated by abdominal ultrasound.	Transversal	To evaluate PWV in patients with NAFLD.	The effect of NAFLD on arterial stiffness was apparent only in subjects with normal glucose tolerance.
Ozturk *et al.*, 2015 [62]	61 biopsy-proven NAFLD patients and 41 controls without NAFLD; adult male patients between 20 and 40 years of age.	Transversal	To evaluate the relationship between NAFLD and subclinical atherosclerosis and to investigate the associations according to the presence or absence of metabolic syndrome.	The presence of NAFLD was associated with endothelial dysfunction and atherosclerosis, independent of metabolic syndrome.
Chung *et al.*, 2015 [63]	2954 healthy individuals; NAFLD detected by ultrasound.	Transversal	To evaluate the association between NAFLD and arterial stiffness (cardio-ankle vascular index).	NAFLD was associated with increased arterial stiffness, independent of cardio-metabolic risk factors.
Li *et al.*, 2015 [64]	728 men and 497 women without hypertension and diabetes; NAFLD detected by ultrasound.	Longitudinal	To evaluate the relationship between the presence of NAFLD at baseline and progression of arterial stiffness (ba-PWV) during follow-up (5 years).	Patients with NAFLD had a faster progression of arterial stiffness, independent of other CV risk factors.
Leite *et al.*, 2015 [65]	291 T2DM patients; NAFLD by abdominal ultrasound or liver biopsy.	Longitudinal	To evaluate the association between progressions of aortic PWV (7 years of follow-up) with advanced liver fibrosis identified by transient elastography.	High or increasing aortic stiffness predicted the development of advanced liver fibrosis on transient elastography.

Abbreviations: T2DM, type-2 diabetes mellitus; NAFLD, non-alcoholic fatty liver disease; cf-PWV, carotid-femoral pulse-wave velocity; ba-PWV, brachial-ankle pulse wave velocity; AIx, arterial augmentation index; IMT, intima media thickness.

5. NAFLD and Arterial Stiffness: Is There an Interplay?

Many studies evaluated if NAFLD contributed to other outcomes, such as cardiovascular mortality; and most of them demonstrated an association, but no causality could be shown [20]. Liver disease and atherogenesis might be mediated by inflamed visceral adipose tissue. In this scenario, the liver might play a role of both the target of the resulting systemic abnormalities and as the source of many proatherogenic variables. In this setting, nonalcoholic steatohepatitis might contribute to the pathogenesis of cardiovascular disease in two ways: first, through the systemic release of several inflammatory, prothrombotic and oxidative-stress substances and, second, through the contribution of nonalcoholic fatty liver disease to insulin resistance and atherogenic dyslipidemia.

Insulin resistance is the utmost important factor that triggers the development of NAFLD. This notwithstanding, insulin resistance is probably one of the mechanisms that is also linked to increased arterial stiffness. Both chronic hyperglycemia, as well as hyperinsulinemia have been demonstrated to increase the local activity of the renin-angiotensin-aldosterone system and also the expression of the angiotensin type I receptor in the vascular milieu, leading to hypertrophy of vascular wall and fibrosis [66–68]. Due to insulin resistance, the proliferative effects of hyperinsulinemia prevails and promotes an impairment of phosphatidylinositol 3 (PI3)-kinase-dependent signaling responsible for the acute metabolic effects of insulin; still preserving the activity of growth promoting mitogen-activated kinase pathways [69]. Triglyceride in the liver has been considered as an epiphenomenon being a marker of a dysmetabolic state, not adding directly to the genesis of the extrahepatic manifestations of this complication.

Omelchenko et al. evaluated the relation between the levels of adiponectin and arterial stiffness parameters using pulse wave velocity (PWV) and the arterial augmentation index (Aix) in NAFLD patients [58]. In their study, adiponectin was positively correlated with Aix ($r = 0.467$; $p < 0.0001$) and with PWV ($r = 0.348$; $p = 0.011$), in spite of a weak correlation coefficient. In a multiple linear regression analysis, adiponectin persisted as a significant predictor of abnormal PWV after controlling for age and gender, suggesting an active role of adiponectin in the pathophysiology of vascular disease in NAFLD patients [58]. Remarkably, it was observed by Kim et al. [53] that NAFLD and arterial stiffness have been related even in the absence of arterial hypertension, diabetes and metabolic syndrome.

Abdominal ultrasound and brachial-ankle pulse wave velocity (ba-PWV) were investigated in 4467 individuals. NAFLD individuals were classified in non-NAFLD, mild and moderate-to-severe NAFLD groups, respectively. The NAFLD group had higher levels of ba-PWV. NAFLD was independently associated with increased ba-PWV ($\geq$1366 cm/s), independent of multiple covariates (OR: 1.24 and 95% CI: 1.05–1.46). Subgroup analyses revealed that there was a significant association between NAFLD and increased ba-PWV only in individuals without metabolic syndrome (OR: 1.27 and 95% CI: 1.07–1.51). The multivariate linear regression models for the overall study population and for individuals without metabolic syndrome also showed a significant association between NAFLD and the absolute values of ba-PWV; however, the result for individuals with metabolic syndrome did not demonstrate an association [53]. This might point to the possibility that NAFLD pathogenetic mechanism per se could be linked to abnormal arterial stiffness not requiring the coexistence of metabolic syndrome for its occurrence. Recently, Chou et al. [61] investigated 4860 subjects who were categorized into normal glucose tolerance, pre-diabetes and newly-diagnosed diabetes groups and, after excluding known diabetes, the independent relationship between non-alcoholic fatty liver disease and arterial stiffness. The severity of non-alcoholic fatty liver disease was divided into mild and moderate-to-severe. Increased arterial stiffness was defined as brachial-ankle pulse wave velocity (ba-PWV) >1400 cm/s. They concluded that the effect of NAFLD on arterial stiffness was apparent in subjects with normal glucose tolerance, but not in diabetes and pre-diabetes [61].

In resume, the possible biological mechanisms linking NAFLD and increased arterial stiffness remain largely unknown, but possibly involve common pathways of chronic low-grade inflammation and adipokines imbalance [70,71]. More prospective studies, including diabetic and non-diabetic patients, are necessary to investigate whether there are causal relationships between them. On the other hand, aortic stiffness, ideally measured by carotid-femoral PWV, may be a useful tool to identify high-risk patients concerning both cardiovascular and liver disease. Its use as a prognostic marker may help define better strategies to slow the progression of both liver and cardiovascular disease. In the future, prospective studies with serial PWV and liver disease severity evaluation may confirm its utility in assessing improvement in both scenarios' outcomes.

Acknowledgments: This study was supported by grants from Conselho Brasileiro de Desenvolvimento Científico e Tecnológico (CNPq-Brazil) and Fundação Carlos Chagas Filho de Amparo à Pesquisa do Estado do Rio de Janeiro (FAPERJ-Brazil).

Author Contributions: Cristiane A. Villela-Nogueira reviewed the literature and drafted the manuscript; Nathalie C. Leite, Claudia R. L. Cardoso and Gil F. Salles revised the manuscript and contributed with important intellectual content.

References

1. Angulo, P. Nonalcoholic fatty liver disease. *N. Engl. J. Med.* **2002**, *346*, 1221–1231. [PubMed]
2. Marchesini, G.; Bugianesi, E.; Forlani, G.; Cerrelli, F.; Lenzi, M.; Manini, R.; Natale, S.; Vanni, E.; Villanova, N.; Melchionda, N.; *et al.* Nonalcoholic fatty liver, steatohepatitis, and the metabolic syndrome. *Hepatology* **2003**, *37*, 917–923. [CrossRef] [PubMed]
3. Bedogni, G.; Miglioli, L.; Masutti, F.; Tiribelli, C.; Marchesini, G.; Bellentani, S. Prevalence of and risk factors for nonalcoholic fatty liver disease: The Dionysos nutrition and liver study. *Hepatology* **2005**, *42*, 44–52. [CrossRef] [PubMed]
4. Bhala, N.; Angulo, P.; van der Poorten, D.; Lee, E.; Hui, J.M.; Saracco, G.; Adams, L.A.; Charatcharoenwitthaya, P.; Topping, J.H.; Bugianesi, E.; *et al.* The natural history of nonalcoholic fatty liver disease with advanced fibrosis or cirrhosis: An international collaborative study. *Hepatology* **2011**, *54*, 1208–1216. [CrossRef] [PubMed]
5. White, D.L.; Kanwal, F.; El-Serag, H.B. Association between nonalcoholic fatty liver disease and risk for hepatocellular cancer, based on systematic review. *Clin. Gastroenterol. Hepatol.* **2012**, *10*, 1342–1359. [CrossRef] [PubMed]
6. Hossain, N.; Afendy, A.; Stepanova, M.; Nader, F.; Srishord, M.; Rafiq, N.; Goodman, Z.; Younossi, Z. Independent predictors of fibrosis in patients with nonalcoholic fatty liver disease. *Clin. Gastroenterol. Hepatol.* **2009**, *7*, 1224–1229. [CrossRef] [PubMed]
7. Prashanth, M.; Ganesh, H.K.; Vima, M.V.; John, M.; Bandgar, T.; Joshi, S.R.; Shah, S.R.; Rathi, P.M.; Joshi, A.S.; Thakkar, H.; *et al.* Prevalence of nonalcoholic fatty liver disease in patients with type 2 diabetes mellitus. *J. Assoc. Physicians India* **2009**, *57*, 205–210. [PubMed]
8. Leite, N.; Villela-Nogueira, C.; Pannain, V.; Bottino, A.; Rezende, G.; Cardoso, C.; Salles, G. Histopathological stages of nonalcoholic fatty liver disease in type 2 diabetes: Prevalences and correlated factors. *Liver Int.* **2011**, *31*, 700–706. [CrossRef] [PubMed]
9. Mittal, S.; El-Serag, H.B.; Sada, Y.H.; Kanwal, F.; Duan, Z.; Temple, S.; May, S.B.; Kramer, J.R.; Richardson, P.A.; Davila, J.A. Hepatocellular carcinoma in the absence of cirrhosis in United States veterans is associated with nonalcoholic fatty liver disease. *Clin. Gastroenterol. Hepatol.* **2016**, *14*, 124–131. [CrossRef] [PubMed]
10. Musso, G.; Gambino, R.; Cassader, M.; Pagano, G. Meta-analysis: Natural history of non-alcoholic fatty liver disease (NAFLD) and diagnostic accuracy of non-invasive tests for liver disease severity. *Ann. Med.* **2011**, *43*, 617–649. [CrossRef] [PubMed]
11. Younossi, Z.M.; Koenig, A.B.; Abdelatif, D.; Fazel, Y.; Henry, L.; Wymer, M. Global Epidemiology of Non-Alcoholic Fatty Liver Disease-Meta-Analytic Assessment of Prevalence, Incidence and Outcomes. *Hepatology* **2015**, in press. [CrossRef] [PubMed]
12. Morita, S.; Neto, D.D.S.; Morita, F.H.; Morita, N.K.; Lobo, S.M. Prevalence of Non-alcoholic Fatty Liver Disease and Steatohepatitis Risk Factors in Patients Undergoing Bariatric Surgery. *Obes. Surg.* **2015**, *25*, 2335–2343. [CrossRef] [PubMed]
13. Matteoni, C.; Younossi, Z.; Gramlich, T.; Boparai, N.; Liu, Y.; McCullough, A. Nonalcoholic fatty liver disease: A spectrum of clinical and pathological severity. *Gastroenterology* **1999**, *116*, 1413–1419. [CrossRef]

14. Brunt, E.M.; Janney, C.G.; Di Bisceglie, A.M.; Neuschwander-Tetri, B.A.; Bacon, B.R. Nonalcoholic steatohepatitis: A proposal for grading and staging the histological lesions. *Am. J. Gastroenterol.* **1999**, *94*, 2467–2474. [CrossRef] [PubMed]

15. Ben-Shlomo, Y.; Spears, M.; Boustred, C.; May, M.; Anderson, S.G.; Benjamin, E.J.; Boutouyrie, P.; Cameron, J.; Chen, C.H.; Cruickshank, J.K.; *et al.* Aortic pulse wave velocity improves cardiovascular event prediction: An individual participant meta-analysis of prospective observational data from 17,635 subjects. *J. Am. Coll. Cardiol.* **2014**, *63*, 636–646. [CrossRef] [PubMed]

16. Cavalcante, J.L.; Lima, J.A.; Redheuil, A.; Al-Mallah, M.H. Aortic stiffness: Current understanding and future directions. *J. Am. Coll. Cardiol.* **2011**, *57*, 1511–1522. [CrossRef] [PubMed]

17. Athyros, V.G.; Tziomalos, K.; Katsiki, N.; Doumas, M.; Karagiannis, A.; Mikhailidis, D.P. Cardiovascular risk across the histological spectrum and the clinical manifestations of non-alcoholic fatty liver disease: An update. *World J. Gastroenterol.* **2015**, *21*, 6820–6834. [PubMed]

18. Targher, G.; Bertolini, L.; Rodella, S.; Tessari, R.; Zenari, L.; Lippi, G.; Arcaro, G. Nonalcoholic fatty liver disease is independently associated with an increased incidence of cardiovascular events in type 2 diabetic patients. *Diabetes Care* **2007**, *30*, 2119–2121. [CrossRef] [PubMed]

19. Targher, G.; Bertolini, L.; Padovani, R.; Rodella, S.; Tessari, R.; Zenari, L.; Day, C.; Arcaro, G. Prevalence of nonalcoholic fatty liver disease and its association with cardiovascular disease among type 2 diabetic patients. *Diabetes Care* **2007**, *30*, 1212–1218. [CrossRef] [PubMed]

20. Targher, G.; Day, C.P.; Bonora, E. Risk of cardiovascular disease in patients with nonalcoholic fatty liver disease. *N. Engl. J. Med.* **2010**, *363*, 1341–1350. [CrossRef] [PubMed]

21. Anstee, Q.M.; Targher, G.; Day, C.P. Progression of NAFLD to diabetes mellitus, cardiovascular disease or cirrhosis. *Nat. Rev. Gastroenterol. Hepatol.* **2013**, *10*, 330–344. [CrossRef] [PubMed]

22. Kim, D.; Choi, S.Y.; Park, E.H.; Lee, W.; Kang, J.H.; Kim, W.; Kim, Y.J.; Yoon, J.H.; Jeong, S.H.; Lee, D.H.; *et al.* Nonalcoholic fatty liver disease is associated with coronary artery calcification. *Hepatology* **2012**, *56*, 605–613. [CrossRef] [PubMed]

23. Oni, E.T.; Agatston, A.S.; Blaha, M.J.; Fialkow, J.; Cury, R.; Sposito, A.; Erbel, R.; Blankstein, R.; Feldman, T.; Al-Mallah, M.; *et al.* A systematic review: Burden and severity of subclinical cardiovascular disease among those with nonalcoholic fatty liver; should we care? *Atherosclerosis* **2013**, *230*, 258–267. [CrossRef] [PubMed]

24. Mellinger, J.L.; Pencina, K.M.; Massaro, J.M.; Hoffmann, U.; Seshadri, S.; Fox, C.S.; O'Donnell, C.J.; Speliotes, E.K. Hepatic steatosis and cardiovascular disease outcomes: An analysis of the Framingham Heart Study. *J. Hepatol.* **2015**, *63*, 470–476. [CrossRef] [PubMed]

25. Moon, S.H.; Noh, T.S.; Cho, Y.S.; Hong, S.P.; Hyun, S.H.; Choi, J.Y.; Kim, B.T.; Lee, K.H. Association between nonalcoholic fatty liver disease and carotid artery inflammation evaluated by 18F-fluorodeoxyglucose positron emission tomography. *Angiology* **2015**, *66*, 472–480. [CrossRef] [PubMed]

26. Targher, G.; Zenari, L.; Bertolini, L.; Cigolini, M.; Padovani, R.; Falezza, G.; Rodella, S.; Arcaro, G.; Zoppini, G. Relations between carotid artery wall thickness and liver histology in subjects with nonalcoholic fatty liver disease. *Diabetes Care* **2006**, *29*, 1325–1330. [CrossRef] [PubMed]

27. Yoneda, M.; Mawatari, H.; Fujita, K.; Iida, H.; Yonemitsu, K.; Kato, S.; Takahashi, H.; Kirikoshi, H.; Inamori, M.; Nozaki, Y.; *et al.* High-sensitivity C-reactive protein is an independent clinical feature of nonalcoholic steatohepatitis (NASH) and also of the severity of fibrosis in NASH. *J. Gastroenterol.* **2007**, *42*, 573–582. [CrossRef] [PubMed]

28. Wieckowska, A.; Papouchado, B.G.; Li, Z.; Lopez, R.; Zein, N.N.; Feldstein, A.E. Increased hepatic and circulating interleukin-6 levels in human nonalcoholic steatohepatitis. *Am. J. Gastroenterol.* **2008**, *103*, 1372–1379. [CrossRef] [PubMed]

29. Thuy, S.; Ladurner, R.; Volynets, V.; Wagner, S.; Strahl, S.; Konigsrainer, A.; Maier, K.P.; Bischoff, S.C.; Bergheim, I. Nonalcoholic fatty liver disease in humans is associated with increased plasma endotoxin and plasminogen activator inhibitor 1 concentrations and with fructose intake. *J. Nutr.* **2008**, *138*, 1452–1455. [PubMed]

30. Cigolini, M.; Targher, G.; Agostino, G.; Tonoli, M.; Muggeo, M.; DeSandre, G. Liver steatosis and its relation to plasma haemostatic factors in apparently healthy men—Role of the metabolic syndrome. *Thromb. Haemost.* **1996**, *76*, 69–73. [PubMed]

31. Targher, G.; Bertolini, L.; Rodella, S.; Lippi, G.; Franchini, M.; Zoppini, G.; Muggeo, M.; Day, C. NASH predicts plasma inflammatory biomarkers independently of visceral fat in men. *Obesity* **2008**, *16*, 1394–1399. [CrossRef] [PubMed]

32. Leung, C.; Herath, C.B.; Jia, Z.; Goodwin, M.; Mak, K.Y.; Watt, M.J.; Forbes, J.M.; Angus, P.W. Dietary glycotoxins exacerbate progression of experimental fatty liver disease. *J. Hepatol.* **2014**, *60*, 832–838. [CrossRef] [PubMed]

33. Pischon, T.; Girman, C.J.; Hotamisligil, G.S.; Rifai, N.; Hu, F.B.; Rimm, E.B. Plasma adiponectin levels and risk of myocardial infarction in men. *J. Am. Med. Assoc.* **2004**, *291*, 1730–1737. [CrossRef] [PubMed]

34. Leite, N.; Salles, G.; Cardoso, C.; Villela-Nogueira, C. Serum biomarkers in type 2 diabetic patients with non-alcoholic steatohepatitis and advanced fibrosis. *Hepatol. Res.* **2013**, *43*, 508–515. [CrossRef] [PubMed]

35. Ekstedt, M.; Franzen, L.; Mathiesen, U.; Thorelius, L.; Holmqvist, M.; Bodemar, G.; Kechagias, S. Long-term follow-up of patients with NAFLD and elevated liver enzymes. *Hepatology* **2006**, *44*, 865–873. [CrossRef] [PubMed]

36. Soderberg, C.; Stal, P.; Askling, J.; Glaumann, H.; Lindberg, G.; Marmur, J.; Hultcrantz, R. Decreased Survival of Subjects with Elevated Liver Function Tests During a 28-Year Follow-Up. *Hepatology* **2010**, *51*, 595–602. [CrossRef] [PubMed]

37. Singh, S.; Allen, A.M.; Wang, Z.; Prokop, L.J.; Murad, M.H.; Loomba, R. Fibrosis progression in nonalcoholic fatty liver *vs.* nonalcoholic steatohepatitis: A systematic review and meta-analysis of paired-biopsy studies. *Clin. Gastroenterol. Hepatol.* **2015**, *13*, 643–654. [CrossRef] [PubMed]

38. Argo, C.K.; Northup, P.G.; Al-Osaimi, A.M.; Caldwell, S.H. Systematic review of risk factors for fibrosis progression in non-alcoholic steatohepatitis. *J. Hepatol.* **2009**, *51*, 371–379. [CrossRef] [PubMed]

39. Pais, R.; Charlotte, F.; Fedchuk, L.; Bedossa, P.; Lebray, P.; Poynard, T.; Ratziu, V.; Group, L.S. A systematic review of follow-up biopsies reveals disease progression in patients with non-alcoholic fatty liver. *J. Hepatol.* **2013**, *59*, 550–556. [CrossRef] [PubMed]

40. Harrison, S.A. Nonalcoholic fatty liver disease and fibrosis progression: The good, the bad, and the unknown. *Clin. Gastroenterol. Hepatol.* **2015**, *13*, 655–657. [CrossRef] [PubMed]

41. Laurent, S.; Cockcroft, J.; van Bortel, L.; Boutouyrie, P.; Giannattasio, C.; Hayoz, D.; Pannier, B.; Vlachopoulos, C.; Wilkinson, I.; Struijker-Boudier, H. European Network for Non-invasive Investigation of Large, A., Expert consensus document on arterial stiffness: Methodological issues and clinical applications. *Eur. Heart J.* **2006**, *27*, 2588–2605. [CrossRef] [PubMed]

42. Laurent, S.; Boutouyrie, P. Recent advances in arterial stiffness and wave reflection in human hypertension. *Hypertension* **2007**, *49*, 1202–1206. [CrossRef] [PubMed]

43. Zieman, S.J.; Melenovsky, V.; Kass, D.A. Mechanisms, pathophysiology, and therapy of arterial stiffness. *Arterioscler. Thromb. Vasc. Biol.* **2005**, *25*, 932–943. [CrossRef] [PubMed]

44. Johnson, C.P.; Baugh, R.; Wilson, C.A.; Burns, J. Age related changes in the tunica media of the vertebral artery: Implications for the assessment of vessels injured by trauma. *J. Clin. Pathol.* **2001**, *54*, 139–145. [CrossRef] [PubMed]

45. Blacher, J.; Guerin, A.P.; Pannier, B.; Marchais, S.J.; Safar, M.E.; London, G.M. Impact of aortic stiffness on survival in end-stage renal disease. *Circulation* **1999**, *99*, 2434–2439. [CrossRef] [PubMed]

46. Laurent, S.; Boutouyrie, P.; Asmar, R.; Gautier, I.; Laloux, B.; Guize, L.; Ducimetiere, P.; Benetos, A. Aortic stiffness is an independent predictor of all-cause and cardiovascular mortality in hypertensive patients. *Hypertension* **2001**, *37*, 1236–1241. [CrossRef] [PubMed]

47. Cardoso, C.R.; Ferreira, M.T.; Leite, N.C.; Salles, G.F. Prognostic impact of aortic stiffness in high-risk type 2 diabetic patients: The Rio deJaneiro Type 2 Diabetes Cohort Study. *Diabetes Care* **2013**, *36*, 3772–3778. [CrossRef] [PubMed]

48. Willum-Hansen, T.; Staessen, J.A.; Torp-Pedersen, C.; Rasmussen, S.; Thijs, L.; Ibsen, H.; Jeppesen, J. Prognostic value of aortic pulse wave velocity as index of arterial stiffness in the general population. *Circulation* **2006**, *113*, 664–670. [CrossRef] [PubMed]

49. Mitchell, G.F.; Hwang, S.J.; Vasan, R.S.; Larson, M.G.; Pencina, M.J.; Hamburg, N.M.; Vita, J.A.; Levy, D.; Benjamin, E.J. Arterial stiffness and cardiovascular events: The Framingham Heart Study. *Circulation* **2010**, *121*, 505–511. [CrossRef] [PubMed]

50. Shiotani, A.; Motoyama, M.; Matsuda, T.; Miyanishi, T. Brachial-ankle pulse wave velocity in Japanese university students. *Intern. Med.* **2005**, *44*, 696–701. [CrossRef] [PubMed]

51. Salvi, P.; Ruffini, R.; Agnoletti, D.; Magnani, E.; Pagliarani, G.; Comandini, G.; Pratico, A.; Borghi, C.; Benetos, A.; Pazzi, P. Increased arterial stiffness in nonalcoholic fatty liver disease: The Cardio-GOOSE study. *J. Hypertens.* **2010**, *28*, 1699–1707. [CrossRef] [PubMed]

52. Vlachopoulos, C.; Manesis, E.; Baou, K.; Papatheodoridis, G.; Koskinas, J.; Tiniakos, D.; Aznaouridis, K.; Archimandritis, A.; Stefanadis, C. Increased arterial stiffness and impaired endothelial function in nonalcoholic Fatty liver disease: A pilot study. *Am. J. Hypertens.* **2010**, *23*, 1183–1189. [CrossRef] [PubMed]

53. Kim, B.J.; Kim, N.H.; Kim, B.S.; Kang, J.H. The association between nonalcoholic fatty liver disease, metabolic syndrome and arterial stiffness in nondiabetic, nonhypertensive individuals. *Cardiology* **2012**, *123*, 54–61. [CrossRef] [PubMed]

54. Huang, Y.; Bi, Y.; Xu, M.; Ma, Z.; Xu, Y.; Wang, T.; Li, M.; Liu, Y.; Lu, J.; Chen, Y.; *et al.* Nonalcoholic fatty liver disease is associated with atherosclerosis in middle-aged and elderly Chinese. *Arterioscler. Thromb. Vasc. Biol.* **2012**, *32*, 2321–2326. [CrossRef] [PubMed]

55. Lee, Y.J.; Shim, J.Y.; Moon, B.S.; Shin, Y.H.; Jung, D.H.; Lee, J.H.; Lee, H.R. The relationship between arterial stiffness and nonalcoholic fatty liver disease. *Dig. Dis. Sci.* **2012**, *57*, 196–203. [CrossRef] [PubMed]

56. Huang, R.C.; Beilin, L.J.; Ayonrinde, O.; Mori, T.A.; Olynyk, J.K.; Burrows, S.; Hands, B.; Adams, L.A. Importance of cardiometabolic risk factors in the association between nonalcoholic fatty liver disease and arterial stiffness in adolescents. *Hepatology* **2013**, *58*, 1306–1314. [CrossRef] [PubMed]

57. Sunbul, M.; Agirbasli, M.; Durmus, E.; Kivrak, T.; Akin, H.; Aydin, Y.; Ergelen, R.; Yilmaz, Y. Arterial stiffness in patients with non-alcoholic fatty liver disease is related to fibrosis stage and epicardial adipose tissue thickness. *Atherosclerosis* **2014**, *237*, 490–493. [CrossRef] [PubMed]

58. Omelchenko, E.; Gavish, D.; Shargorodsky, M. Adiponectin is better predictor of subclinical atherosclerosis than liver function tests in patients with nonalcoholic fatty liver disease. *J. Am. Soc. Hypertens* **2014**, *8*, 376–380. [CrossRef] [PubMed]

59. Yu, X.Y.; Zhao, Y.; Song, X.X.; Song, Z.Y. Association between non-alcoholic fatty liver disease and arterial stiffness in the non-obese, non-hypertensive, and non-diabetic young and middle-aged Chinese population. *J. Zhejiang Univ. Sci. B* **2014**, *15*, 879–887. [CrossRef] [PubMed]

60. Chen, Y.; Xu, M.; Wang, T.; Sun, J.; Sun, W.; Xu, B.; Huang, X.; Xu, Y.; Lu, J.; Li, X.; *et al.* Advanced fibrosis associates with atherosclerosis in subjects with nonalcoholic fatty liver disease. *Atherosclerosis* **2015**, *241*, 145–150. [CrossRef] [PubMed]

61. Chou, C.Y.; Yang, Y.C.; Wu, J.S.; Sun, Z.J.; Lu, F.H.; Chang, C.J. Non-alcoholic fatty liver disease associated with increased arterial stiffness in subjects with normal glucose tolerance, but not pre-diabetes and diabetes. *Diabetes Vasc. Dis. Res.* **2015**, *12*, 359–365. [CrossRef] [PubMed]

62. Ozturk, K.; Uygun, A.; Guler, A.K.; Demirci, H.; Ozdemir, C.; Cakir, M.; Sakin, Y.S.; Turker, T.; Sari, S.; Demirbas, S.; *et al.* Nonalcoholic fatty liver disease is an independent risk factor for atherosclerosis in young adult men. *Atherosclerosis* **2015**, *240*, 380–386. [CrossRef] [PubMed]

63. Chung, G.E.; Choi, S.Y.; Kim, D.; Kwak, M.S.; Park, H.E.; Kim, M.K.; Yim, J.Y. Nonalcoholic fatty liver disease as a risk factor of arterial stiffness measured by the cardioankle vascular index. *Medicine* **2015**, *94*, e654. [CrossRef] [PubMed]

64. Li, N.; Zhang, G.W.; Zhang, J.R.; Jin, D.; Li, Y.; Liu, T.; Wang, R.T. Non-alcoholic fatty liver disease is associated with progression of arterial stiffness. *Nutr. Metab. Cardiovasc. Dis.* **2015**, *25*, 218–223. [CrossRef] [PubMed]

65. Leite, N.C.; Villela-Nogueira, C.A.; Ferreira, M.T.; Cardoso, C.R.; Salles, G.F. Increasing aortic stiffness is predictive of advanced liver fibrosis in patients with type 2 diabetes: The Rio-T2DM cohort study. *Liver. Int.* **2015**. [CrossRef] [PubMed]

66. Nickenig, G.; Roling, J.; Strehlow, K.; Schnabel, P.; Bohm, M. Insulin induces upregulation of vascular AT1 receptor gene expression by posttranscriptional mechanisms. *Circulation* **1998**, *98*, 2453–2460. [CrossRef] [PubMed]

67. Jesmin, S.; Sakuma, I.; Salah-Eldin, A.; Nonomura, K.; Hattori, Y.; Kitabatake, A. Diminished penile expression of vascular endothelial growth factor and its receptors at the insulin-resistant stage of a type II diabetic rat model: A possible cause for erectile dysfunction in diabetes. *J. Mol. Endocrinol.* **2003**, *31*, 401–418. [CrossRef] [PubMed]

68. Rizzoni, D.; Porteri, E.; Guelfi, D.; Muiesan, M.L.; Valentini, U.; Cimino, A.; Girelli, A.; Rodella, L.; Bianchi, R.; Sleiman, I.; *et al.* Structural alterations in subcutaneous small arteries of normotensive and hypertensive patients with non-insulin-dependent diabetes mellitus. *Circulation* **2001**, *103*, 1238–1244. [CrossRef] [PubMed]

69. Cusi, K.; Maezono, K.; Osman, A.; Pendergrass, M.; Patti, M.E.; Pratipanawatr, T.; DeFronzo, R.A.; Kahn, C.R.; Mandarino, L.J. Insulin resistance differentially affects the PI 3-kinase- and MAP kinase-mediated signaling in human muscle. *J. Clin. Investig.* **2000**, *105*, 311–320. [CrossRef] [PubMed]

70. Jain, S.; Khera, R.; Corrales-Medina, V.F.; Townsend, R.R.; Chirinos, J.A. Inflammation and arterial stiffness in humans. *Atherosclerosis* **2014**, *237*, 381–390. [CrossRef] [PubMed]

71. Fargion, S.; Porzio, M.; Fracanzani, A.L. Nonalcoholic fatty liver disease and vascular disease: State-of-the-art. *World J. Gastroenterol.* **2014**, *20*, 13306–13324. [CrossRef] [PubMed]

11

Non-Alcoholic Fatty Liver Disease and Metabolic Syndrome after Liver Transplant

Stefano Gitto and Erica Villa *

Department of Gastroenterology, Azienda Ospedaliero-Universitaria and University of Modena and Reggio Emilia, Via del Pozzo 1, 41124 Modena, Italy; stefano.gitto@studio.unibo.it
* Correspondence: erica.villa@unimore.it

Academic Editors: Amedeo Lonardo and Giovanni Targher

Abstract: Liver transplant is the unique curative therapy for patients with acute liver failure or end-stage liver disease, with or without hepatocellular carcinoma. Increase of body weight, onset of insulin resistance and drug-induced alterations of metabolism are reported in liver transplant recipients. In this context, post-transplant diabetes mellitus, hyperlipidemia, and arterial hypertension can be often diagnosed. Multifactorial illnesses occurring in the post-transplant period represent significant causes of morbidity and mortality. This is especially true for metabolic syndrome. Non-alcoholic steatosis and steatohepatitis are hepatic manifestations of metabolic syndrome and after liver transplant both recurrent and *de novo* steatosis can be found. Usually, post-transplant steatosis shows an indolent outcome with few cases of fibrosis progression. However, in the post-transplant setting, both metabolic syndrome and steatosis might play a key role in the stratification of morbidity and mortality risk, being commonly associated with cardiovascular disease. The single components of metabolic syndrome can be treated with targeted drugs while lifestyle intervention is the only reasonable therapeutic approach for transplant patients with non-alcoholic steatosis or steatohepatitis.

Keywords: liver transplant; multifactorial disease; metabolic syndrome; non-alcoholic fatty liver disease; non-alcoholic steatohepatitis

1. Introduction

Liver transplant (LT) represents the curative treatment for patients with acute liver failure, end-stage liver disease and/or non-resectable hepatocellular carcinoma worldwide. After surgery, transplanted patients often develop an increase of body weight, insulin resistance (IR) and metabolic alterations [1]. Multifactorial disease such as diabetes mellitus (DM), hyperlipidemia and arterial hypertension are common complications after LT, all negatively affecting quality of life, morbidity and mortality [1]. Consolidated immunosuppressant drugs such as corticosteroids, calcineurin inhibitors (CNIs) (cyclosporine (CSA) and tacrolimus (TAC)) and mammalian target of rapamycin inhibitors (mTORs) (such as sirolimus (SIR)) play a key role in the metabolic balance, favoring hyperglycemia, arterial hypertension and hyperlipidemia [2]. In this context, a significant amount of transplanted patients fulfill the criteria of metabolic syndrome (MS) which is strongly associated with an increased cardiovascular risk [1]. Since non-alcoholic fatty liver disease (NAFLD) and non-alcoholic steatohepatitis (NASH) are considered the liver expression of MS, it is not surprising that both recurrent and *de novo* NAFLD/NASH can be found after LT [3]. Although post-LT steatosis shows an indolent outcome in terms of fibrosis progression, NAFLD/NASH should be considered for the stratification of morbidity and mortality risk of transplant patients. Notably, cardiovascular disease represents the major cause of death unrelated to liver disease and the third most common cause of mortality among transplant patients, accounting for 12%–16% of deaths. Today, targeted drugs for MS and NAFLD/NASH do not exist. Clinicians can use specific drugs against the single components of MS while a strong improvement of behavior in terms of diet and aerobic exercise is the only reasonable approach for recurrent or *de novo* NAFLD/NASH [1].

This review article focuses on the current literature regarding the main metabolic diseases affecting transplanted patients, the clinical impact of post-LT MS and NAFLD/NASH and, finally, the feasible therapeutic strategies.

2. Multifactorial Disease after Liver Transplant

The majority of transplant patients develop a rise in body weight after surgery. The highest weight increase occurs after the first six months and at one and three years from LT, and the median weight gain is 5.1 and 9.5 kg, respectively. Notably, at one and three years, 24% and 31% of transplant patients become obese [4]. However, the above-cited authors [4] reported that the vast part of enrolled patients were also obese before LT. Considering only patients who were not obese at the time of surgery, 15.5% at one year and 26.3% at three years had a body mass index (BMI) >30 [4]. In a further study, 23 patients were followed for nine months after LT. At the end of the study, 87 of the subjects were overweight or obese with a significant increase in fat mass and a minor improvement in lean mass [5]. Another study [6] showed progressive weight gain in the first year after LT, with one-third of patients becoming obese at the end of observation. Considering a follow-up of four years, overweight and obesity were found in 58% and 21% of cases and high BMI before LT was the main risk factor of post-LT obesity [7].

In this context, DM, hyperlipidemia and arterial hypertension can be often diagnosed after LT [1] (see Table 1).

Table 1. Multifactorial conditions affecting transplant patients.

Disease	Incidence	Risk Factors	References
Diabetes mellitus	10%–64%	Male gender, high pre-LT BMI, family history, hepatitis C, older age, immunosuppressants, rapamycin gene polymorphisms, *TCF7L2* gene polymorphisms (donor)	[8–11]
Hyperlipidemia	45%–69%	Diet, older age, high BMI, DM, renal impairment, immunosuppressants, low-density lipoprotein receptor gene polymorphism (donor)	[12–15]
Arterial hypertension	50%–100%	Obesity, older age, impaired glycemia, immunosuppressants	[9,16,17]

LT: liver transplant; BMI, body mass index; TCF7L2, Transcription factor 7-like 2; DM, diabetes mellitus.

Post-LT DM is associated with more significant morbidity with respect to pre-LT disease, determining an increased risk of post-operative infection and cardiovascular events [8,18]. The incidence of post-LT DM ranges from 10% to 64% [9]. Ahn *et al.* [19] showed that among 74 patients transplanted with post-LT DM, post-LT DM was transient in 56.8%, while in the others it was persistent. Although the underlying mechanisms are not yet clear, the main risk factors for the onset of post-LT DM are the following: male gender, high pre-LT BMI, positive family history, hepatitis C virus infection, older age, high dosage of immunosuppressant drugs and rapamycin gene polymorphisms [8]. A meta-analysis confirmed that male gender, high pre-LT BMI and positive family history are predictive of post-LT DM development [10]. Transcription factor 7-like 2 (TCF7L2) protein regulates cell proliferation and differentiation modifying the insulin secretion [20]. Notably, it was reported that polymorphisms of the *TCF7L2* gene in LT donors are another independent risk factor of post-LT DM [11].

Among transplanted patients, a percentage ranging from 45% to 69% develops hyperlipidemia, which is a significant risk factor for cardiovascular morbidity and mortality [12]. Increased nutrient intake, older age, body weight, presence of DM, renal impairment, immunosuppressive drugs, such as steroids, CSA, TAC, and SIR, are risk factors for post-LT hyperlipidemia [13,14].

Interestingly, the polymorphism of the low-density lipoprotein receptor gene in the donor may facilitate the development of hyperlipidemia in the recipient [15].

Arterial hypertension, an uncommon feature in subjects with chronic liver disease, arises in 50%–100% of patients after LT [9,16]. Post-LT hypertension usually develops in the first six months after LT as a consequence of systemic vasoconstriction, elevation in plasma endothelin-1 concentrations, and increased arterial stiffness [21]. Occurrence of post-LT hypertension is favored by obesity and older age and is often associated with impaired glycemia. Moreover, it is well known that both CNIs and corticosteroids have negative effects on pressure control [17].

3. Metabolic Impact of Immunosuppressant Drugs

It is well known that immunosuppressive agents might exert negative metabolic effects [22] (see Table 2).

Table 2. Most used immunosuppressant drugs and main metabolic side effects.

Drug	Side Effects	References
Corticosteroids	Increased fat depositions, decreased fat oxidation, increased proteolysis, reduced protein synthesis, IR, hyperlipidemia, sodium retention, NAFLD	[23–25]
CSA	Decreased energy metabolism and muscle mass, weight gain, hyperlipidemia, arterial hypertension	[26–30]
TAC	DM, hyperlipidemia, arterial hypertension	[10,27–30]
SIR	Decreased muscle mass, hyperlipidemia, glycemic alteration	[31–33]

CSA: cyclosporine; TAC: tacrolimus; SIR: sirolimus; IR, insulin resistance; NAFLD, non-alcoholic fatty liver disease; DM, diabetes mellitus.

Corticosteroids represent a key component of the immunosuppressant protocol in the first months after LT but are also necessary in the long-term management of patients transplanted for autoimmune or cholestatic liver disease. Corticosteroids show dose-related metabolic side effects. They increase appetite and fat depositions, drop fat oxidation, and lead to increased proteolysis and reduced protein synthesis [23,24]. Moreover, high doses of corticosteroids determine the rise of both IR and gluconeogenesis [25]. Corticosteroids also negatively alter lipid metabolism and steroid-free protocols might lead to a significant decrease in hypertriglyceridemia [34]. Corticosteroids also influence mineralocorticoid metabolism, causing sodium retention. Interestingly, steroids directly correlate with NAFLD/NASH occurrence in liver allografts [35].

CNIs may negatively affect energy metabolism and muscle mass [26] and CSA represents an independent predictor of post-LT weight gain [36]. Through a meta-analysis including 10 studies, Li et al. [10] demonstrated that TAC is an independent risk factor for post-LT DM. Regarding lipid metabolism, CSA has a more negative effect in comparison with TAC. The incidence of hyperlipidemia is higher in patients treated with CSA than with TAC (14% versus 5% and 49% versus 17%) [27,28]. CNIs also favor the onset of arterial hypertension determining arterial vasoconstriction. Among CNIs, TAC seems to have a lesser impact on arterial pressure in comparison to CSA, but data are not conclusive [29,30]. As expected, minimizing the use of CNIs improves their metabolic profile and, consequently, the long-term outcome of patients [37,38].

SIR increases triglyceride production, being the most dangerous immunosuppressant in terms of lipid alteration. Among patients treated with SIR, 55% develop hyperlipidemia [31]. In addition, SIR alters the insulin signaling pathway [31] and negatively affects muscle mass status [32]. Recently, Zimmermann et al. [33] conducted a study involving 92 transplant patients, reporting that patients treated with mTORs were at higher risk of hyperlipidemia and glycemic alteration with respect to patients under CNIs.

4. Metabolic Syndrome after Transplant

The definition of MS includes a combination of at least three of the following factors: arterial hypertension, IR, hypertriglyceridemia, low high-density lipoprotein and obesity [39]. In the post-LT period, MS can be found in 50%–60% of patients. MS represents a relevant risk factor for atherosclerosis and cardiovascular disease, which are the main causes of post-LT morbidity and mortality [39]. Interestingly, the prevalence of post-LT MS is about twice that of the general North American population [40]. Older age, obesity, pre-LT DM, genetic polymorphisms in the living donor and the use of high-dosage immunosuppressive drugs are risk factors for post-LT MS [9]. Sprinzl *et al.* [41] analyzed a cohort of 170 transplant patients with a follow-up of two years. The authors showed that *de novo* MS was present in one-third of patients and glycosylated hemoglobin ≥5% and arterial hypertension were independent risk factors for it. Moreover, the authors demonstrated a negative dose-dependent role for steroids. It was also confirmed that in the post-LT period, MS could be considered as a link toward NAFLD/NASH. Interestingly, it was reported that changes in intestinal microbiota might also play a relevant role in the development of MS after LT [42]. Fussner *et al.* [43] retrospectively analyzed 455 consecutive LT recipients with a long follow-up (8–12 years), suggesting that increased BMI was a strong predictor of MS at one year from the LT. Consequently, the authors suggested that preventing weight gain in the early months after LT might decrease the probability of MS. However, the authors suggested that older age, post-LT DM, prior family history of cardiovascular disease, altered serum troponin, but not MS, were independent predictors of cardiovascular events. It has to be underlined that specific treatments for MS are not yet available, while the only feasible way to manage it is to treat its single components [44].

5. Post-Transplant Non-Alcoholic Fatty Liver Disease

In the pre-LT period, NAFLD and NASH represent the liver expression of altered metabolic status being associated in a large number of cases to IR, dyslipidemia and obesity. Considering the significant prevalence of metabolic diseases after LT, it is clear why both recurrent and *de novo* NAFLD/NASH can be found in transplant patients [41].

Burra *et al.* [45] reported that NASH recurrence ranges from 20% to 40%, this wide variability depending on the methodology used for the diagnosis. Notably, in the majority of cases the outcome of recurrent NAFLD/NASH is harmless, without an evolution toward cirrhosis [46]. Nevertheless, patients with recurrent NAFLD/NASH more frequently show cardiovascular disease and worse infection-related morbidity and mortality. This is evident considering that the recurrence of NASH is associated with DM, weight gain, and dyslipidemia [47]. Interestingly, genetic predisposition might play a role in the recurrence of NAFLD and NASH. The presence of the rs738409-G allele of the Patatin-like phospholipase in the LT recipients represents an independent risk factor for post-LT obesity, DM and steatosis [48,49].

The leading risk factors for the development of *de novo* NAFLD/NASH are the following: obesity, hyperlipidemia, DM, arterial hypertension, TAC-based immunosuppression, pre-LT alcoholic cirrhosis and liver graft steatosis [50]. Sprinzl *et al.* [41] analyzed the association between MS and post-LT NAFLD/NASH. Mixed vesicular steatosis was observed in 34.1% of patients. Hepatic steatosis was mild, moderate, and severe in 16.5%, 7.1%, and 2.9% of cases. Among patients with MS and steatosis, NASH was diagnosed only in 5.4% of patients, confirming that post-LT metabolic liver disease might be relevant not as a primary liver disease but as an indicator of cardiovascular risk. Remarkably, NAFLD/NASH patients showed higher triglyceride levels, elevated uric acid and higher BMI with respect to patients with MS but without liver disease. The authors demonstrated that obesity and dyslipidemia but not arterial hypertension and DM favored the onset of NAFLD/NASH among transplanted patients with MS. Another interesting assumption was that a BMI greater than 28.9 was the only specific risk factor for histological NASH. Mikolasevic *et al.* [51] identified the association between NAFLD/NASH and the development of post-LT cardiovascular and chronic kidney disease.

Consequently, according to these authors, diagnosing NAFLD/NASH in the post-LT period might improve the stratification of cardiovascular and kidney damage risk.

6. Therapeutic Approach against Post-Transplant Dysmetabolism

The knowledge of pathogenesis is central for understanding the rationale of the therapeutic approach against MS and NAFLD/NASH. The onset of IR represents a true turning point. In fact, IR determines a status of chronic inflammation that favors the other metabolic alterations [52]. The molecular basis of IR depends on both genetic and non-genetic mechanisms. IR determines a chain of events involving inflammation, hypercoagulability, and atherogenesis. Notably, IR occurs firstly in the vascular structures, and this is one of the main reasons for its association with cardiovascular disease [53]. Regarding the NAFLD/NASH, the latest proposed model is the "multiparallel hits" [54]. According to this hypothesis, many events happen in parallel, and all are potential therapeutic targets. The main pathological characters are IR, oxidative stress, adipose and pancreatic tissues, altered lipid metabolism, bile acids, gut microbiota, and bacterial endotoxins.

As we reported, transplant patients often develop IR and an increase in body weight [1]. Interestingly, Kouz et al. [55] demonstrated that in patients transplanted for NASH-cirrhosis, most of the weight gain occurs in the first year after LT, while the increase of the weight is more progressive in subjects with a different etiology. However, regardless of the kind of pre-LT liver disease, after LT a relevant increase in dietary intake can be found, especially in patients with pre-LT severe dietary restrictions, gastrointestinal symptoms or anorexia. In detail, from the pre-LT period to one year after LT, calories rise from 27 to 32 kCal/kg and proteins from 0.8 to 1.3 g/kg per day [56]. Richardson et al. [5] showed that in overweight or obese transplant patients, more significant energy intake, higher consumption of both proteins and carbohydrates and doubled intake of fat can be found with respect to the pre-LT period.

The feasible pharmacological tools for treating the single metabolic disease, associated or not with NAFLD/NASH, should be used with caution for the possible drug-drug interactions [57]. Notably, a single drug for post-LT MS is not available. Based on these considerations, the main intervention after surgery should be a strong lifestyle control for both prevention and treatment of MS. However, the only randomized trial of exercise and dietary counseling after LT published in 2006 did not show a real advantage with this approach [58]. In this study, 151 liver transplant patients, randomized into exercise and dietary counseling or usual care, showed a similar increase in body weight, fat mass and lean mass. It should be underlined that full adherence to exercise and nutrition was obtained only in 37% of subjects.

Many drugs have been proposed for the treatment of NAFLD/NASH, but lifestyle intervention should be the first-line therapy. In particular, lifestyle modification is the standard of care according to the Italian, European, Asian-Pacific and North American guidelines [59–62]. The main targets for the usefulness evaluation should be a weight loss of 7% and 150 min/week of physical activity [63,64]. In particular, a weight loss of 7% has been seen to significantly decrease fat accumulation and reduce necroinflammation in non-transplanted patients with NAFLD/NASH [63]. Markedly, aerobic and resistance physical activity have an independent positive effect in decreasing fat in the liver, regardless of the weight loss [65,66]. Furthermore, clinicians should take into account that the physical activity per se improves cardio-respiratory fitness [67,68]. Vitamin E and pioglitazone represent the first-line pharmacological options. Both vitamin E and pioglitazone improve fat accumulation and liver inflammation. However, the use of vitamin E is limited to patients without DM and it has no clear effects on fibrosis. On the other hand, pioglitazone shows a negative impact on patients' weight. In addition, the long-term safety of these drugs is uncertain. Many other drugs such as metformin, ursodeoxycholic acid, statins, pentoxifylline, and orlistat have been tested in pilot studies or randomized clinical trials with few results in terms of efficacy. Telmisartan, a safe antihypertensive drug, is an emerging drug with an interesting preliminary effect on NAFLD/NASH. It seems to have a positive impact on IR, liver steatosis, inflammation, and fibrosis [52]. As recently reported in a review article by Lassailly *et al.* [69], many other drugs are in progress for the treatment of NAFLD/NASH, including obeticholic acid, liraglutide and elafibranor. Authors also suggest that bariatric surgery may be successful in well-selected obese patients with NAFLD/NASH.

Concerning the transplanted patient, none of the cited therapeutic options have been validated.

7. Conclusions

Starting in the first months after surgery, transplant patients tend to develop overweight or obesity, IR and, consequently, multifactorial diseases. Consequently, a high prevalence of multifactorial disease such as DM, hyperlipidemia and arterial hypertension can be found. All these metabolic features negatively influence the outcome of transplant patients in terms of quality of life, morbidity and mortality.

All the main immunosuppressant drugs, such as corticosteroids, CSA, TAC and SIR, favor the onset of metabolic alterations. Corticosteroids are surely very important in the first months after LT but also in the long-term in selected cases. They lead to weight gain and fat accumulation negatively affecting lipid, glycemic and pressure profiles. Moreover, they directly increase the risk of steatosis development. CNIs have a negative metabolic impact since they increase weight gain and reduce muscle mass. TAC seems to be superior compared to CSA concerning the metabolic risk in terms of the alteration of lipid and arterial pressure. It should be the first choice among CNIs. SIR is the immunosuppressant with the worst lipid profile. Moreover, SIR shows a worse glycemic profile with respect to CNIs and has a negative effect on the muscle mass status. The choice of immunosuppressant is central and related to many aspects and evaluations such as the cardiovascular and renal risks. In general, one of the main aims of clinicians should be to minimize the dosage of immunosuppressants. This last assumption is true especially in the long-term period and in patients with pre-LT etiology different from autoimmune or cholestatic disease and without a history of graft rejection.

The presence of criteria for MS is frequent in the post-LT period and represents the main indicator of cardiovascular-related morbidity and mortality. NAFLD and its progressive form, represented by NASH, can be considered the liver expression of MS. Indeed, both recurrent and *de novo* NAFLD can be diagnosed in transplanted patients. The hepatic outcome of steatosis after surgery is generally not very aggressive, with few percentages of advanced fibrosis, in comparison with the pre-LT phase. However, together with MS, steatosis is a relevant indicator of increased cardiovascular risk. This assumption is important if we consider that cardiovascular disease is found in 10.6%, 20.7%, and 30.3% of recipients at one, five, and eight years from the LT [43]. Interestingly, post-LT NAFLD/NASH is also associated with an increased risk of infections and renal injury.

Clinicians might definitely use the diagnosis of NAFLD in the post-LT period as an indicator of increased cardiovascular and renal risk. Transplant patients with a first diagnosis of NAFLD should be closely monitored regarding peripheral atherosclerotic signs and kidney function. In this direction, the development of diagnostic algorithms with the use non-invasive tools is warranted. Karlas *et al.* [70] demonstrated that modern non-invasive liver graft assessments such as hepatic ultrasound and transient elastography might be able to properly detect both steatosis and graft fibrosis.

Specific therapeutic options against post-LT MS or NAFLD are not available. Targeted pharmacological tools can be used for each component of MS. So far, a strong behavioral change in terms of diet and aerobic exercise is the only reasonable approach for transplant patients for both primary and secondary care. Transplant patients should be educated starting from the first weeks after surgery for preventing the development of multifactorial diseases, MS and metabolic liver illness. A well-done stratification of the cardiovascular risk should be developed as soon as possible after LT. In the next years, the genetic study of recipients and donors might improve the quality of organ allocation, decreasing the metabolic complications after LT.

Author Contributions: Stefano Gitto and Erica Villa conceived and designed the article; Stefano Gitto wrote the paper; Erica Villa reviewed the manuscript and performed a critical revision.

Abbreviations

LT	Liver Transplant
IR	insulin resistance
DM	Diabetes mellitus
CNIs	calcineurin inhibitors
CSA	cyclosporine
TAC	tacrolimus
mTORs	mammalian target of rapamycin inhibitors
SIR	sirolimus
MS	Metabolic Syndrome
NAFLD	Non-alcoholic fatty liver disease
NASH	Non-alcoholic steatohepatitis
BMI	body mass index
TCF7L2	Transcription factor 7-like 2

References

1. Watt, K.D.; Pedersen, R.A.; Kremers, W.K.; Heimbach, J.K.; Charlton, M.R. Evolution of causes and risk factors for mortality post-liver transplant: Results of the NIDDK long-term follow-up study. *Am. J. Transplant.* **2010**, *10*, 1420–1427. [CrossRef] [PubMed]
2. Charco, R.; Cantarell, C.; Vargas, V.; Capdevila, L.; Lázaro, J.L.; Hidalgo, E.; Murio, E.; Margarit, C. Serum cholesterol changes in long-term survivors of liver transplantation: A comparison between cyclosporine and tacrolimus therapy. *Liver Transpl. Surg.* **1999**, *5*, 204–208. [CrossRef] [PubMed]
3. Bhagat, V.; Mindikoglu, A.L.; Nudo, C.G.; Schiff, E.R.; Tzakis, A.; Regev, A. Outcomes of liver transplantation in patients with cirrhosis due to nonalcoholic steatohepatitis *versus* patients with cirrhosis due to alcoholic liver disease. *Liver Transplant.* **2009**, *15*, 1814–1820. [CrossRef] [PubMed]
4. Richards, J.; Gunson, B.; Johnson, J.; Neuberger, J. Weight gain and obesity after liver transplantation. *Transpl. Int.* **2005**, *18*, 461–466. [CrossRef] [PubMed]
5. Richardson, R.A.; Garden, O.J.; Davidson, H.I. Reduction in energy expenditure after liver transplantation. *Nutrition* **2001**, *17*, 585–589. [CrossRef]
6. Ferreira, L.G.; Santos, L.F.; Anastácio, L.R.; Lima, A.S.; Correia, M.I. Resting energy expenditure, body composition, and dietary intake: A longitudinal study before and after liver transplantation. *Transplantation* **2013**, *96*, 579–585. [CrossRef] [PubMed]
7. Anastácio, L.R.; Ferreira, L.G.; de Sena Ribeiro, H.; Lima, A.S.; Vilela, E.G.; Toulson Davisson Correia, M.I. Body composition and over-weight of liver transplant recipients. *Transplantation* **2011**, *92*, 947–951. [CrossRef] [PubMed]
8. Lane, J.T.; Dagogo-Jack, S. Approach to the patient with new-onset diabetes after transplant (NODAT). *J. Clin. Endocrinol. Metab.* **2011**, *96*, 3289–3297. [CrossRef] [PubMed]
9. Parekh, J.; Corley, D.A.; Feng, S. Diabetes, hypertension and hyperlipidemia: Prevalence over time and impact on long-term survival after liver transplantation. *Am. J. Transplant.* **2012**, *12*, 2181–2187. [CrossRef] [PubMed]
10. Li, D.W.; Lu, T.F.; Hua, X.W.; Dai, H.J.; Cui, X.L.; Zhang, J.J.; Xia, Q. Risk factors for new onset diabetes mellitus after liver transplantation: A meta-analysis. *World J. Gastroenterol.* **2015**, *21*, 6329–6340. [CrossRef] [PubMed]
11. Ling, Q.; Xie, H.; Lu, D.; Wei, X.; Gao, F.; Zhou, L.; Xu, X.; Zheng, S. Association between donor and recipient *TCF7L2* gene polymorphisms and the risk of new-onset diabetes mellitus after liver transplantation in a Han Chinese population. *J. Hepatol.* **2013**, *58*, 271–277. [CrossRef] [PubMed]

12. Bianchi, G.; Marchesini, G.; Marzocchi, R.; Pinna, A.D.; Zoli, M. Metabolic syndrome in liver transplantation: Relation to etiology and immunosuppression. *Liver Transplant.* **2008**, *14*, 1648–1654. [CrossRef] [PubMed]

13. Singh, S.; Watt, K.D. Long-term medical management of the liver transplant recipient: What the primary care physician needs to know. *Mayo Clin. Proc.* **2012**, *87*, 779–790. [CrossRef] [PubMed]

14. Morrisett, J.D.; Abdel-Fattah, G.; Hoogeveen, R.; Mitchell, E.; Ballantyne, C.M.; Pownall, H.J.; Opekun, A.R.; Jaffe, J.S.; Oppermann, S.; Kahan, B.D. Effects of sirolimus on plasma lipids, lipoprotein levels, and fatty acid metabolism in renal transplant patients. *J. Lipid Res.* **2002**, *43*, 1170–1180. [PubMed]

15. Nikkilä, K.; Åberg, F.; Isoniemi, H. Transmission of LDLR mutation from donor through liver transplantation resulting in hypercholesterolemia in the recipient. *Am. J. Transplant.* **2014**, *14*, 2898–2902. [CrossRef] [PubMed]

16. Hryniewiecka, E.; Zegarska, J.; Paczek, L. Arterial hypertension in liver transplant recipients. *Transplant. Proc.* **2011**, *43*, 3029–3034. [CrossRef] [PubMed]

17. Zheng, J.; Wang, W.L. Risk factors of metabolic syndrome after liver transplantation. *Hepatobiliary Pancreat. Dis. Int.* **2015**, *14*, 582–587. [CrossRef]

18. Wilkinson, A.; Davidson, J.; Dotta, F.; Home, P.D.; Keown, P.; Kiberd, B.; Jardine, A.; Levitt, N.; Marchetti, P.; Markell, M.; *et al.* Guidelines for the treatment and management of new-onset diabetes after transplantation. *Clin. Transplant.* **2005**, *19*, 291–298. [CrossRef] [PubMed]

19. Ahn, H.Y.; Cho, Y.M.; Yi, N.J.; Suh, K.S.; Lee, K.U.; Park, K.S.; Kim, S.Y.; Lee, H.K. Predictive factors associated with the reversibility of post-transplantation diabetes mellitus following liver transplantation. *J. Korean Med. Sci.* **2009**, *24*, 567–570. [CrossRef] [PubMed]

20. Musavi, Z.; Azarpira, N.; Sangtarash, M.H.; Kordi, M.; Kazemi, K.; Geramizadeh, B.; Malek-Hosseini, S.A. Polymorphism of transcription factor-7-Like 2 (*TCF7L2*) gene and new-onset diabetes after liver transplantation. *Int. J. Organ Transplant. Med.* **2015**, *6*, 14–22. [PubMed]

21. Neal, D.A.; Brown, M.J.; Wilkinson, I.B.; Alexander, G.J. Mechanisms of hypertension after liver transplantation. *Transplantation* **2005**, *79*, 935–940. [CrossRef] [PubMed]

22. Giusto, M.; Lattanzi, B.; Di Gregorio, V.; Giannelli, V.; Lucidi, C.; Merli, M. Changes in nutritional status after liver transplantation. *World J. Gastroenterol.* **2014**, *20*, 10682–10690. [CrossRef] [PubMed]

23. Van den Ham, E.C.; Kooman, J.P.; Christiaans, M.H.; Leunissen, K.M.; van Hooff, J.P. Posttransplantation weight gain is predominantly due to an increase in body fat mass. *Transplantation* **2000**, *70*, 241–242. [PubMed]

24. Mercier, J.G.; Hokanson, J.F.; Brooks, G.A. Effects of cyclosporine A on skeletal muscle mitochondrial respiration and endurance time in rats. *Am. J. Respir. Crit. Care Med.* **1995**, *151*, 1532–1536. [CrossRef] [PubMed]

25. Rodríguez-Perálvarez, M.; Germani, G.; Darius, T.; Lerut, J.; Tsochatzis, E.; Burroughs, A.K. Tacrolimus trough levels, rejection and renal impairment in liver transplantation: A systematic review and meta-analysis. *Am. J. Transplant.* **2012**, *12*, 2797–2814. [CrossRef] [PubMed]

26. Sakuma, K.; Yamaguchi, A. The functional role of calcineurin in hypertrophy, regeneration, and disorders of skeletal muscle. *J. Biomed. Biotechnol.* **2010**, *2010*. [CrossRef] [PubMed]

27. Rabkin, J.M.; Corless, C.L.; Rosen, H.R.; Olyaei, A.J. Immunosuppression impact on long-term cardiovascular complications after liver transplantation. *Am. J. Surg.* **2002**, *183*, 595–599. [CrossRef]

28. Manzarbeitia, C.; Reich, D.J.; Rothstein, K.D.; Braitman, L.E.; Levin, S.; Munoz, S.J. Tacrolimus conversion improves hyperlipidemic states in stable liver transplant recipients. *Liver Transplant.* **2001**, *7*, 93–99. [CrossRef] [PubMed]

29. Ojo, A.O.; Held, P.J.; Port, F.K.; Wolfe, R.A.; Leichtman, A.B.; Young, E.W.; Arndorfer, J.; Christensen, L.; Merion, R.M. Chronic renal failure after transplantation of a nonrenal organ. *N. Engl. J. Med.* **2003**, *349*, 931–940. [CrossRef] [PubMed]

30. Rossetto, A.; Bitetto, D.; Bresadola, V.; Lorenzin, D.; Baccarani, U.; de Anna, D.; Bresadola, F.; Adani, G.L. Cardiovascular risk factors and immunosuppressive regimen after liver transplantation. *Transplant. Proc.* **2010**, *42*, 2576–2578. [CrossRef] [PubMed]

31. Neff, G.W.; Montalbano, M.; Tzakis, A.G. Ten years of sirolimus therapy in orthotopic liver transplant recipients. *Transplant. Proc.* **2003**, *35*, 209S–216S. [CrossRef]

32. Miyabara, E.H.; Conte, T.C.; Silva, M.T.; Baptista, I.L.; Bueno, C.; Fiamoncini, J.; Lambertucci, R.H.; Serra, C.S.; Brum, P.C.; Curi, T.; *et al.* Mammalian target of rapamycin complex 1 is involved in differentiation of regenerating myofibers *in vivo Muscle Nerve* **2010** *42*, 778–787. [CrossRef] [PubMed]

33. Zimmermann, A.; Zobeley, C.; Weber, M.M.; Lang, H.; Galle, P.R.; Zimmermann, T. Changes in lipid and carbohydrate metabolism under mTOR- and calcineurin-based immunosuppressive regimen in adult patients after liver transplantation. *Eur. J. Intern. Med.* **2016**, *29*, 104–109. [CrossRef] [PubMed]

34. Klintmalm, G.B.; Washburn, W.K.; Rudich, S.M.; Heffron, T.G.; Teperman, L.W.; Fasola, C.; Eckhoff, D.E.; Netto, G.J.; Katz, E. Corticosteroid-free immunosuppression with daclizumab in HCV+ liver transplant recipients: 1-Year interim results of the HCV-3 study. *Liver Transplant.* **2007**, *13*, 1521–1531. [CrossRef] [PubMed]

35. Contos, M.J.; Cales, W.; Sterling, R.K.; Luketic, V.A.; Shiffman, M.L.; Mills, A.S.; Fisher, R.A.; Ham, J.; Sanyal, A.J. Development of nonalcoholic fatty liver disease after orthotopic liver transplantation for cryptogenic cirrhosis. *Liver Transplant.* **2001**, *7*, 363–373. [CrossRef] [PubMed]

36. Iadevaia, M.; Giusto, M.; Giannelli, V.; Lai, Q.; Rossi, M.; Berloco, P.; Corradini, S.G.; Merli, M. Metabolic syndrome and cardiovascular risk after liver transplantation: A single-center experience. *Transplant. Proc.* **2012**, *44*, 2005–2006. [CrossRef] [PubMed]

37. Rodríguez-Perálvarez, M.; Germani, G.; Papastergiou, V.; Tsochatzis, E.; Thalassinos, E.; Luong, T.V.; Rolando, N.; Dhillon, A.P.; Patch, D.; O'Beirne, J.; et al. Early tacrolimus exposure after liver transplantation: Relationship with moderate/severe acute rejection and long-term outcome. *J. Hepatol.* **2013**, *58*, 262–270. [CrossRef] [PubMed]

38. Heisel, O.; Heisel, R.; Balshaw, R.; Keown, P. New onset diabetes mellitus in patients receiving calcineurin inhibitors: A system-atic review and meta-analysis. *Am. J. Transplant.* **2004**, *4*, 583–595. [CrossRef] [PubMed]

39. Watt, K.D.; Charlton, M.R. Metabolic syndrome and liver transplantation: A review and guide to management. *J. Hepatol.* **2010**, *53*, 199–206. [CrossRef] [PubMed]

40. Ford, E.S.; Giles, W.H.; Dietz, W.H. Prevalence of the metabolic syndrome among US adults: Findings from the third National Health and Nutrition Examination Survey. *JAMA* **2002**, *287*, 356–359. [CrossRef] [PubMed]

41. Sprinzl, M.F.; Weinmann, A.; Lohse, N.; Tönissen, H.; Koch, S.; Schattenberg, J.; Hoppe-Lotichius, M.; Zimmermann, T.; Galle, P.R.; Hansen, T.; et al. Metabolic syndrome and its association with fatty liver disease after orthotopic liver transplantation. *Transpl. Int.* **2013**, *26*, 67–74. [CrossRef] [PubMed]

42. Qin, N.; Yang, F.; Li, A.; Prifti, E.; Chen, Y.; Shao, L.; Guo, J.; Le Chatelier, E.; Yao, J.; Wu, L.; et al. Alterations of the human gut microbiome in liver cirrhosis. *Nature* **2014**, *513*, 59–64. [CrossRef] [PubMed]

43. Fussner, L.A.; Heimbach, J.K.; Fan, C.; Dierkhising, R.; Coss, E.; Leise, M.D.; Watt, K.D. Cardiovascular disease after liver transplantation: When, what, and who is at risk. *Liver Transplant.* **2015**, *21*, 889–896. [CrossRef] [PubMed]

44. Pagadala, M.; Dasarathy, S.; Eghtesad, B.; McCullough, A.J. Posttransplant metabolic syndrome: An epidemic waiting to happen. *Liver Transplant.* **2009**, *15*, 1662–1670. [CrossRef] [PubMed]

45. Burra, P.; Germani, G. Orthotopic liver transplantation in non-alcoholic fatty liver disease patients. *Rev. Recent Clin. Trials* **2014**, *9*, 210–216. [CrossRef] [PubMed]

46. Dureja, P.; Mellinger, J.; Agni, R.; Chang, F.; Avey, G.; Lucey, M.; Said, A. NAFLD recurrence in liver transplant recipients. *Transplantation* **2011**, *91*, 684–689. [CrossRef] [PubMed]

47. Malik, S.M.; de Vera, M.E.; Fontes, P.; Shaikh, O.; Sasatomi, E.; Ahmad, J. Recurrent disease following liver transplantation for nonalcoholic steatohepatitis cirrhosis. *Liver Transplant.* **2009**, *15*, 1843–1851. [CrossRef] [PubMed]

48. Finkenstedt, A.; Auer, C.; Glodny, B.; Posch, U.; Steitzer, H.; Lanzer, G.; Pratschke, J.; Biebl, M.; Steurer, M.; Graziadei, I.; et al. Patatin-like phospholipase domain-containing protein 3 rs738409-G in recipients of liver transplants is a risk factor for graft steatosis. *Clin. Gastroenterol. Hepatol.* **2013**, *11*, 1667–1672. [CrossRef] [PubMed]

49. Watt, K.D.; Dierkhising, R.; Fan, C.; Heimbach, J.K.; Tillman, H.; Goldstein, D.; Thompson, A.; Krishnan, A.; Charlton, M.R. Investigation of PNPLA3 and IL28B genotypes on diabetes and obesity after liver transplantation: Insight into mechanisms of disease. *Am. J. Transplant.* **2013**, *13*, 2450–2457. [CrossRef] [PubMed]

50. Dumortier, J.; Giostra, E.; Belbouab, S.; Morard, I.; Guillaud, O.; Spahr, L.; Boillot, O.; Rubbia-Brandt, L.; Scoazec, J.Y.; Hadengue, A. Non-alcoholic fatty liver disease in liver transplant recipients: Another story of "seed and soil". *Am. J. Gastroenterol.* **2010** *105*, 613–620. [CrossRef] [PubMed]

51. Mikolasevic, I.; Orlic, L.; Hrstic, I.; Milic, S. Metabolic syndrome and non-alcoholic fatty liver disease after liver or kidney transplantation. *Hepatol. Res.* **2015**. [CrossRef] [PubMed]

52. Gitto, S.; Vitale, G.; Villa, E.; Andreone, P. Treatment of nonalcoholic steatohepatitis in adults: Present and future. *Gastroenterol. Res. Pract.* **2015**, *2015*. [CrossRef] [PubMed]

53. Kim, F.; Pham, M.; Maloney, E.; Rizzo, N.O.; Morton, G.J.; Wisse, B.E.; Kirk, E.A.; Chait, A.; Schwartz, M.W. Vascular inflammation, insulin resistance, and reduced nitric oxide production precede the onset of peripheral insulin resistance. *Arterioscler. Thromb. Vasc. Biol.* **2008**, *28*, 1982–1988. [CrossRef] [PubMed]

54. Tilg, H.; Moschen, A.R. Evolution of inflammation in nonalcoholic fatty liver disease: The multiple parallel hits hypothesis. *Hepatology* **2010**, *52*, 1836–1846. [CrossRef] [PubMed]

55. Kouz, J.; Vincent, C.; Leong, A.; Dorais, M.; Räkel, A. Weight gain after orthotopic liver transplantation: Is nonalcoholic fatty liver disease cirrhosis a risk factor for greater weight gain? *Liver Transplant.* **2014**, *20*, 1266–1274. [CrossRef] [PubMed]

56. Merli, M.; Giusto, M.; Riggio, O.; Gentili, F.; Molinaro, A.; Attili, A.F.; Ginanni Corradini, S.; Rossi, M. Improvement of nutritional status in malnourished cirrhotic patients one year after liver transplantation. *e-SPEN* **2011**, *6*, e142–e147. [CrossRef]

57. Charlton, M. Evolving aspects of liver transplantation for nonalcoholic steatohepatitis. *Curr. Opin. Organ Transplant.* **2013**, *18*, 251–258. [CrossRef] [PubMed]

58. Krasnoff, J.B.; Vintro, A.Q.; Ascher, N.L.; Bass, N.M.; Paul, S.M.; Dodd, M.J.; Painter, P.L. A randomized trial of exercise and dietary counseling after liver transplantation. *Am. J. Transplant.* **2006**, *6*, 1896–1905. [CrossRef] [PubMed]

59. Loria, P.; Adinolfi, L.E.; Bellentani, S.; Bugianesi, E.; Grieco, A.; Fargion, S.; Gasbarrini, A.; Loguercio, C.; Lonardo, A.; Marchesini, G.; *et al.* Practice guidelines for the diagnosis and management of nonalcoholic fatty liver disease: A decalogue from the Italian Association for the Study of the Liver (AISF) Expert Committee. *Dig. Liver Dis.* **2010**, *42*, 272–282. [CrossRef] [PubMed]

60. Ratziu, V.; Bellentani, S.; Cortez-Pinto, H.; Day, C.; Marchesini, G. A position statement on NAFLD/NASH based on the EASL 2009 special conference. *J. Hepatol.* **2010**, *53*, 372–384. [CrossRef] [PubMed]

61. Farrell, G.C.; Chitturi, S.; Lau, G.K.; Sollano, J.D.; Asia-Pacific Working Party on NAFLD. Guidelines for the assessment and management of non-alcoholic fatty liver disease in the Asia-Pacific region: Executive summary. *J. Gastroenterol. Hepatol.* **2007**, *22*, 775–777. [CrossRef] [PubMed]

62. Chalasani, N.; Younossi, Z.; Lavine, J.E.; Diehl, A.M.; Brunt, E.M.; Cusi, K.; Charlton, M.; Sanyal, A.J.; American Gastroenterological Association; American Association for the Study of Liver Diseases; *et al.* The diagnosis and management of non-alcoholic fatty liver disease: Practice guideline by the American Gastroenterological Association, American Association for the Study of Liver Diseases, and American College of Gastroenterology. *Gastroenterology* **2012**, *142*, 1592–1609. [PubMed]

63. Promrat, K.; Kleiner, D.E.; Niemeier, H.M.; Jackvony, E.; Kearns, M.; Wands, J.R.; Fava, J.L.; Wing, R.R. Randomized controlled trial testing the effects of weight loss on nonalcoholic steatohepatitis. *Hepatology* **2010**, *51*, 121–129. [CrossRef] [PubMed]

64. Diabetes Prevention Program (DPP) Research Group. The Diabetes Prevention Program (DPP): Description of lifestyle intervention. *Diabetes Care* **2002**, *25*, 2165–2171.

65. George, A.; Bauman, A.; Johnston, A.; Farrell, G.; Chey, T.; George, J. Independent effects of physical activity in patients with nonalcoholic fatty liver disease. *Hepatology* **2009**, *50*, 68–76. [CrossRef] [PubMed]

66. Hallsworth, K.; Fattakhova, G.; Hollingsworth, K.G.; Thoma, C.; Moore, S.; Taylor, R.; Day, C.P.; Trenell, M.I. Resistance exercise reduces liver fat and its mediators in non-alcoholic fatty liver disease independent of weight loss. *Gut* **2011**, *60*, 1278–1283. [CrossRef] [PubMed]

67. Kantartzis, K.; Thamer, C.; Peter, A.; Machann, J.; Schick, F.; Schraml, C.; Königsrainer, A.; Königsrainer, I.; Kröber, S.; Niess, A.; *et al.* High cardiorespiratory fitness is an independent predictor of the reduction in liver fat during a lifestyle intervention in non-alcoholic fatty liver disease. *Gut* **2009**, *58*, 1281–1288. [CrossRef] [PubMed]

68. Targher, G.; Marra, F.; Marchesini, G. Increased risk of cardiovascular disease in non-alcoholic fatty liver disease: Causal effect or epiphenomenon? *Diabetologia* **2008**, *51*, 1947–1953. [CrossRef] [PubMed]

69. Lassailly, G.; Caiazzo, R.; Pattou, F.; Mathurin, P. Perspectives on treatment for nonalcoholic steatohepatitis. *Gastroenterology* **2016**. [CrossRef] [PubMed]

70. Karlas, T.; Kollmeier, J.; Böhm, S.; Müller, J.; Kovacs, P.; Tröltzsch, M.; Weimann, A.; Bartels, M.; Rosendahl, J.; Mössner, J.; *et al.* Noninvasive characterization of graft steatosis after liver transplantation. *Scand. J. Gastroenterol.* **2015**, *50*, 224–232. [CrossRef] [PubMed]

12

NAFLD and NASH in HCV Infection: Prevalence and Significance in Hepatic and Extrahepatic Manifestations

Luigi Elio Adinolfi *, Luca Rinaldi, Barbara Guerrera, Luciano Restivo, Aldo Marrone, Mauro Giordano and Rosa Zampino

Department of Medical, Surgical, Neurological, Metabolic, and Geriatric Sciences, Second University of Naples, Naples 80100, Italy; lucarinaldi@hotmail.it (L.R.); barbara.guerrera@alice.it (B.G.); luciano.restivo@gmail.it (L.R.); Aldo.marrone@unina2.it (A.M.); mauro.giordano@unina2.it (M.G.); rosa.zampino@unina2.it (R.Z.)
* Correspondence: luigielio.adinolfi@unina2.it

Academic Editors: Amedeo Lonardo and Giovanni Targher

Abstract: The aim of this paper is to review and up to date the prevalence of hepatitis C virus (HCV)-associated non-alcoholic fatty liver disease (NAFLD) and non-alcoholic steatohepatitis (NASH) and their significance in both accelerating progression of HCV-related liver disease and development of HCV-associated extrahepatic diseases. The reported mean prevalence of HCV-related NAFLD was 55%, whereas NASH was reported in 4%–10% of cases. HCV genotype 3 directly induces fatty liver deposition, namely "viral steatosis" and it is associated with the highest prevalence and degree of severity, whereas, HCV non-3 genotype infection showed lower prevalence of steatosis, which is associated with metabolic factors and insulin resistance. The host's genetic background predisposes him or her to the development of steatosis. HCV's impairment of lipid and glucose metabolism causes fatty liver accumulation; this seems to be a viral strategy to optimize its life cycle. Irrespective of insulin resistance, HCV-associated NAFLD, in a degree-dependent manner, contributes towards accelerating the liver fibrosis progression and development of hepatocellular carcinoma by inducing liver inflammation and oxidative stress. Furthermore, NAFLD is associated with the presence of metabolic syndrome, type 2 diabetes, and atherosclerosis. In addition, HCV-related "metabolic steatosis" impairs the response rate to interferon-based treatment, whereas it seems that "viral steatosis" may harm the response rate to new oral direct antiviral agents. In conclusion, a high prevalence of NAFLD occurs in HCV infections, which is, at least in part, induced by the virus, and that NAFLD significantly impacts progression of the liver disease, therapeutic response, and some extrahepatic diseases.

Keywords: HCV-associated NAFLD; insulin resistance; liver fibrosis; HCC; metabolic syndrome; diabetes; atherosclerosis

1. Introduction

Non-alcoholic fatty liver disease (NAFLD) is a condition characterized by fatty liver accumulation with a spectrum of liver damage ranging from simple steatosis to non-alcoholic steatohepatitis (NASH). The latter accounted for one third of cases [1] and it is a common cause of chronic liver diseases, including cirrhosis and hepatocellular carcinoma (HCC) [2]. NAFLD is strictly associated with metabolic syndrome in the general population and can be considered as a multisystem disease associated with inflammation, oxidative stress, and insulin resistance with an increasing risk of type 2 diabetes mellitus, cardiovascular diseases, and chronic kidney diseases [1]. Moreover, irrespective of metabolic syndrome, recently, several host genetic backgrounds have been reported as potential risk factors for development of NAFLD [1].

NAFLD is a prominent feature of chronic hepatitis C virus (HCV) infection [3]. Both viral and host factors contribute to the development of steatosis. NAFLD in HCV genotype 3 infected patients is strictly associated with serum viral load [3–7], thus steatosis in this setting is considered to be of viral origin and it is namely "viral steatosis"; whereas in HCV non-3 genotype infected patients, NAFLD is mainly linked to host factors such as body mass index (BMI), obesity, particular visceral obesity [8], insulin resistance, and type 2 diabetes mellitus, and it is called "metabolic steatosis". Accordingly, liver steatosis localization in HCV non-3 genotypes infected patients is similar to that observed in NAFLD/NASH (*i.e.*, mostly in the centrolobular zone (acinar 3)) [9], whereas in genotype 3 infection steatosis is localized mainly in the periportal zone (acinar 1) [10]. With respect to the sustained virologic response rate to interferon-based treatment, a substantial difference in the behavior of the two types of HCV-associated NAFLD has been reported. Metabolic steatosis significantly reduces response rate to interferons [6,11–14], whereas virologic steatosis does not impact the interferon response rate and it even disappears following HCV clearance with reappearance in relapse cases [5,15]. In addition, HCV-related metabolic steatosis is strictly associated with insulin resistance; although HCV *per sé* induces insulin resistance, which predates the development of steatosis, that, in turn, aggravates insulin resistance [16,17]. Furthermore, it has been demonstrated that HCV-associated steatosis induces hepatic and systemic inflammation and oxidative stress [18,19].

The mechanisms by which HCV induces steatosis are complex and specific for genotype 3 (viral steatosis) and non-3 genotypes (metabolic steatosis). However, the two forms of steatosis share some mechanisms and overlapping conditions may occur. Recently, we reviewed the main molecular mechanisms by which HCV induces steatosis [20] and in Figure 1 the chief genotype-specific mechanisms are reported.

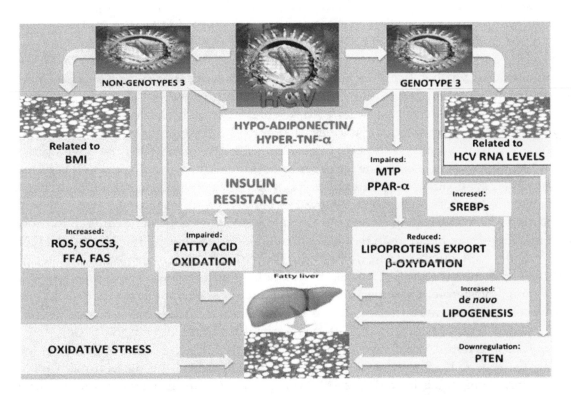

Figure 1. Schematically are illustrated the mains HCV genotype-specific molecular mechanisms of steatogenesis. Abbreviations used: HCV: hepatitis C virus; BMI: body mass index; MTP: microsomal triglyceride transfer protein; PPAR-α: peroxisome proliferator-activated receptor α; SREBPs: sterol regulatory element-binding proteins; ROS: reactive oxygen species; SOCS3: suppressor of cytokine signaling 3; FFA: free fatty acid; FAS: fatty acid synthase; PTEN: phosphatase and tensin homolog.

Chronic HCV infection is considered a systemic disease and there is evidence that steatosis may change the natural history of both HCV-related hepatic and extrahepatic diseases, and that host genetic backgrounds may promote HCV-associated steatosis and progression of liver disease.

In this paper we reviewed the prevalence and associated factors which promote NAFLD/NASH in chronic HCV infections and the evidence that highlights the role of steatosis in both accelerating the progression of HCV-related liver disease and the development of HCV-associated extrahepatic diseases.

2. Prevalence of NAFLD/NASH and Associated Conditions in Chronic HCV Infection

In chronic HCV infection, NAFLD has been reported with a mean prevalence of about 55%, ranging from 40% to 86% [3,5,6,21–30] depending on HCV genotype and local prevalence of metabolic syndrome. HCV genotype 3 infected patients showed the highest prevalence of steatosis (up to 86%), whereas in HCV genotype 1 and 2 the mean reported prevalence was about 40% and 50%, respectively. The above reported prevalence of NAFLD-associated to HCV infection is higher than the rates observed in non-HCV infected subjects in the general population (*i.e.*, 20%–30%) [31], and of the rates reported for other hepatic diseases, such as HBV infection (about 22%) and autoimmune hepatitis (about 16%) [17].

Data on the prevalence of NASH in chronic hepatitis C cases are less consistent than those reported for NAFLD. The published data reported an occurrence of NASH from 4% to 10% [25,32–35]. Risk factors associated with development of HCV-associated NASH include BMI and, for HCV genotype 1, triglyceride and HDL-cholesterol levels, whereas for genotype 3, aspartate transaminase levels are a contributing factor [35,36].

A strict association between HCV-associated NAFLD and insulin resistance has been reported. However, insulin resistance can be both a direct consequence of HCV infection and a result of NAFLD, and *vice versa* [17]. Overall, insulin resistance has been reported with high prevalence in chronic hepatitis C infection cases (up to 80%) and it is commonly observed in HCV non-3 genotypes infected patients, whereas it is not a feature of HCV genotype 3 infection [19].

Overweight and obese BMI levels significantly contribute to the development of HCV-associated NAFLD, in particular, it has been demonstrated that visceral obesity has a preeminent role [2]. Visceral obesity plays an important role in the regulation of glucose and lipid metabolism in chronic HCV infection. In HCV-infected patients with visceral obesity, it has been reported that there are increased levels of pro-inflammatory cytokines (IL-6 and TNF-α) that inhibit insulin signaling and the secretion of adiponectin, which results in corresponding consequences for the development of liver steatosis and insulin resistance [37]. The latter represents the pathophysiological link between steatosis and the metabolic syndrome. Despite chronic HCV patients showing a high prevalence of insulin resistance, an overall low prevalence of full-blown metabolic syndrome was reported [38]. Patients with HCV-associated steatosis presented a higher prevalence of metabolic syndrome than those without steatosis, but a lower prevalence than that observed in NAFLD patients [38]. However, HCV infection is associated with multiple metabolic derangements, which has been termed hepatitis C associated dysmetabolic syndrome (HCADS) [20]. Such metabolic derangements are characterized by insulin resistance, hypocholesterolemia, hyperuricemia, and altered body fat distribution [20].

It has been demonstrated that oxidative stress occurs with high prevalence in chronic HCV infection (e.g., greater that 60% [18]), and that it contributes to the development of NAFLD in HCV non-3 genotypes, but not in "viral steatosis" associated with HCV genotype 3 infections.

The host's genetic background has an important impact on the development of NAFLD in chronic HCV infections. It has been demonstrated that microsomal triglyceride transfer protein (MTP) polymorphism (493GT) was associated with a higher prevalence of NAFLD in HCV genotype 3 [39]; methylene tetrahydrofolate reductase (MTHFR) polymorphism (C677T) [40] was correlated with an increased prevalence of NAFLD in chronic HCV infections as well as an increased risk to develop severe steatosis (*i.e.*, 6-fold higher for hosts with a MTHFR "CT" genotype and 20-fold higher for those with a "TT" genotype) [40]. The patatin-like phospholipase domain-containing 3 (PNPLA3) gene, in particular, its I148M variant, has been linked with an increased prevalence of HCV-related

NAFLD and with visceral obesity [41,42]. Recently, we demonstrated that the TM6SF2, E167K variant, contributes to liver steatosis in chronic hepatitis C [43].

3. HCV-Induces Steatosis: Is It a Finalistic Condition?

A characteristic feature of HCV infections is the strict association between viral factors and host metabolic factors (*i.e.*, lipid and glucose metabolism), which are involved in the development of liver steatosis. Experimental and clinical evidence showed that HCV core proteins, in a genotype-specific manner, cause hepatic fat accumulation by activating SREBP-1 and 2 [44], inhibiting MTP activity [45], impairing peroxisome proliferator-activated receptor (PPAR) expression, and promoting de novo lipid synthesis [46], which harms assembly, excretion, and uptake of very low density lipoprotein (VLDL).

The interaction between HCV and the host's lipid metabolism seems to be crucial for the viral life cycle. It is reported that triglyceride-rich VLDL represents an essential role in the assembly and secretion of HCV. Elements of infective HCV circulate in patient sera as lipo-viro particles (LVPs) in association with ApoB- and ApoE-containing lipoproteins, which suggests the association of viral particles with LDL and VLDL. It was reported that the interaction with the LDL receptor is important for HCV entry into hepatocytes [47]. Similarly, synthesis of farnesyl pyrophosphate and geranylgeranyl pyrophosphate are essential for HCV replication [48]. On the bases of this evidence it has been hypothesized that the abnormalities of hepatic lipid content are essential to perpetuate the HCV life cycle [49].

4. HCV-Associated Steatosis and Progression of Liver Damage

One important question was to define if NAFLD/NASH could impact hepatic fibrosis progression in chronic hepatitis C infections through modifying the natural history of liver damage. Earlier cross-sectional studies demonstrated an association between NAFLD and advanced liver fibrosis [3,8] as well as an association between NAFLD and liver inflammation, which was also strictly associated with progression of fibrosis [50]. Such data were confirmed by prospective studies using paired liver biopsies. A study by Westin *et al.* [25] that featured paired liver biopsies for98 HCV patients showed that steatosis, especially in genotype 3, was an independent factor associated with fibrosis progression. Similarly, Castera *et al.* [28] evaluated the fibrosis progression in 96 chronic hepatitis C patients by means of paired liver biopsy with a mean interval of four years, and found that steatosis was an independent factor associated with fibrosis progression via performing a multivariate analysis (odds ratio (OR) = 4.7%–95% CI = 1.3–10.8; $p = 0.0001$). In addition, Cross *et al.* [51] also used multivariate analysis tin a study involving 112 chronic hepatitis C patients with serial liver biopsy to show that fibrosis progression was associated with steatosis (OR: 14.3; 95% CI: 2.1–1110; $p = 0.006$).

Twenty-eight other cross-sectional or prospective studies, carefully reviewed by Lonardo *et al.* [20], evaluated the association between steatosis and fibrosis confirming that steatosis is strictly associated with liver fibrosis in chronic HCV infections. However, there were some studies that reported an association between steatosis and liver fibrosis that was genotype-dependent [7,25,29,51,52].

A meta-analysis, including data from 10 centers in Europe, Australia, and North America for 3068 individuals with chronic hepatitis C, analyzed the independent factors associated with liver fibrosis [53]. The meta-analysis showed that steatosis was independently associated with liver fibrosis (OR: 1.66; 1.27–2.18: $p < 0.001$) and with liver inflammation. The data of the meta-analysis also reinforce the hypothesis that inflammation is the link between steatosis and liver fibrosis progression.

It is important to underline that there were a marginal number of studies that were not able to demonstrate an association between liver fibrosis and steatosis [22,29,53–56]. The discrepancy of such results may be explained by differences in study design, patient demographic characteristics, differences in histological grading of steatosis/fibrosis, type of statistical analysis performed, and confounding variables, in particular, insulin resistance which has been reported to be independently associated with both steatosis and liver fibrosis progression [53,57–59]. Overall, the majority of the studies evaluated the role of steatosis without considering insulin resistance or *vice versa*, due to the overlapping conditions, thus their independent role in the progression of liver fibrosis has not yet been adequately assessed. However, Moucari *et al.* [60] evaluated 500 patients with chronic hepatitis C and the multivariate analysis showed that both steatosis (adjusted OD 1.95, 1.24–3.06, p = 0.004) and insulin resistance (adjusted OD: 1.80, 1.15–2.81, p = 0.009) were independently associated with advanced liver fibrosis. Hu *et al.* [61], in a retrospective study including 460 patients with chronic hepatitis C, also showed that grade 2 and 3 levels of steatosis were independently associated with liver fibrosis.

The mechanisms by which steatosis and insulin resistance induce progression of liver fibrosis seem to be different. On the basis of the data within the literature [17,52,62,63], in Figure 2 we schematically reported such mechanisms. Both steatosis and insulin resistance activate connective tissue growth factor (CTGF), but steatosis does so by increasing inflammation [17,53] while insulin resistance does so by increasing glucose and insulin levels [62,63].

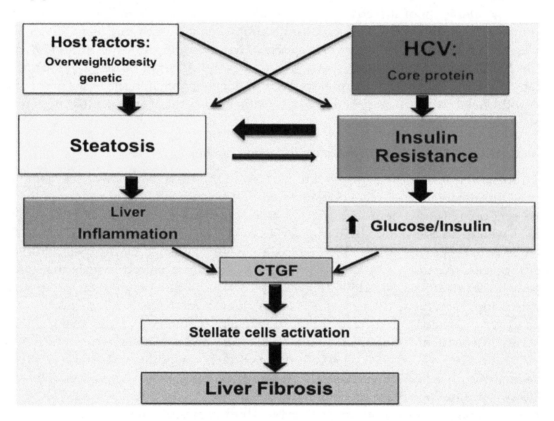

Figure 2. Schematic representation of factors and mechanisms involved in the progression of liver fibrosis in chronic hepatitis C patients. HCV: hepatitis C virus: CTGF: connective tissue growth factor.

Fartoux *et al.* [64] showed that the cumulative probability of progression of fibrosis in mild chronic hepatitis C during a follow up period of more than 90 months was strictly associated with the presence of steatosis. In Fartoux's study, patients with less than 5% steatosis showed a negligible progression of liver fibrosis; patients with steatosis greater than 30% showed the highest (and statistically significant) progression of fibrosis (p < 0.0001), and patients with steatosis between 5% and 30% showed an intermediate progression of liver fibrosis.

It has been reported that similar to patients with HCV-associated NAFLD, those with NASH showed advanced fibrosis [32]. The data seem to suggest that the biological significance of NASH-associated with HCV infection is similar to that observed for cases with a high-degree of steatosis.

In conclusion, there is significant evidence that steatosis is strictly associated with faster progression of liver fibrosis in chronic hepatitis C. The fibrogenic effect of HCV-associated steatosis seems to be multi-factorial involving pro-inflammatory cytokines, oxidative stress, insulin resistance, glucose levels, and increased susceptibility to apoptosis.

There is experimental and clinical evidence supporting a role of HCV-related steatosis in the development of HCC. In experimental models, using transgenic mice, HCV core proteins showed a causative role in the development of steatosis and HCC [65–68]. The experimental evidence has been confirmed in the majority of clinical studies performed [67,69–76]. Both retrospective and prospective studies, with only a few exceptions, showed that HCV-related steatosis was strictly associated with the development of HCC and that the amount of fatty liver deposition was an important risk factor for HCC [67,69–76]. Thus, HCV patients with the highest degree of steatosis carry a higher risk of HCC. Accordingly, HCV genotype 3 infection has been reported to convey the highest risk to develop HCC [67]. However, at present, direct evidence supporting a role for viral steatosis in inducing HCC is lacking. It has also been shown that patients with HCV-related steatosis and diabetes have an enhanced risk of HCC [77]. The data underline the necessity to increase surveillance for HCC in patients with HCV-related steatosis and advanced liver disease.

It seems that HCV-related steatosis may influence the development of HCC by several mechanisms. Among these, it has been suggested that oxidative stress may have a role through reactive oxygen species inducing mutagenesis [78] and both insulin resistance and lipid metabolic alterations are considered hepato-carcinogenic factors in HCV-related steatosis [79].

5. HCV-Associated Steatosis, Diabetes, Metabolic Syndrome, and Atherosclerosis

HCV infection is associated with an increased risk of type 2 diabetes [80]; HCV patients showed a 12 times higher risk to develop type 2 diabetes [81]. Similarly, diabetes patients had a 5–10 times increased risk of being HCV positive [82]. It has been demonstrated that, in predisposed individuals, chronic HCV infection accelerates the appearance of type 2 diabetes by at least 10 years [81]. The mechanism involved in HCV-induced diabetes is insulin resistance, which is strictly associated with both viral infection and steatosis. It has been reported that 75% of HCV patients with diabetes have steatosis [83] and that HCV-related steatosis is associated with diabetes [53]. Thus, HCV-related steatosis may influence diabetes by aggravating insulin resistance. Otherwise, it is also possible that both insulin resistance and type 2 diabetes can increase or aggravate steatosis in chronic HCV infection.

The presence of steatosis, insulin resistance, and diabetes are associated with advanced liver fibrosis, HCC, and poor outcome of chronic hepatitis C infections [84–86].

The prevalence of metabolic syndrome in chronic hepatitis C patients was about 5% and was similar to that observed in the general population [37]. However, metabolic syndrome was significantly higher in patients with HCV-related steatosis as compared with HCV patients without steatosis (13.3% vs. 1.8%) [50]. The data indicate that in chronic hepatitis C patients the presence of liver steatosis predicts metabolic syndrome.

There is a consistent body of literature demonstrating that chronic HCV infection is a risk factor for atherosclerosis, cardiovascular diseases, and related forms of mortality [18]. It has been demonstrated that HCV may live and replicate within carotid plaque [87]. Moreover, chronic HCV infection is associated with many pro-atherogenic conditions such as inflammation, hypoadiponectinemia, hyperhomocysteinemia, increased oxidative stress, insulin resistance, and diabetes [18]. HCV-related steatosis was associated with the above reported pro-atherogenic conditions [50]. Thus, it was anticipated that hepatic steatosis might predict the presence of atherosclerosis in chronic hepatitis C patients. Accordingly, it has been demonstrated that in HCV patients, steatosis is an independent factor associated with the highest prevalence of atherosclerosis [50]. Steatosis predicted, with a good specificity (81.7%) and sensitivity (74.2%), both early (intima-media thickness) and advanced (plaques) lesions of carotid atherososclerosis. It has been suggested that steatosis may modulate atherogenic factors; such as inflammation and metabolic elements favoring the development of atherosclerosis and that patients with HCV-associated steatosis should be screened for atherosclerosis [50].

6. HCV-Associated Steatosis and Response to Antiviral Treatments

HCV-related "metabolic steatosis" has been reported as a negative predictor of response to interferon-based antiviral therapy in genotypes 1 and 2 infections [6,11–14]. In this setting of treatment, patients with "viral steatosis" associated with HCV genotype 3 infection were considered easy to treat.

In the last few years, the new oral direct antiviral agents (DAAs) are becoming the standard of HCV treatment. The impact of steatosis on DAAs treatment has been scantly evaluated. However, there is an agreement that the HCV genotype 3 showed lower response rate to DAAs and now it has been considered to be difficult to treat. It has been proposed that steatosis could partly explain the lower response rate in HCV genotype 3 infections [88]. Thus, specific studies are needed to evaluate the impact of steatosis and metabolic factors on the response rate of the new DAAs.

7. Conclusions

The data demonstrate that hepatic steatosis is a feature of chronic HCV infections and that liver fatty accumulation seems to be a finalistic condition favoring the persistence and replication of HCV. HCV-associated steatosis, in a degree-dependent fashion, producing hepatic inflammation and oxidative stress, induces a more rapid progression of liver fibrosis and increases the risk of the development of HCC. HCV-associated steatosis also influences the development of some extrahepatic manifestations of chronic HCV infection such as diabetes, metabolic syndrome, and atherosclerosis. In addition, the presence of steatosis impairs the response rate to interferons based anti-HCV treatments and could have a role in the lower response rate observed in HCV genotype 3 treated with new DAAs. Thus, steatosis should be regarded as a marker to individuate patients at higher risk of progression of HCV-associated liver disease, development of extrahepatic diseases, and lower therapeutic response rate, perhaps even in the era of new DAAs.

Author Contributions: All authors equally contributed to this review.

References

1.   Christopher, D.; Byrne, C.D.; Targher, G. NAFLD: A multisystem disease. *J. Hepatol.* **2015**, *62*, S47–S64.
2.   Baffy, G.; Brunt, E.M.; Caldwell, S.H. Hepatocellular carcinoma in non-alcoholic fatty liver disease: An emerging menace. *J. Hepatol.* **2012**, *56*, 1384–1391. [CrossRef] [PubMed]
3.   Adinolfi, L.E.; Gambardella, M.; Andreana, A.; Tripodi, M.F.; Utili, R.; Ruggiero, G. Steatosis accelerates the progression of liver damage of chronic hepatitis C patients and correlates with specific HCV genotype and visceral obesity. *Hepatology* **2001**, *33*, 1358–1364. [CrossRef] [PubMed]
4.   Adinolfi, L.E.; Utili, R.; Ruggiero, G. Body composition and hepatic steatosis as precursors of fibrosis in chronic hepatitis C patients. *Hepatology* **1999**, *30*, 1530–1531. [CrossRef] [PubMed]
5.   Rubbia-Brandt, L.; Quadri, R.; Abid, K.; Giostra, E.; Malé, P.J.; Mentha, G.; Spahr, L.; Zarski, J.P.; Borisch, B.; Hadengue, A.; *et al.* Hepatocyte steatosis is a cytopathic effect of hepatitis C virus genotype 3. *J. Hepatol.* **2000**, *33*, 106–115. [CrossRef]
6.   Poynard, T.; Ratziu, V.; McHutchison, J.; Manns, M.; Goodman, Z.; Zeuzem, S.; Younossi, Z.; Albrecht, J. Effect of treatment with peginterferon or interferon alfa-2b and ribavirin on steatosis in patients infected with hepatitis C. *Hepatology* **2003**, *38*, 75–85. [CrossRef] [PubMed]
7.   Patton, H.M.; Patel, K.; Behling, C.; Bylund, D.; Blatt, L.M.; Vallée, M.; Heaton, S.; Conrad, A.; Pockros, P.J.; McHutchison, J.G. The impact of steatosis on dise. *J. Hepatol.* **2004**, *40*, 484–490. [CrossRef] [PubMed]
8.   Hickman, I.J.; Powell, E.E.; Prins, J.B.; Clouston, A.D.; Ash, S.; Purdie, D.M.; Jonsson, J.R. In overweight patients with chronic hepatitis C, circulating insulin is associated with hepatic fibrosis: Implications for therapy. *J. Hepatol.* **2003**, *39*, 1042–1048. [CrossRef]
9.   Zubair, A.; Jamal, S.; Mubarik, A.; Saudi, J. Morphometric analysis of hepatic steatosis in chronic hepatitis C infection. *Saudi J. Gastroenterol.* **2009**, *15*, 11–14. [PubMed]
10.   Pazienza, V.; Clément, S.; Pugnale, P.; Conzelman, S.; Foti, M.; Mangia, A.; Negro, F. The hepatitis C virus core protein of genotypes 3A and 1b downregulates insulin receptor substrate 1 through genotype-specific mechanisms. *Hepatology* **2007**, *45*, 1164–1171. [CrossRef] [PubMed]

11. Hwang, S.J.; Luo, J.C.; Chu, C.W.; Lai, C.R.; Lu, C.L.; Tsay, S.H.; Wu, J.C.; Chang, F.Y.; Lee, S.D. Hepatic steatosis in chronic hepatitis C virus infection: Prevalence and clinical correlation. *J. Gastroenterol. Hepatol.* **2001**, *16*, 190–195. [CrossRef] [PubMed]

12. Zeuzem, S.; Hultcrantz, R.; Bourliere, M.; Goeser, T.; Marcellin, P.; Sanchez-Tapias, J.; Sarrazin, C.; Harvey, J.; Brass, C.; Albrecht, J. Peginterferon alfa-2b plus ribavirin for treatment of chronic hepatitis C in previously untreated patients infected with HCV genotypes 2 or 3. *J. Hepatol.* **2004**, *40*, 993–999. [CrossRef] [PubMed]

13. Harrison, S.A.; Brunt, E.M.; Qazi, R.A.; Oliver, D.A.; Neuschwander-Tetri, B.A.; Di Bisceglie, A.M.; Bacon, B.R. Effect of significant histologic steatosis or steatohepatitis on response to antiviral therapy in patients with chronic hepatitis C. *Clin. Gastroenterol. Hepatol.* **2005**, *3*, 604–609. [CrossRef]

14. Romero-Gómez, M.; del Mar Viloria, M.; Andrade, R.J.; Salmerón, J.; Diago, M.; Fernández-Rodríguez, C.M.; Corpas, R.; Cruz, M.; Grande, L.; Vázquez, L.; *et al.* Insulin resistance impairs sustained response rate to peginterferon plus ribavirin in chronic hepatitis C patients. *J. Gastroenterol.* **2005**, *128*, 636–641. [CrossRef]

15. Kumar, D.; Farrell, G.C.; Fung, C.; George, J. Hepatitis C virus genotype 3 is cytopathic to hepatocytes: Reversal of hepatic steatosis after sustained therapeutic response. *Hepatology* **2002**, *36*, 1266–1272. [CrossRef] [PubMed]

16. Shintani, Y.; Fujie, H.; Miyoshi, H.; Tsutsumi, T.; Tsukamoto, K.; Kimura, S.; Moriya, K.; Koike, K. Hepatitis C virus infection and diabetes: Direct involvement of the virus in the development of insulin resistance. *Gastroenterology* **2004**, *126*, 840–848. [CrossRef] [PubMed]

17. Lonardo, A.; Adinolfi, L.E.; Loria, P.; Carulli, N.; Ruggiero, G.; Day, C.P. Steatosis and hepatitis C virus: Mechanisms and significance for hepatic and extrahepatic disease. *Gastroenterology* **2004**, *126*, 586–597. [CrossRef] [PubMed]

18. Adinolfi, L.E.; Zampino, R.; Restivo, L.; Lonardo, A.; Guerrera, B.; Marrone, A.; Nascimbeni, F.; Florio, A.; Loria, P. Chronic hepatitis C virus infection and atherosclerosis: Clinical impact and mechanisms. *World J. Gastroenterol.* **2014**, *20*, 3410–3417. [CrossRef] [PubMed]

19. Vidali, M.; Tripodi, M.F.; Ivaldi, A.; Zampino, R.; Occhino, G.; Restivo, L.; Sutti, S.; Marrone, A.; Ruggiero, G.; Albano, E.; *et al.* Interplay between oxidative stress and hepatic steatosis in the progression of chronic hepatitis C. *J. Hepatol.* **2008**, *48*, 399–406. [CrossRef] [PubMed]

20. Lonardo, A.; Adinolfi, L.E.; Restivo, L.; Ballestri, S.; Romagnoli, D.; Baldelli, E.; Nascimbeni, F.; Loria, P. Pathogenesis and significance of hepatitis C virus steatosis: An update on survival strategy of a successful pathogen. *World J. Gastroenterol.* **2014**, *23*, 7089–7103. [CrossRef] [PubMed]

21. Mihm, S.; Fayyazi, A.; Hartmann, H.; Ramadori, G. Analysis of histopathological manifestations of chronic hepatitis C virus infection with respect to virus genotype. *Hepatology* **1997**, *25*, 735–739. [CrossRef] [PubMed]

22. Czaja, A.J.; Carpenter, H.A.; Santrach, P.J.; Moore, S.B. Host- and disease-specific factors affecting steatosis in chronic hepatitis C. *J. Hepatol.* **1998**, *29*, 198–206. [CrossRef]

23. Hourigan, L.F.; Macdonald, G.A.; Purdie, D.; Whitehall, V.H.; Shorthouse, C.; Clouston, A.; Powell, E.E. Fibrosis in chronic hepatitis C correlates significantly with body mass index and steatosis. *Hepatology* **1999**, *29*, 1215–1219. [CrossRef] [PubMed]

24. Serfaty, L.; Andreani, T.; Giral, P.; Carbonell, N.; Chazouillères, O.; Poupon, R. Hepatitis C virus induced hypobetalipoproteinemia: A possible mechanism for steatosis in chronic hepatitis C. *J. Hepatol.* **2001**, *34*, 428–434. [CrossRef]

25. Monto, A.; Alonzo, J.; Watson, J.J.; Grunfeld, C.; Wright, T.L. Steatosis in chronic hepatitis C: Relative contributions of obesity, diabetes mellitus, and alcohol. *Hepatology* **2002**, *36*, 729–736. [CrossRef] [PubMed]

26. Westin, J.; Nordlinder, H.; Lagging, M.; Norkrans, G.; Wejstål, R. Steatosis accelerates fibrosis development over time in hepatitis C virus genotype 3 infected patients. *J. Hepatol.* **2002**, *37*, 837–842. [CrossRef]

27. Hui, J.M.; Kench, J.; Farrell, G.C.; Lin, R.; Samarasinghe, D.; Liddle, C.; Byth, K.; George, J. Genotype-specific mechanisms for hepatic steatosis in chronic hepatitis C infection. *J. Gastroenterol. Hepatol.* **2002**, *17*, 873–881. [CrossRef] [PubMed]

28. Castéra, L.; Hézode, C.; Roudot-Thoraval, F.; Bastie, A.; Zafrani, E.S.; Pawlotsky, J.M.; Dhumeaux, D. Worsening of steatosis is an independent factor of fibrosis progression in untreated patients with chronic hepatitis C and paired liver biopsies. *Gut* **2003**, *52*, 288–292. [CrossRef] [PubMed]

29.   Asselah, T.; Boyer, N.; Guimont, M.C.; Cazals-Hatem, D.; Tubach, F.; Nahon, K.; Daïkha, H.; Vidaud, D.; Martinot, M.; Vidaud, M.; *et al.* Liver fibrosis is not associated with steatosis but with necroinflammation in French patients with chronic hepatitis C. *Gut* **2003**, *52*, 1638–1643. [CrossRef] [PubMed]

30.   Rubbia-Brandt, L.; Fabris, P.; Paganin, S.; Leandro, G.; Male, P.J.; Giostra, E.; Carlotto, A.; Bozzola, L.; Smedile, A.; Negro, F. Steatosis affects chronic hepatitis C progression in a genotype specific way. *Gut* **2004**, *53*, 406–412. [CrossRef] [PubMed]

31.   Clark, J.M.; Brancati, F.L.; Diehl, A.M. Nonalcoholic fatty liver disease. *Gastroenterology* **2002**, *122*, 1649–1657. [CrossRef] [PubMed]

32.   Ong, J.P.; Younossi, Z.M.; Speer, C.; Olano, A.; Gramlich, T.; Boparai, N. Chronic hepatitis C and superimposed nonalcoholic fatty liver disease. *Liver* **2001**, *21*, 266–271. [CrossRef] [PubMed]

33.   Brunt, E.M.; Ramrakhiani, S.; Cordes, B.G.; Neuschwander-Tetri, B.A.; Janney, C.G.; Bacon, B.R.; di Bisceglie, A.M. Concurrence of histologic features of steatohepatitis with other forms of chronic liver disease. *Mod. Pathol.* **2003**, *16*, 49–56. [CrossRef] [PubMed]

34.   Liu, C.J.; Jeng, Y.M.; Chen, P.J.; Lai, M.Y.; Yang, H.C.; Huang, W.L.; Kao, J.H.; Chen, D.S. Influence of metabolic syndrome, viral genotype and antiviral therapy on superimposed fatty liver disease in chronic hepatitis C. *Antivir. Ther.* **2005**, *10*, 405–415. [PubMed]

35.   Bedossa, P.; Moucari, R.; Chelbi, E.; Asselah, T.; Paradis, V.; Vidaud, M.; Cazals-Hatem, D.; Boyer, N.; Valla, D.; Marcellin, P. Evidence for a role of nonalcoholic steatohepatitis in hepatitis C: A prospective study. *Hepatology* **2007**, *46*, 380–387. [CrossRef] [PubMed]

36.   Solis-Herruzo, J.A.; Pérez-Carreras, M.; Rivas, E.; Fernández-Vázquez, I.; Garfia, C.; Bernardos, E.; Castellano, G.; Colina, F. Factors associated with the presence of nonalcoholic steatohepatitis in patients with chronic hepatitis C. *Am. J. Gastroenterol.* **2005**, *100*, 1091–1098. [CrossRef] [PubMed]

37.   Jonsson, J.R.; Barrie, H.D.; O'Rourke, P.; Clouston, A.D.; Powell, E.E. Obesity and steatosis influence serum and hepatic inflammatory markers in chronic hepatitis C. *Hepatology* **2008**, *48*, 80–87. [CrossRef] [PubMed]

38.   Lonardo, A.; Ballestri, S.; Adinolfi, L.E.; Violi, E.; Carulli, L.; Lombardini, S.; Scaglioni, F.; Ricchi, M.; Ruggiero, G.; Loria, P. Hepatitis C virus-infected patients are "spared" from the metabolic syndrome but not from insulin resistance. A comparative study of nonalcoholic fatty liver disease and hepatitis C virus-related steatosis. *Can. J. Gastroenterol.* **2009**, *23*, 273–278. [CrossRef] [PubMed]

39.   Zampino, R.; Ingrosso, D.; Durante-Mangoni, E.; Capasso, R.; Tripodi, M.F.; Restivo, L.; Zappia, V.; Ruggiero, G.; Adinolfi, L.E. Microsomal triglyceride transfer protein (MTP)-493G/T gene polymorphism contributes to fat liver accumulation in HCV genotype 3 infected patients. *J. Viral. Hepat.* **2008**, *10*, 740–746. [CrossRef] [PubMed]

40.   Adinolfi, L.E.; Ingrosso, D.; Cesaro, G.; Cimmino, A.; D'Antò, M.; Capasso, R.; Zappia, V.; Ruggiero, G. Hyperhomocysteinemia and the MTHFR C677T polymorphism promote steatosis and fibrosis in chronic hepatitis C patients. *Hepatology* **2005**, *41*, 995–1003. [CrossRef] [PubMed]

41.   Valenti, L.; Fargion, S. Patatin-like phospholipase domain containing-3 Ile148Met and fibrosis progression after liver transplantation. *Hepatology* **2011**, *54*, 1484. [CrossRef] [PubMed]

42.   Zampino, R.; Coppola, N.; Cirillo, G.; Boemio, A.; Grandone, A.; Stanzione, M.; Capoluongo, N.; Marrone, A.; Macera, M.; Sagnelli, E.; *et al.* Patatin-like phospholipase domain-containing 3 I148M variant is associated with liver steatosis and fat distribution in chronic hepatitis B. *Dig. Dis. Sci.* **2015**, *60*, 3005–3010. [CrossRef] [PubMed]

43.   Coppola, N.; Rosa, Z.; Cirillo, G.; Stanzione, M.; Macera, M.; Boemio, A.; Grandone, A.; Pisaturo, M.; Marrone, A.; Adinolfi, L.E.; *et al.* TM6SF2 E167K variant is associated with severe steatosis in chronic hepatitis C, regardless of PNPLA3 polymorphism. *Liver Int.* **2015**, *35*, 1959–1963. [CrossRef] [PubMed]

44.   Oem, J.K.; Jackel-Cram, C.; Li, Y.P.; Zhou, Y.; Zhong, J.; Shimano, H.; Babiuk, L.A.; Liu, Q. Activation of sterol regulatory element-binding protein 1C and fatty acid synthase transcription by hepatitis C virus non-structural protein 2. *J. Gen. Virol.* **2008**, *89*, 1225–1230. [CrossRef] [PubMed]

45.   Perlemuter, G.; Sabile, A.; Letteron, P.; Vona, G.; Topilco, A.; Chrétien, Y.; Koike, K.; Pessayre, D.; Chapman, J.; Barba, G.; *et al.* Hepatitis C virus core protein inhibits microsomal triglyceride transfer protein activity and very low density lipoprotein secretion: A model of viral-related steatosis. *FASEB J.* **2002**, *16*, 185–194. [CrossRef] [PubMed]

46.   De Gottardi, A.; Pazienza, V.; Pugnale, P.; Bruttin, F.; Rubbia-Brandt, L.; Juge-Aubry, C.E.; Meier, C.A.; Hadengue, A.; Negro, F. Peroxisome proliferator-activated receptor-α and -γ mRNA levels are reduced in

chronic hepatitis C with steatosis and genotype 3 infection. *Aliment. Pharmacol. Ther.* **2006**, *23*, 107–114. [CrossRef] [PubMed]

47. Burlone, M.E.; Budkowska, A. Hepatitis C virus cell entry: Role of lipoproteins and cellular receptors. *J. Gen. Virol.* **2009**, *90*, 1055–1070. [CrossRef] [PubMed]

48. Kapadia, S.B.; Chisari, F.V. Hepatitis C virus RNA replication is regulated by host geranylgeranylation and fatty acids. *Proc. Natl. Acad. Sci. USA* **2005**, *102*, 2561–2566. [CrossRef] [PubMed]

49. Westin, J.; Lagging, M.; Dhillon, A.P.; Norkrans, G.; Romero, A.I.; Pawlotsky, J.M.; Zeuzem, S.; Schalm, S.W.; Verheij-Hart, E.; Negro, F.; *et al.* Impact of hepatic steatosis on viral kinetics and treatment outcome during antiviral treatment of chronic HCV infection. *J. Viral Hepat.* **2007**, *14*, 29–35. [CrossRef] [PubMed]

50. Adinolfi, L.E.; Restivo, L.; Guerrera, B.; Sellitto, A.; Ciervo, A.; Iuliano, N.; Rinaldi, L.; Santoro, A.; li Vigni, G.; Marrone, A. Chronic HCV infection is a risk factor of ischemic stroke. *Atherosclerosis* **2013**, *23*, 22–26. [CrossRef] [PubMed]

51. Cross, T.J.; Quaglia, A.; Hughes, S.; Joshi, D.; Harrison, P.M. The impact of hepatic steatosis on the natural history of chronic hepatitis C infection. *J. Viral Hepat.* **2009**, *16*, 492–499. [CrossRef] [PubMed]

52. Nieminen, U.; Arkkila, P.E.; Kärkkäinen, P.; Färkkilä, M.A. Effect of steatosis and inflammation on liver fibrosis in chronic hepatitis C. *Liver Int.* **2009**, *29*, 153–158. [CrossRef] [PubMed]

53. Leandro, G.; Mangia, A.; Hui, J.; Fabris, P.; Rubbia-Brandt, L.; Colloredo, G.; Adinolfi, L.E.; Asselah, T.; Jonsson, J.R.; Smedile, A.; *et al.* Relationship between steatosis, inflammation, and fibrosis in chronic hepatitis C: A meta-analysis of individual patient data. *Gastroenterology* **2006**, *130*, 1636–1642. [CrossRef] [PubMed]

54. Sterling, R.K.; Wegelin, J.A.; Smith, P.G.; Stravitz, R.T.; Luketic, V.A.; Fuchs, M.; Puri, P.; Shiffman, M.L.; Contos, M.A.; Mills, A.S.; *et al.* Similar progression of fibrosis between HIV/HCV-infected and HCV-infected patients: Analysis of paired liver biopsy samples. *Clin. Gastroenterol. Hepatol.* **2010**, *8*, 1070–1076. [CrossRef] [PubMed]

55. Matos, C.A.; Perez, R.M.; Pacheco, M.S.; Figueiredo-Mendes, C.G.; Lopes-Neto, E.; Oliveira, E.B.; Lanzoni, V.P.; Silva, A.E.; Ferraz, M.L. Steatosis in chronic hepatitis C: Relationship to the virus and host risk factors. *J. Gastroenterol. Hepatol.* **2006**, *21*, 1236–1239. [CrossRef] [PubMed]

56. Macías, J.; Berenguer, J.; Japón, M.A.; Girón, J.A.; Rivero, A.; López-Cortés, L.F.; Moreno, A.; González-Serrano, M.; Iribarren, J.A.; Ortega, E.; *et al.* Fast fibrosis progression between repeated liver biopsies in patients coinfected with human immunodeficiency virus/hepatitis C virus. *Hepatology* **2009**, *50*, 1056–1063. [CrossRef] [PubMed]

57. Taura, N.; Ichikawa, T.; Hamasaki, K.; Nakao, K.; Nishimura, D.; Goto, T.; Fukuta, M.; Kawashimo, H.; Fujimoto, M.; Kusumoto, K.; *et al.* Association between liver fibrosis and insulin sensitivity in chronic hepatitis C patients. *Am. J. Gastroenterol.* **2006**, *101*, 2752–2759. [CrossRef] [PubMed]

58. Fartoux, L.; Poujol-Robert, A.; Guéchot, J.; Wendum, D.; Poupon, R.; Serfaty, L. Insulin resistance is a cause of steatosis and fibrosis progression in chronic hepatitis C. *Gut* **2005**, *54*, 1003–1008. [CrossRef] [PubMed]

59. Perumalswami, P.; Kleiner, D.E.; Lutchman, G.; Heller, T.; Borg, B.; Park, Y.; Liang, T.J.; Hoofnagle, J.H.; Ghany, M.G. Steatosis and progression of fibrosis in untreated patients with chronic hepatitis C infection. *Hepatology* **2006**, *43*, 780–787. [CrossRef] [PubMed]

60. Moucari, R.; Asselah, T.; Cazals-Hatem, D.; Voitot, H.; Boyer, N.; Ripault, M.P.; Sobesky, R.; Martinot-Peignoux, M.; Maylin, S.; Nicolas-Chanoine, M.H.; *et al.* Insulin resistance in chronic hepatitis C: Association with genotypes 1 and 4, serum HCV RNA level, and liver fibrosis. *Gastroenterology* **2008**, *134*, 416–423. [CrossRef] [PubMed]

61. Hu, S.X.; Kyulo, N.L.; Xia, V.W.; Hillebrand, D.J.; Hu, K.Q. Factors associated with hepatic fibrosis in patients with chronic hepatitis C: A retrospective study of a large cohort of U.S. patients. *J. Clin. Gastroenterol.* **2009**, *43*, 758–764. [CrossRef] [PubMed]

62. Paradis, V.; Perlemuter, G.; Bonvoust, F.; Dargere, D.; Parfait, B.; Vidaud, M.; Conti, M.; Huet, S.; Ba, N.; Buffet, C.; *et al.* High glucose and hyperinsulinemia stimulate connective tissue growth factor expression: A potential mechanism involved in progression to fibrosis in nonalcoholic steatohepatitis. *Hepatology* **2001**, *34*, 738–744. [CrossRef] [PubMed]

63. Ratziu, V.; Munteanu, M.; Charlotte, F.; Bonyhay, L.; Poynard, T. LIDO Study Group. Fibrogenic impact of high serum glucose in chronic hepatitis C. *J. Hepatol.* **2003** *39*, 1049–1055. [CrossRef]

64. Fartoux, L.; Chazouillères, O.; Wendum, D.; Poupon, R.; Serfaty, L. Impact of steatosis on progression of fibrosis in patients with mild hepatitis C. *Hepatology* **2005**, *41*, 82–87. [CrossRef] [PubMed]

65. Moriya, K.; Fujie, H.; Shintani, Y.; Yotsuyanagi, H.; Tsutsumi, T.; Ishibashi, K.; Matsuura, Y.; Kimura, S.; Miyamura, T.; Koike, K. The core protein of hepatitis C virus induces hepatocellular carcinoma in transgenic mice. *Nat. Med.* **1998**, *4*, 1065–1067. [CrossRef] [PubMed]

66. Kanwal, F.; Kramer, J.R.; Ilyas, J.; Duan, Z.; El-Serag, H.B. HCV genotype 3 is associated with an increased risk of cirrhosis and hepatocellular cancer in a national sample of U.S. Veterans with HCV. *Hepatology* **2014**, *60*, 98–105. [CrossRef] [PubMed]

67. Nkontchou, G.; Ziol, M.; Aout, M.; Lhabadie, M.; Baazia, Y.; Mahmoudi, A.; Roulot, D.; Ganne-Carrie, N.; Grando-Lemaire, V.; Trinchet, J.C.; *et al.* HCV genotype 3 is associated with a higher hepatocellular carcinoma incidence in patients with ongoing viral C cirrhosis. *J. Viral Hepat.* **2011**, *18*, e516–e522. [CrossRef] [PubMed]

68. van der Meer, A.J.; Veldt, B.J.; Feld, J.J.; Wedemeyer, H.; Dufour, J.F.; Lammert, F.; Duarte-Rojo, A.; Heathcote, E.J.; Manns, M.P.; Kuske, L.; *et al.* Association between sustained virological response and all-cause mortality among patients with chronic hepatitis C and advanced hepatic fibrosis. *JAMA* **2012**, *308*, 2584–2593. [CrossRef] [PubMed]

69. Asahina, Y.; Tsuchiya, K.; Nishimura, T.; Muraoka, M.; Suzuki, Y.; Tamaki, N.; Yasui, Y.; Hosokawa, T.; Ueda, K.; Nakanishi, H.; *et al.* α-fetoprotein levels after interferon therapy and risk of hepatocarcinogenesis in chronic hepatitis C. *Hepatology* **2013**, *58*, 1253–1262. [CrossRef] [PubMed]

70. Salomao, M.; Yu, W.M.; Brown, R.S.; Emond, J.C.; Lefkowitch, J.H. Steatohepatitic hepatocellular carcinoma (SH-HCC): A distinctive histological variant of HCC in hepatitis C virus-related cirrhosis with associated NAFLD/NASH. *Am. J. Surg. Pathol.* **2010**, *34*, 1630–1636. [CrossRef] [PubMed]

71. Nojiri, K.; Sugimoto, K.; Shiraki, K.; Kusagawa, S.; Tanaka, J.; Beppu, T.; Yamamoto, N.; Takei, Y.; Hashimoto, A.; Shimizu, A.; *et al.* Development of hepatocellular carcinoma in patients with chronic hepatitis C more than 10 years after sustained virological response to interferon therapy. *Oncol. Lett.* **2010**, *1*, 427–430. [PubMed]

72. Tanaka, A.; Uegaki, S.; Kurihara, H.; Aida, K.; Mikami, M.; Nagashima, I.; Shiga, J.; Takikawa, H. Hepatic steatosis as a possible risk factor for the development of hepatocellular carcinoma after eradication of hepatitis C virus with antiviral therapy in patients with chronic hepatitis C. *World J. Gastroenterol.* **2007**, *13*, 5180–5187. [CrossRef] [PubMed]

73. Takuma, Y.; Nouso, K.; Makino, Y.; Saito, S.; Takayama, H.; Takahara, M.; Takahashi, H.; Murakami, I.; Takeuchi, H. Hepatic steatosis correlates with the postoperative recurrence of hepatitis C virus-associated hepatocellular carcinoma. *Liver Int.* **2007**, *27*, 620–626. [CrossRef] [PubMed]

74. Pekow, J.R.; Bhan, A.K.; Zheng, H.; Chung, R.T. Hepatic steatosis is associated with increased frequency of hepatocellular carcinoma in patients with hepatitis C-related cirrhosis. *Cancer* **2007**, *109*, 2490–2496. [CrossRef] [PubMed]

75. Kumar, D.; Farrell, G.C.; Kench, J.; George, J. Hepatic steatosis and the risk of hepatocellular carcinoma in chronic hepatitis C. *J. Gastroenterol. Hepatol.* **2005**, *20*, 1395–1400. [CrossRef] [PubMed]

76. Ohata, K.; Hamasaki, K.; Toriyama, K.; Matsumoto, K.; Saeki, A.; Yanagi, K.; Abiru, S.; Nakagawa, Y.; Shigeno, M.; Miyazoe, S.; *et al.* Hepatic steatosis is a risk factor for hepatocellular carcinoma in patients with chronic hepatitis C virus infection. *Cancer* **2003**, *97*, 3036–3043. [CrossRef] [PubMed]

77. Tazawa, J.; Maeda, M.; Nakagawa, M.; Ohbayashi, H.; Kusano, F.; Yamane, M.; Sakai, Y.; Suzuki, K. Diabetes mellitus may be associated with hepatocarcinogenesis in patients with chronic hepatitis C. *Dig. Dis. Sci.* **2002**, *47*, 710–715. [CrossRef] [PubMed]

78. Jahan, S.; Ashfaq, U.A.; Qasim, M.; Khaliq, S.; Saleem, M.J.; Afzal, N. Hepatitis C virus to hepatocellular carcinoma. *Infect. Agents Cancer* **2012**, *7*. [CrossRef] [PubMed]

79. Koike, K. Hepatitis C virus contributes to hepatocarcinogenesis by modulating metabolic and intracellular signaling pathways. *J. Gastroenterol. Hepatol.* **2007**, *22*, S108–S111. [CrossRef] [PubMed]

80. Adinolfi, L.E.; Restivo, L.; Zampino, R.; Lonardo, A.; Loria, P. Metabolic alterations and chronic hepatitis C: Treatment strategies. *Expert Opin. Pharmacother.* **2011**, *12*, 2215–2234. [CrossRef] [PubMed]

81. Mehta, S.H.; Brancati, F.L.; Sulkowski, M.S.; Strathdee, S.A.; Szklo, M.; Thomas, D.L. Prevalence of type 2 diabetes mellitus among persons with hepatitis C virus infection in the United States. *Ann. Intern. Med.* **2000** *133*, 592–599. [CrossRef] [PubMed]

82. Simó, R.; Hernández, C.; Genescà, J.; Jardí, R.; Mesa, J. High prevalence of hepatitis C virus infection in diabetic patients. *Diabetes Care* **1996**, *19*, 998–1000. [CrossRef] [PubMed]

83. Hadziyannis, S.J. The spectrum of extrahepatic manifestations in hepatitis C virus infection. *J. Viral Hepat.* **1997**, *4*, 9–28. [CrossRef] [PubMed]

84. Petta, S.; Cammà, C.; di Marco, V.; Alessi, N.; Cabibi, D.; Caldarella, R.; Licata, A.; Massenti, F.; Tarantino, G.; Marchesini, G.; *et al.* Insulin resistance and diabetes increase fibrosis in the liver of patients with genotype 1 HCV infection. *Am. J. Gastroenterol.* **2008**, *103*, 1136–1144. [CrossRef] [PubMed]

85. Kwon, S.Y.; Kim, S.S.; Kwon, O.S.; Kwon, K.A.; Chung, M.G.; Park, D.K.; Kim, Y.S.; Koo, Y.S.; Kim, Y.K.; Choi, D.J.; *et al.* Prognostic significance of glycaemic control in patients with HBV and HCV-related cirrhosis and diabetes mellitus. *Diabet. Med.* **2005**, *22*, 1530–1535. [CrossRef] [PubMed]

86. Chen, C.L.; Yang, H.I.; Yang, W.S.; Liu, C.J.; Chen, P.J.; You, S.L.; Wang, L.Y.; Sun, C.A.; Lu, S.N.; Chen, D.S.; *et al.* Metabolic factors and risk of hepatocellular carcinoma by chronic hepatitis B/C infection: A follow-up study in Taiwan. *Gastroenterology* **2008**, *135*, 111–121. [CrossRef] [PubMed]

87. Boddi, M.; Abbate, R.; Chellini, B.; Giusti, B.; Giannini, C.; Pratesi, G.; Rossi, L.; Pratesi, C.; Gensini, G.F.; Paperetti, L.; *et al.* Hepatitis C virus RNA localization in human carotid plaques. *J. Clin. Virol.* **2010**, *47*, 72–75. [CrossRef] [PubMed]

88. Ampuero, J.; Romero-Gómez, M.; Reddy, K.R. HCV genotype 3. The new treatment challenge. *Aliment. Pharmacol. Ther.* **2014**, *39*, 686–698. [CrossRef] [PubMed]

13

Relevant Aspects of Nutritional and Dietary Interventions in Non-Alcoholic Fatty Liver Disease

Maria Catalina Hernandez-Rodas [1], Rodrigo Valenzuela [1,*] and Luis A. Videla [2]

[1] Department of Nutrition, Faculty of Medicine, University of Chile, Santiago 8380453, Chile; cata.hernandezr@gmail.com

[2] Molecular and Clinical Pharmacology Program, Institute of Biomedical Sciences, Faculty of Medicine, University of Chile, Santiago 8380453, Chile; lvidela@med.uchile.cl

* Author to whom correspondence should be addressed; rvalenzuelab@med.uchile.cl

Academic Editors: Amedeo Lonardo and Giovanni Targher

Abstract: Non-alcoholic fatty liver disease (NAFLD) is the main cause of liver disease worldwide. NAFLD is linked to circumstances such as type 2 diabetes, insulin resistance, obesity, hyperlipidemia, and hypertension. Since the obesity figures and related comorbidities are increasing, NAFLD has turned into a liver problem that has become progressively more common. Currently, there is no effective drug therapy for NAFLD; therefore, interventions in lifestyles remain the first line of treatment. Bearing in mind that adherence rates to this type of treatment are poor, great efforts are currently focused on finding novel therapeutic agents for the prevention in the development of hepatic steatosis and its progression to nonalcoholic steatohepatitis and cirrhosis. This review presents a compilation of the scientific evidence found in the last years showing the results of interventions in lifestyle, diet, and behavioral therapies and research results in human, animal and cell models. Possible therapeutic agents ranging from supplementation with vitamins, amino acids, prebiotics, probiotics, symbiotics, polyunsaturated fatty acids and polyphenols to interventions with medicinal plants are analyzed.

Keywords: NAFLD; lifestyle; diet; exercise; vitamins; amino acids; prebiotics; polyunsaturated fatty acids; polyphenols; medicinal plants

1. Introduction

The burden of nonalcoholic fatty liver disease (NAFLD) has a clinical significance in the health system and is a public health problem affecting about a third of the Western population [1]. NAFLD afflicts 30% of the adult population [2] and the majority of obese individuals [3], making obesity the main promoter disease condition. In the pediatric population, NAFLD has also begun to be a relevant problem in public health due to the etiology and pathogenesis are not fully understood, the significant increase in prevalence and the impact of its progression in level of hepatic dysfunction and associated diseases such as diabetes and cardiovascular diseases [4]. Traditionally, the NAFLD has been considered the hepatic manifestation of the metabolic syndrome. However, recently, researchers indicated that this conventional view of NAFLD is outdated and it has been suggested that NAFLD is a precondition to the development of type 2 diabetes mellitus and metabolic syndrome [5]. Lonardo *et al.* [5] in a systematic review found that in 28 longitudinal studies provided sufficient evidence to consider NAFLD as a risk factor for the emergence of future metabolic syndrome and in 19 longitudinal studies reported that NAFLD precedes the metabolic syndrome and is a risk factor for its development [5]. Liver steatosis is mainly a consequence of excess caloric intake and lack of physical activity, which points to the correction of unhealthy lifestyles as first step to follow in the prevention and handling of NAFLD. When such intervention is inefficient or inadequate, then drug therapy becomes the second strategy; however, the efficacy and safety of the proposed drug treatments for treating NAFLD are still unclear [6].

2. Lifestyle Intervention and NAFLD

Today, the therapeutic strategies are aimed at reducing the incidence of risk factors involved in the progression of the hepatic disease and comorbidities associated with NAFLD [7]. Nowadays, all the international guidelines report that lifestyle changes that include diet are the only therapeutic approach recommended (Figure 1). As can be observed in Table 1, a variety of human trials and reviews have evaluated the effects of lifestyle interventions in NAFLD. There are limited data on details of how much and how fast weight loss through diet modification must be attained [8], and, besides, extrahepatic and benefits in the liver granted by weight loss are not well explained [9]. The quality and speed of weight loss have been reported to be important, but not explicitly beneficial [10]. In this regard, a moderate weight loss in the same way that physical activity induces a reduction in insulin resistance, and both behaviors are considered as the current therapeutic strategy for patients with NAFLD who are overweight or obese. However, it has been observed that liver biochemistry (alanine aminotransferase (ALT) serum) and the hepatic steatosis share is modified in the presence of dietary treatment, but inflammation and fibrosis are unchanged [9]. Likewise, physical inactivity and type of physical activity are factors that have different effects on the health of the liver and the achievement and maintenance of a healthy body weight. In this regard, vigorous physical exercise reduces insulin resistance, helps maintain weight loss over time and improves hepatic histology. However, mild or moderate exercise intensity does not provide a significant benefit over protection in the development of NAFLD [11]. Similarly, intervention studies looking to increase adherence to the Mediterranean diet and level of physical activity have reported that adherence to the Mediterranean diet is considered a significant predictor of changes in liver fat content in patients with fatty liver, who are non-alcoholic and overweight and that the effect of the diet is gradual and favorable and it is independent of other changes in lifestyle; so the qualitative profile of the intervention from the diet is responsible for the benefits and instead the concurrent weight loss is negligible [12]. Therefore, weight loss and calorie restriction can be a poor approach for the problem of metabolic liver disease, since other factors like the quality of food, lifestyle and exercise, have a significant impact on non-alcoholic fatty liver and these have been less studied.

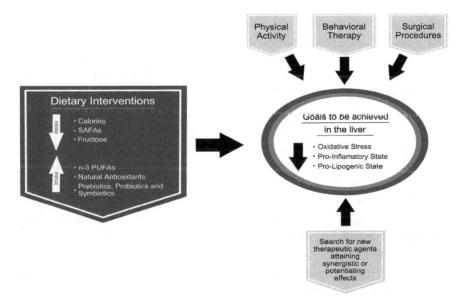

Figure 1. Interventions for the prevention and treatment of non-alcoholic fatty liver disease (NAFLD). *Abbreviations*: n-3 PUFAs, n-3 polyunsaturated fatty acids; SAFAs, saturated fatty acids.

Since there is no consensus about weight loss in the NAFLD treatment, Ghaemi *et al.* [13] implemented a pilot study that assessed the effects of weight loss on characteristics of NAFLD and associated conditions. For this purpose, 44 NAFLD patients received a diet including a reduction in the daily intake from 1000 to 500 kcal, with a distribution with respect to the total caloric value of 30% fat, 15% protein and 55% carbohydrate for six months. At the end of follow-up period, patients were classified as adherent or non-adherent to treatment according to a weight loss ≥5% or <5% of initial body weight, respectively. After the intervention, 56.8% of patients were classified as adherent group and the 43.2% as non-adherent group, and significant reductions were found in the adherent group in relation to diastolic blood pressure (80.2 to 76.9 mmHg) and the serum levels of total cholesterol (TC), low-density lipoprotein LDL cholesterol (LDL-C), triglycerides (TGs), alanine aminotransferase (ALT), aspartate aminotransferase (AST) and gamma-glutamyl transpeptidase (GGT) activities. These results suggest that reduction in weight is a good therapeutic strategy for obese patients with NAFLD, which reach a weight loss of 9.7% of initial body weight after six months of dietary therapy [13]. Similarly, a systematic review of the impact of non-surgical treatments currently available for liver disease and NASH was conducted in order to determine the metabolic risk in publications, which included a total of 78 randomized trials (30 in nonalcoholic steatohepatitis (NASH) and 40 in NAFLD) [14]. It was found that weight loss was safe, improved the cardiometabolic risk profile, and that a weight loss of ≥7% recovered the histological features of the disease; however, this weight loss was only achieved in less than 50% of patients [14].

The interventions focused on changes in lifestyle are considered a key element for the treatment of NAFLD and metabolic syndrome, and although the optimal strategy has not been developed, and that weight loss and exercise are essential, the long-term sustainability of any intervention is a key factor for this to be successful [15]. While interventions aimed at weight loss are recommended, the reduction in weight by dietary restriction is on average unsustainable in the long term, considering that weight loss usually returns to the initial weight over time [16]. Therefore, appropriate strategies to reduce NAFLD that not only include weight loss are necessary, physical activity being an important factor playing a protective healthy role in NAFLD [17] (Figure 1).

Few studies have demonstrated the efficacy of physical activity, in combination with a diet and weight loss. In a prospective study of 141 individuals with NAFLD who were approached in interventions in lifestyle with mild or moderate intensity, those who increased or maintained their physical activity at a level of 150 min/week or more had greater improvement in liver enzymes, regardless of changes in the weight [18]. In another study of 44 patients who completed a regular exercise program, serum ALT was normalized in 55% of patients, whereas 34% that did not meet the exercise program did not present any standardization [19]. Even small gains in fitness and physical activity can have significant health benefits for patients with NAFLD, as found when practiced training exercise by a very short period (4 weeks) attained decreased liver lipids in obese patients without changes in body weight [20].

However, as the success in changing lifestyle is influenced by personal beliefs and values, it becomes complex to encourage patients to make changes in unhealthy behaviors. Accordingly, behavioral and psychological strategies are considered necessary [6]. Behavioral treatments are global therapeutic approaches that give patients practical tools to achieve their goals of intake and exercise [21]. Few studies have evaluated the effects of behavioral approaches in patients with NAFLD; two out of 10 were controlled trials [22]. These studies compared the effects of Vitamin E and Orlistat against behavioral treatments, and both were in favor of the behavioral approach, with an added effect of Orlistat in weight loss. More recently, intensive interventions of lifestyles in patients with different backgrounds of disease (28 with suspected of fatty liver) were shown to be more effective than the prescription of a dietary standard, both in terms of weight loss and in liver enzymes [23].

Few randomized controlled trials (RCTs) have evaluated the effectiveness of treatments for NAFLD in pediatric population. At present, weight loss by controlling caloric intake, the improvement in the quality of diet and exercise are considered the first line of treatment [24]. An analysis of the current management of pediatric NAFLD showed bariatric surgery and drug treatment with Orlistat and insulin sensitizers are not recommended as first or second line treatment for NAFLD. Thus, interventions focused on changes in lifestyle through diet and exercise remain the first line treatment of NAFLD in children population [5]. Trials have shown that treatments with cysteamine bitartrate, probiotics, polyunsaturated fatty acids (PUFAs) and pentoxifylline have beneficial effects. However, few RCTs with powered statistical that have evaluated the impact of these treatments on histological changes. In the case of vitamin E, it was shown to have beneficial effects and was able to improve liver morphology in children with non-alcoholic steatohepatitis. In conclusion, in pediatric patients the interventions in lifestyle are the first choice of treatment and vitamin E should be considered for children with demonstrated NASH or for those at risk of NASH who have failed to the first choice of treatment. While other therapies show promising results, large RCTs with persuasive endpoints are needed [5].

Table 1. Studies on lifestyle interventions in non-alcoholic fatty liver disease (NAFLD).

Intervention	Findings	Reference
Weight loss ≥5% of initial body weight	Significant reduction in systolic blood pressure, total cholesterol, low-density lipoprotein cholesterol, triglycerides, alanine aminotransferase (ALT), aspartate aminotransferase, and γ-glutamyl transferase in the adherent group (weight loss ≥5% of initial body weight)	[13]
Weight loss (≥7%)	Weight loss is safe and improves liver histology and cardiometabolic profile, but it is only achieved in <50% of patients	[16]
Increasing or maintaining the level of physical activity in 150 min/week or more	Greater improvement in levels of liver enzymes, independently of changes in weight	[18]
Complete a regular exercise program	ALT normalization	[19]
Training exercises for 4 weeks	Reduction in liver lipids in obese patients even in the absence of changes in body weight	[20]
Intensive lifestyle interventions	Intensive lifestyle interventions were more effective than the prescription of dietary standard, both in weight loss and in liver enzymes	[23]
Review of the current management of pediatric NAFLD	Lifestyle interventions should be the first line treatment for pediatric NAFLD. Vitamin E could be considered for those with non-alcoholic steatohepatitis (NASH) demonstrated by biopsy or those at risk for NASH where the first line therapy has failed. Other therapies require large RCTs in pediatric population	[5]

3. Dietary Interventions

Various changes in dietary intake have occurred in recent years, which are characterized by an increase in energy intake (24%) due to enhancements in the consumption of flour, cereal products, added sugar and fats, and/or in total fat and fruit intake [25]. The use of corn syrup or high fructose as sweeteners in beverages has increased to comprise 41% of the total sweeteners, with added sucralose accounting for 45%, changes that have undoubtedly helped to increase the prevalence of NAFLD, in association with enhanced obesity and fructose intake from soft drinks [26]. Consequently, a number of diet interventions in different models of NAFLD have been evaluated, as shown in Table 2. In Addition, given the high prevalence of NAFLD in adolescents and its close relationship with cardiovascular disease (CVD), it is imperative to implement strategies focused on prevention through diet and changes in lifestyle, and the validation of effective treatment options [27].

3.1. Caloric Restriction and Macronutrient Distribution

With the central point that insulin resistance is one of the main problems in NAFLD, a diet with low carbohydrate intake could be considered a reasonable treatment option for these patients

(Figure 1). Similarly, studies have reported the benefits of a diet with caloric restriction independent of macronutrients distribution [28], and soy products also have been considered as an important component in the diet for the treatment of NAFLD in the animal model [29], since soy isoflavones increase the antioxidant capacity and reduce hepatic lipid deposits [30]. The latter effect may be related to inhibition of lipogenic transcription factor sterol regulatory element binding protein 1c (SREBP-1c) and activation of peroxisome proliferator-activated receptor alpha (PPAR-α), upregulating fatty acids (FA) oxidation enzymes in the liver [30]. Kani *et al.* [31] evaluated the effects of a diet low in calories and low in carbohydrate containing soy in patients with NAFLD through a RCT of 45 patients with NAFLD who received three different diets: The low calorie diet (restriction of 200–500 calories according to the requirements of each participant and a distribution of 55% of calories from carbohydrates, 15% from proteins and 30% from fat), the low-calorie and low-carbohydrate diet (the same calorie restriction but the distribution was 45% carbohydrates, 35% fat and 25% protein), or a diet low in carbohydrates and in calories, containing soy (the same calorie restriction, the distribution was 45% carbohydrates, 35% fat and 25% protein, but 30 g of soy nut was incorporated instead of 30 g of red meat) for 6 weeks. It was found that changes in both weight and in lipid profile were not significantly different between the 3 groups, but the low-calorie, low-carbohydrate containing soy diet could reduce further the levels of serum ALT, AST, fibrinogen, and of the lipid peroxidation indicator malondialdehyde (MDA), over those achieved by the low-calorie diet [31].

Few studies have evaluated the relationship between protein intake and NAFLD. Protein supplements have offered short-term benefits against hepatic steatosis and lipid profile in sedentary and obese women [32]. In this regard, the research focus has been on the functional properties of soy intake and nitrogen, because soy protein has been shown to be successful in this scenario [33]. In this respect, dietary recommendations in NAFLD patients are 1.000/1.200 kcal/day for overweight women and 1.200/1.600 kcal/day for overweight men. Ideal diet: 50% carbohydrates, 30% lipids (7%–10% saturated fatty acids), and 20% proteins. Diets are developed to provide a calorie deficit of approximately 500 kcal from usual food consumption causing a weight loss of 0.5–1.0 kg/week [34]. Facts interventions with this type of diet (25% of the caloric value from fat (7% saturated fat, 10% monounsaturated fat and 8% polyunsaturated fat), 35% from protein (animal and plant) and 40% from carbohydrates (50% from whole grains, sugar 25 g and 20 g protein/day)) show that the body mass index (BMI), waist circumference, and body fat mass remained relatively stable, whereas high-density lipoprotein HDL cholesterol (HDL-C) increased significantly and TC, LDL-C, VLDL cholesterol (VLDL-C), TGs, AST, GGT, alkaline phosphatase (ALP), fasting blood glucose, and glycosylated hemoglobin (HbA1c) decreased significantly [34]. When stratify patients according to the increase or reduction in BMI, an association between weight loss and liver profit reflected through the ALP and ALT markers was found, and the AST/ALT ratio was observed, with failure to show any changes in patients that increased their weight. Multivariate analysis showed that waist circumference, ferritin, TGs and markers of glucose homeostasis were the parameters most associated with liver enzymes [34].

Studies in an animal model with high-protein diets have also been developed, evaluating whether a high-protein diet prevents the development of steatosis in C57BL/6 male mice with or without pre-existing liver failure, using diets including low-fat or high-fat, low in protein (11% protein) or high in protein (35% protein), high fat/high protein (42% fat and 35% protein), or high fat/low protein (42% fat and 11% protein) for 3 weeks [35]. The results indicate that diets high in protein decreased the hepatic lipid content to ~40% of the corresponding low protein diets, high protein diets being more effective in this regard that reducing energy intake by 80%, which were able to reverse the steatosis induced by pre-existing diet. Compared to diets with low protein, mice fed high protein diets showed increased mitochondrial oxidative capacity and elongation of long chain fatty acids (LCFA), a selective enhancement in plasma branched chain amino acids (BCAA) levels, stellate cells diminution, and a trend towards reduced inflammation [35].

3.2. Fructose Restriction

The fructose intake in American adolescents (mainly as soft drink) representing the 12% of daily calories, this high fructose intake exceeds current recommendations and is considered as one of the components dietary responsible for promoting NAFLD in this demographic group [36]. In studies of short-term feeding in experimental animals and humans, fructose intake increases the accumulation of fats in the liver and of TGs in plasma due in part to increased *de novo* lipogénesis [37]. In this sense, it has been seen that patients with NAFLD have a fructose intake 2-fold greater than the average intake in control patients, according to population studies, exhibited significant increases in the hepatic mRNA expression of fructokinase and FA synthase, suggesting a high pro-lipogenic potential with consequent ATP depletion that can promote necroinflammation [38]. Also, fructose is involved in oxidative damage through the reduction of antioxidant defense and improvement in the production of reactive oxygen species (ROS) [39]. Both lipid overload and oxidative stress promote the fructose as a triggering factor in the onset and progression of NAFLD [40]. Dyslipidemia, insulin resistance and oxidative damage induced by high fructose intake may contribute to increased risk of CVD that is evident in patients with NAFLD [41]; it makes lack direct evidence demonstrating the benefits of the restriction of fructose in the liver steatosis and CVD. An intervention double-blind, controlled, randomized trial in 24 Hispanic-American adolescents with overweight who had a frequent intake of sweet drinks and a content of liver fat greater than 8% as determined by magnetic resonance spectroscopy, showed that when patients were submitted to take only beverages with fructose or glucose only (33 g of sugar that match the standard amount of sugar in a typical drink) for four weeks, no significant changes in liver fat or body weight in either group were found. However, in the glucose drinking group there was a significant progress in adipose tissue insulin sensitivity, high-sensitivity C-reactive protein (hs-CRP), and in LDL oxidation, suggesting that fructose reduction improves markers of CVD despite the lack of recovery in hepatic steatosis [27].

3.3. Mediterranean Diet

The Mediterranean diet has been extensively investigated in terms of benefits with regard to cardiovascular risk reduction and improved insulin sensitivity. However, studies have specifically examined their effects on NAFLD are scarce.

Protective effects have been attributed to the Mediterranean diet because of the high intake of antioxidants; vegetables are the main source of phenolic compounds on this diet. Moreover, polyunsaturated fatty acids of the n-3 series from fish regulate haemostatic factors that induce protection against a variety of chronic diseases, and besides, the olive oil represents a high intake of monounsaturated fatty acids and a good source of phytochemicals, and some protective properties of the Mediterranean diet on human health have been granted to the polyphenols present in wine [42].

A recent meta-analysis showed that n-3 PUFAs found in the Mediterranean diet were beneficial in reducing hepatic steatosis [43]. In order to evaluate whether intervention with Mediterranean diet could improve insulin sensitivity in individuals with NAFLD and reduce steatosis to a greater extent than current dietary recommendations, 12 nondiabetic subjects (six males and six females) with biopsy-proven NAFLD were enrolled for a transverse randomized dietary intervention for 6 weeks. All participants were subjected to the Mediterranean diet and to a control diet (low in fat and high in carbohydrates) in a random order with a period of six weeks of washing between each of the diets. As a result, the weight loss was not different between the two types of diet; there was a significant reduction in relative hepatic steatosis after the Mediterranean diet compared to control diet, with improved insulin sensitivity being observed only with the Mediterranean diet [44]. However, this diet should be further investigated in subjects with NAFLD since the size of the groups evaluated was very small in this investigation.

Table 2. Studies on dietary interventions in non-alcoholic fatty liver disease (NAFLD).

Intervention	Model	Conclusions	Reference
Diets restricted in calories and carbohydrates with soy protein addition	Human	Intervention can have beneficial effects on serum levels of liver enzymes, malonaldehyde and fibrinogen in patients with NAFLD	[31]
Low calorie diet rich in proteins	Human	A protein diet is associated with improved lipid profile, glucose homeostasis, and improved liver enzymes in NAFLD, independently of decreases in body mass index (BMI) or in body fat mass	[34]
High protein diet	Animal	The high-protein diet prevents and reverses the steatosis, regardless of fat and carbohydrate intake, and is more efficient than a 20% reduction in energy intake	[35]
Soft drinks with fructose compared to glucose sodas	Human	Reducing fructose improves several important factors to cardiovascular disease, despite the lack of appreciable improvement in hepatic steatosis in overweight adolescents	[27]
Mediterranean diet	Human	The Mediterranean diet reduces hepatic steatosis and improves insulin sensitivity in insulin-resistant people with NAFLD compared to current dietary recommendations, even in the absence of weight loss	[44]

4. Therapeutic Agents

As mentioned above, fatty liver is mainly generated from the excessive caloric intake and lack of physical activity, pointing to correction of unhealthy styles as the first line approach in the prevention and treatment of NAFLD, which when this intervention is insufficient, drug therapy becomes a strategic line [6] (Figure 1). Because weight loss has been reported to have a low rate of success in the long term [45], research has focused on the development and validation of new dietary therapies aimed at preventing the hepatic steatosis and its progression to NASH [46]. The challenge for the development of therapies for NASH is related to the complexity of the disease, which is directly associated with to visceral obesity, dyslipidemia, hyperglycemia, insulin resistance, and oxidative stress [47,48]. Effective treatments are needed in order to prevent progression of simple steatosis to chronic liver disease [49], considering that fatty liver disease is a reversible condition which if not treated early can lead to a terminal liver disease [50]. Although the pathophysiology of NASH is still not fully understood and the treatments available are not entirely satisfactory, therapies that limit liver injury and the occurrence of inflammation and fibrosis are particularly attractive for this condition [51]. Currently, it is a great challenge for the pharmaceutical industry to develop a combined therapy that is effective in NAFLD patients exhibiting obesity, insulin resistance, dyslipidemia, and oxidative stress. Therefore, serious efforts have been directed to explore novel therapeutic agents that may be directed to multiple targets [52], natural products extracted from medicinal plants being rich sources of biologically active substances having effects on health benefits and disease prevention in humans [53]. Accordingly, current investigations have focused on herbal extracts and natural products with antihyperlipidemic and hepatoprotective effects against NAFLD [54], particularly potential sources of antioxidants [55] (Table 3).

4.1. Amino Acid Supplementation Interventions

4.1.1. Tryptophan

Earlier studies conducted in hens have suggested that supplementation with the amino acid tryptophan (Trp) reduces hepatic lipid accumulation [56]. Recently, the influence of Trp supplementation on NAFLD induced by a fructose-rich diet was studied in C57BL/6J mice, as precursor of serotonin, a regulator of the intestinal motility and permeability [51]. Under these conditions, NAFLD underlying lipid accumulation and increased portal plasma lipopolysaccharide (LPS) concentrations, resulted in derangement of intestinal barrier functions, as evidenced by depressed expression of the tight-junction protein occluding and the serotonin re-uptake transporter (SERT), changes that were attenuated or abolished by Trp. The authors suggested that modulation of the intestinal barrier and the serotonergic system by Trp supplementation may be of importance as a protective mechanism against development of NAFLD in mice [57], although further studies are required to validate this proposal in humans.

4.1.2. Glutamine

In recent years, glutamine was shown to improve hepatic ischemia-reperfusion injury, alcohol-induced liver injury, and gut-derived endotoxemia, promoting resistance to oxidative stress, reducing inflammatory cytokine release, and regulating immune reactions [58]. Assessment of the influence of glutamine on NAFLD induced in rats by a high fat diet (HFD) revealed that hepatic steatosis was accompanied by significant increased liver lipid peroxidation, tumor necrosis factor α (TNF-α) levels, and of p65 NF-κB expression, with concomitant glutathione (GSH) depletion.

Glutamine supplementation reduced the oxidative status of the liver and inhibited NF-κB expression, in association with improvement of hepatic steatosis, suggesting a protective effect of glutamine in NAFLD [58].

4.1.3. L-Carnitine Intervention

L-carnitine plays a critical role in lipid metabolism as it acts as an essential cofactor for β-oxidation of PUFAs by facilitating their transport into the mitochondrial matrix associated with carnitine palmitoyltransferase I (CPT-I) activation, thus converting fat into energy [59]. In recent years, L-carnitine has been proposed as a treatment option for various diseases including liver disease [59]. Using a NASH model mouse subjected to either HFD, HFD plus L-carnitine, or HFD with α-tocopherol, L-carnitine induced an enhancement in the hepatic expression of genes implicated in the transport of long chain PUFAs, mitochondrial β-oxidation, and antioxidant enzymes, with suppression of markers of oxidative stress and inflammatory cytokines in NASH, changes that were similar to those elicited by α-tocopherol. It was concluded that L-carnitine acts as a protective agent to prevent progression of NASH by favoring mitochondrial β-oxidation and redox systems [59].

4.2. n-3 Polyunsaturated Fatty Acids (n-3 PUFAs) Interventions

The n-3 PUFAs are crucial structural components of cellular lipids, substrates for the biosynthesis of physiological mediators, and signaling molecules regulating liver lipid metabolism. The latter feature is achieved by (i) transcriptional activation of the expression of enzymes involved in FA oxidation acting as ligands of PPAR-α; and (ii) suppression of de novo lipogenesis by down-regulation of SREBP-1c [60]. Therefore, n-3 PUFA depletion in the liver of NAFLD patients favoring FA and TGs formation over FA oxidation [61] points n-3 PUFAs as specific anti-steatotic drugs for NAFLD (Figure 1) [62]. A systematic review by Parker et al. [43] on studies pertaining to the effect of n-3 PUFA supplementation in NAFLD patients, including 9 reports and 355 individuals who were administered either n-3 PUFA treatment or placebo, confirmed a significant reduction in hepatic lipid content. Although there was significant heterogeneity between studies, pooled data suggest that supplementation of n-3 PUFAs reduces liver fat, an effect that persists when data from RCTs are analyzed; however, the optimal dose remains to be established. Interestingly, n-3 PUFAs also improved circulating liver functions markers, TGs and TNF-α level, and hepatic microcirculatory function [43]. It was suggested that future designs of RCTs quantifying the magnitude of the effects of n-3 PUFA supplementation on liver fat are necessary [43], which are also important for liver inflammation and fibrosis outcomes [63].

Studies in pediatric patients with NAFLD have also been developed, the most prominent being the RCT of Nobili *et al.* [64] using docosahexaenoic acid (DHA) treatment (250 and 500 mg/day) *versus* placebo in 60 pediatric patients with NAFLD, with evaluation of the changes in the fat liver content by ultrasonography after 6, 12, 18 and 24 months of intervention, and changes in TGs, ALT, BMI, and the homeostatic model assessment (HOMA) index of insulin resistance. Data reported indicate that DHA decreased liver fat content after 6 months of supplementation, an effect that persists up to 24 months and is equally effective at the two dosages studied, when compared with the placebo group. Furthermore, TGs were lower in DHA-treated children than in controls at any time intervention, ALT was lower in groups with 12 months of DHA treatment onwards, and HOMA was lower in the group given 250 mg DHA/day *versus* placebo group at 6 and 12 months [64], in agreement with the positive outcomes reported in adult NAFLD patients.

4.3. Vitamin Supplementation Interventions

4.3.1. Niacin

Niacin is the precursor of nicotinamide coenzymes acting either as oxidants $(NAD(P)^+)$ in catabolic processes or as reductants (NADPH) in anabolic reactions or in the recovery of the reduced form of antioxidant components, thus decreasing oxidative stress [65]. It has been used for the treatment of dyslipidemia and CVD [66], and proposed to prevent hepatic steatosis and delay NASH induced by HFD [67]. This proposal was tested in Sprague-Dawley rats fed either a standard rodent diet, HFD, or HFD containing 0.5% or 1.0% niacin for 4 weeks. Under these conditions, niacin supplementation in the HFD significantly decreased the content of liver fat, liver weight, liver oxidative products, preventing fatty liver [67]. While niacin had no effect on the mRNA expression of enzymes related to FA synthesis and oxidation including acetyl CoA carboxylase 1 (ACC-1), FAS, and CPT-1, and lipogenic transcription factor SREBP-1c, it significantly down-regulated the mRNA and protein expression and the activity of diacylglycerol acyltransferase (DGAT), a key enzyme in triglyceride synthesis, thus in agreement with its receding effect on steatosis [67].

4.3.2. Vitamin E

Natural vitamin E is fat soluble tocopherol comprising eight isomers including four tocopherols and four tocotrienols, RRR-α-tocopherol being the most abundant and with the highest biological activity, which is mainly related to antioxidation by avoid the propagation of free radical reactions at the cell membrane level [68,69]. The potential role of vitamin E in preventing fat infiltration in the liver was assessed in Wistar rats fed either a standard diet (SD), a diet high in cholesterol and saturated fat (HCSF), or a diet high in cholesterol and saturated fat with added of water soluble vitamin E (10 IU/kg/day; HCSF-E) for ten weeks. The results indicate that vitamin E exerted hypolipidemic and hepatoprotective effects, as evidenced by the lower levels of total cholesterol found in HCSF-E treated rats over the HCSF group, in addition to lower serum glutamic oxaloacetic transaminase (SGOT) and steatosis scores at the end of the study compared with the initial values [70]. However, no significant differences between the different experimental groups were observed in relation to blood glucose and serum lipids [70]. In addition, it has been found that when vitamin E is supplied for a period of 2 years to patients with NAFLD, the histological features of the disease improve but, in turn, an increase in insulin resistance and plasma levels of TGs was observed [14].

4.4. Interventions with Prebiotics, Probiotics, and Synbiotics

Current evidence suggests that the accumulation of triglycerides in the liver responds not only to obesity, but also, the intestinal microbiota plays a key role in the development of insulin resistance, fatty liver, fibrosis and necroinflammatory score, and thereby becomes an endogenous factor that favors the development of NAFLD [71,72]. The link between the liver-intestinal axis and NAFLD is associated with bacterial overgrowth in the small intestine and increased intestinal permeability [73].

The intestine has a complex array of species of microorganisms, wherein the concentration and type of these microorganisms is mainly influenced by the host genotype and availability nutrient [74]. The liver is susceptible to exposure to intestinal bacterial-derived products through a functional and anatomical connection with the intestinal lumen via the portal vein system [75]. The contribution of the microflora in the progression of NAFLD is given mainly by the improvement in hepatic oxidative stress as a result of increased ethanol production and LPS in the intestinal lumen, and the subsequent release of inflammatory cytokines from the inflammatory cells [76]. High concentrations of cytokines may increase intestinal permeability via disruption of intercellular tight junctions, resulting in progressive inflammation and fibrosis within the liver [77], TNF-α plays a critical role in both insulin resistance and uptake by the liver of inflammatory cells in NAFLD [78]. In recent years, it became clear that a high degree of inflammation due to metabolic endotoxemia has an implication in various diseases, including that induced by high fructose intake that changes the intestinal microbiota and intestinal barrier permeability, resulting in increased bacteria derived LPS [79]. As the various species of the gut microbiota are involved in different intestinal biological functions, such as the defense against colonization by opportunistic pathogens, development of a suitable gut architecture can contribute to immune system homeostasis [80]. In this respect, it has been found that manipulating the enteric flora may represent a key therapeutic strategy in the treatment of NASH. Intake of probiotics (living microorganisms), prebiotics (oligosaccharides), and symbiotics (mixture of probiotics and prebiotics) has been reported by their ability to modify the composition of the microbiota and thereby restore the microbial balance. So, exert benefits for health protection [81] (Figure 1).

Animal model studies have shown that probiotics can reduce the progression of NAFLD. Among these, one study evaluated the effect of supplementation with the mixture VSL Pharmaceuticals, Inc., Ft. Lauderdale, FL, USA (VSL#3); a probiotic containing 450 billion bacteria in various strains (three types of bacteria: *Streptococcus*, *Bifidobacterium* and *Lactobacillus*), to ob/ob mice for a period of four weeks and showed that in response to supplementation was observed a reduction in hepatic fatty acid content, in liver inflammation and, in addition to an improvement in the insulin resistance in the liver [82]. It has also been shown that treatment with probiotics lead to a direct reduction in the release of pro-inflammatory cytokines by a down-regulation in the activity of transcription factor NF-κB [83]. In the model of NASH induced by HFD in rats, the treatment with VSL#3 resulted in a reduction in the expression of markers of lipid peroxidation, TNF-α, inducible nitric oxide synthase (iNOS) and cyclooxygenase 2 (COX-2), when compared with the control group [84]. Similarly, treatment with VSL#3 resulted in a minor insulin resistance in liver and adipose tissue, thus counteracting the development of NASH and atherosclerosis in genetically dyslipidemic ApoE($-/-$) mice [85]. Moreover, Ritze *et al.* [86] studied whether supplementation with *Lactobacillus* rhamnosus (LGG) could alleviate experimental NAFLD in C57BL/J6 mice, through administration of fructose via drinking water containing 30% fructose with or without LGG at a concentration of 5×10^7 colony-forming units (cfu) per g body weight. Upon completion of the intervention period, it was found that treatment with LLG generated an increase of beneficial bacteria in the small intestine as well as a restoration in the duodenal tight-junction protein concentration and reduced of portal LPS levels. In addition, attenuation in the hepatic mRNA expression of TNF-α, interleukin-8 (IL-8), and IL-1β, liver fat accumulation, and portal ALT levels were observed in animals fed the high fructose diet plus LGG [86]. Similar studies with *Lactobacillus casei* strain Shirota (LcS) given orally to mice fed a methionine-choline-deficient diet (MCD) that reduces lactic acid bacteria such as *Lactobacillus* and *Bifidobacterium* in feces, increased not only the LcS subgroup but also the lactic acid types, with concomitant suppression of MCD-diet-induced NASH development [87].

In agreement with experimental studies [82], the use of the probiotic VSL#3 in NAFLD patients for 2 to 3 months improved routine liver damage tests and oxidative stress-related indicators, without improvement in pro-inflammatory cytokines, suggesting that manipulation of intestinal flora should be taken into consideration as adjunctive therapy in NAFLD [88]. Two randomized placebo-controlled double-blind studies showed a significant decrease in liver AST with the administration of probiotics in children [89] and in adults [90]. Also, symbiotic studies have been developed in humans, which are included in a recent meta-analysis reporting favorable results in four RCTs, two of which involved the use of symbiotic by co-treatment of probiotics with fructo-oligosaccharides (FOS), the latter prebiotics being potentially promoters of the growth of beneficial bifidobacteria in the intestinal tract [91]. It is noteworthy that one of the previous trials in patients with NASH including liver biopsies showed improvement in liver histology after 6 months of symbiotic treatment containing *Bifidobacterium longum* and FOS [92]. With the intention of defining whether treatment with symbiotics imply greater effectiveness on changes in lifestyle for the treatment of NAFLD, Eslamparast *et al.* [78] designed a RCT with 52 NAFLD patients treated with either a symbiotic or placebo for 28 days, concomitantly with diet and physical activity recommendations. It was found that symbiotic supplementation with lifestyle modification is a better strategy than life style adjustment alone in NAFLD treatment, leading to attenuation of markers of liver damage, inflammation, and fibrosis [78].

4.5. Interventions with Polyphenols

Polyphenols are natural compounds produced by plants comprising a heterogeneous group of agents characterized by hydroxylated phenyl moieties. Among them, two types of compounds are distinguished, namely (i) flavonoids containing a common diphenylpropane skeleton (e.g., flavonoids, flavones, flavonols, flavanols, isoflavones, proanthocyanidins, and anthocyanins); and (ii) non flavonoids mainly comprising mono-phenols alcohols (e.g., hydroxytyrosol), or stilbene phenolic acids (e.g., resveratrol) [93]. Several polyphenols have beneficial actions on human health, with potential mechanisms including (i) non-specific antioxidant action due to the existence of a phenol group capable of scavenging free radicals (Figure 1); and (ii) certain mechanisms focused on interactions of particular structural characteristics of polyphenols with proteins or defined membrane domains [94].

4.5.1. Resveratrol, Catechin and Quercetin

The cardioprotective, anti-cancer, and anti-inflammatory properties of resveratrol have been well characterized, a polyphenol that has been reported to present suitable protective effects on the liver against the hepatic lipid accumulation in response to a HFD [95]. The beneficial effects attributed to resveratrol have been awarded mainly to its antioxidant and anti-inflammatory effects that exert protective tissues such as the liver, kidney and brain against a variety of damage caused by oxidative stress and inflammation [96], raising the proposal that resveratrol can be used in the treatment for metabolic disorders including fatty liver disease [97]. In this context, resveratrol was reported to activate sirtuin 1 (SIRT1) with the consequent stimulation of AMP-activated protein kinase (AMPK) [98] through phosphorylation mediated by liver kinase B1 (LKB1) that protects against liver lipid accumulation by down-regulation of FAS expression induced by high glucose [97]. Similarly, resveratrol also blocks the expression of SREBP-1 through the SIRT1/forkhead box O1 (FOXO1) pathway leading to a lipid-lowering effect in HepG2 cells treated with palmitate [99]. A recent randomized, double-blind, placebo-controlled study assessed the scope of resveratrol supplementation in 50 individuals with NAFLD over subjects given placebo for 12 weeks, both groups being subjected to lifestyle improvement. In both groups, the anthropometric measurements, liver enzymes, and degree of steatosis improved. However, resveratrol supplementation was associated with a significant reduction in liver ALT, inflammatory cytokines, NF-κβ activity, serum cytokeratin 18, and grade of hepatic steatosis, compared to placebo-supplemented group. The authors concluded that resveratrol supplementation along with lifestyle modification is a better treatment for NAFLD than lifestyle improvement alone, which is mainly due to attenuation of inflammation and hepatocyte apoptosis [100]. Diminutions in hepatic inflammation and lipogenesis are also observed in HFD fed mice given 30 mg resveratrol/kg/day for 60 days over control values, as evidenced by significant decreases in mRNA expression of either TNF-α, interleukin-6 (IL-6) and NF-κB or the lipogenic factors PPAR-γ, SREBP-1, and ACC-1 [101].

Epidemiological evidence has reported that intake of green tea (Camellia sinensis) may protect against liver injury due to inverse association with lipid profile and serum ALT [102]. While this approach has not yet been confirmed through RCTs in humans, epigallocatechin gallate (EGCG), the main polyphenol catechin in green tea, have been shown to generate a reduction in hepatic lipid accumulation and serum monocyte chemoattractant protein-1 (MCP-1) levels, in a mouse model of diet-induced NASH [103]. Liver protection against HFD-induced NASH in rats was also attained by a green tea extract after 8 weeks supplementation, as shown by an increase in glutathione status related with the inhibition of liver and adipose tissue inflammatory responses mediated by NF-κβ [46].

Quercetin is a flavonoid present in the human diet with a variety of preventive effects in typical human diseases [104], through mechanisms that include a down-regulation in the activation of NF-κB, inducible nitric oxide synthase expression in IL-1β activated rat hepatocytes [105] and also in the improvement in hepatic damage in rats with biliary obstruction [106]. Other significant beneficial effects of quercetin include a reduction in plasma concentrations of oxidized LDL in patients with overweight [107] and a decreased hepatic steatosis induced by Western diet in C57BL/6J mice [108] and attenuation of inflammation and fibrosis in a mouse model of NASH by MCD [51].

4.5.2. Proanthocyanidins and Anthocyanidins

Proanthocyanidins from grape seeds (GSP) are a complex mixture of polyphenolic bioflavonoids having high antioxidant activity, with preventive effects in some forms of cancer and oxidative injury [109]. In a recent study, the effects of GSP and the insulin sensitizer metformin were assessed individually or in combination in a diet-induced NAFLD in Wistar rats subjected to a high fat and high fructose diet (HFFD) [110]. GSP (100 mg/kg/day) and metformin (50 mg/kg/day) were given orally once a day and for the combined treatment, GSP and metformin was administered at 4 h intervals. HFFD resulted in an abnormal plasma lipid profile, with liver inflammation and steatosis, hepatic TGs levels being reduced by 69%, 23%, and 63% after GSP, metformin, and combined treatment, respectively. Accordingly, GSP reduced the mRNA expression of SREBP-1c and increased that of PPAR-α more effectively compared to metformin in HFFD-treated rats; however, no additive effect restoring lipid levels was observed when GSP and metformin were combined [110].

Anthocyanidins (ACNs) are hydrosoluble flavonoids within the polyphenol class, which are responsible for the red, purple, and blue colors of many flowers, cereal grains, fruits, and vegetables [111]. ACNs alleviate hyperglycemia, modulate endothelial function, and reduce inflammation [112], and are able to modulate lipid metabolism and fat deposits in various tissues including the liver [113]. Since the impact of ACNs on NAFLD is not well defined, a literature search grouping experimental in vitro and in vivo models and human trials was conducted [111]. Although the interpretation of the evidence from in vitro studies is hampered by differences in cell models, experimental protocols, and molecular pathways evaluated, most studies are consistent in that ACNs reduced hepatocellular accumulation of lipids by inhibiting lipogenesis and possibly by promoting lipolysis. In addition, interpretation of the data from in vivo studies is difficult, due to the large difference in experimental models of NASH used and the utilization of animals exposed to either synthetic ACNs (e.g., Cyanidin-3-o-β-glucoside) or to extracts of foods rich in ACNs (e.g., sweet potato, berries, and oranges). Nonetheless, these studies reported an improvement in systemic and hepatic insulin resistance and serum lipids, sometimes related to weight loss and increased PPAR-α activation inducing lipolysis and diminished lipogenesis, thus decreasing hepatic fat content [111]. Finally, a clinical trial enrolling 48 adult borderline hepatitis patients with increased liver enzymes supplemented with 200 mg ANCs of purple sweet potato (PSP) or placebo twice a day for 8 weeks showed that ACNs are associated with reduced levels of liver enzymes, particularly GGT [114]. Although this feature was not associated with liver damage and liver fat was not confirmed by direct imaging, the researchers suggest that the PSP beverage can offer potential activity hepatoprotective against oxidative stress [114]. The final conclusion of the literature search by Valenti et al. [111] is that ACNs can prevent the progression of liver damage related to NAFLD by three independent mechanisms, namely, inhibition of lipogenesis by decrease of SREBP-1c, lipolysis promotion by induction of PPAR-α activity, and reduction of oxidative stress, pointing to foods rich in ACNs as a promising strategy for preventing NAFLD and its complications, however future RCTs are needed to test their hepatoprotective efficacy in NAFLD [113].

4.6. Medicinal Plants Interventions

For centuries, products made from natural herbs derived from Traditional Chinese Medicine have been used to treat almost all types of diseases in China [115]. Natural products extracted from medicinal plants are rich sources of biologically active substances and have desirable effects on health benefits and disease prevention in humans [53]; therefore, an increasing number of investigations has been focused on extracts of herbs or natural products with anti-hyperlipidemic and hepatoprotectives effects against NAFLD. Considering the above and also that the use of medicinal herbs is becoming increasingly common for handling of NAFLD, Liu et al. [50] conducted a systematic review in order to evaluate both beneficial and detrimental effects of them. The study included 77 randomized trials covering 6753 participants with fatty liver disease, the average sample size was 88 participants per test, and 75 different herbal products were evaluated including single herb products, commercially available proprietary medicinal herbs, and combination formulas prescribed by physicians. It was found that (i) six trials showed a statistically significant effect on hepatic B-ultrasound; (ii) four trials showed a significant increase on liver/spleen computed tomography ratio; and (iii) forty two trials showed reduction in AST levels, forty nine trials in ALT, three trials in ALP, and thirty-two in GGT levels in the herbal group. Overall, these findings indicate that herbal medicines may have positive consequences on fatty liver disease, However, there is insufficient evidence to recommend these medicinal herbs for the management of NAFLD because of the high risk of bias and lack of homogeneous data in studies [50].

4.6.1. Tamarindus Indica Linn

At present time, Tamarindus indica Linn is one of the most important resources of plants for supply of foods and materials [52]. Considering that the seed coat of tamarind contains polyphenols including tannins, anthocyanins, and anthocyanidin oligomers, Sasidharan et al. [52] evaluated the ameliorative potential of seed coat of Tamarindus indica (ETS) extracts on HFD-induced NAFLD in rats. At dosages of 45, 90, and 180 mg/kg ETS significantly attenuated the pathological changes associated with NAFLD induced by HFD, namely, hepatomegaly, elevated liver lipids and lipid peroxides, serum ALT levels, free fatty acids, and macro and micro hepatic steatosis. In addition, ETS treatment markedly reduced body weight and adiposity, probably acting in part through anti-obesity, insulin sensitizing, and antioxidant mechanisms [52].

4.6.2. Salvia-Nelumbinis Naturalis (SNN)

Salvia-Nelumbinis naturalis (SNN) formulae (initially called Jiangzhi Granula) was designed, in which Salvia as being the principal element and Nelumbinis, Rhizoma Polygoni Cuspidati, Herba Artemisiae Scopariae the ancillary components [115]. In a study of in vivo and in vitro model the researchers found that intervention with SNN components in HepG2 cells decreased lipid accumulation and in rats the SNN extract improved the steatohepatitis and conferred a normal lipoproteinemia profile in rats fed high-calorie diet, where the effectiveness of the extract SNN to improve liver function and insulin sensitivity was comparable with medications such as simvastatin and pioglitazone [115].

4.6.3. Ostol Treatment

Ostol is the active compound of Cnidium monnieri extract. Ostol has been described by its anti-inflammatory and cytoprotective effects to promote the oxidation of fat. In an animal model of fatty liver in rats, the ostol treatment induced a decrease in fasting glucose levels and hepatic fat content, besides, resulted in improved insulin resistance [116]. Another study reported that treatment with ostol decreased liver fat content by increasing in the hepatic expression of PPAR-α/γ [117]. Similarly, in a model of NASH, ostol treatment led to an increase in the activation of superoxide dismutase (SOD) and decrease in oxidative stress [118]. Nam *et al.* [119] treated rats Sprague-Dawley with HFD plus ostol (20 mg/kg) 5 times a week and found that compared with the group only HFD, HFD plus ostol group showed a significant decrease in intrahepatic fat (39.4% *versus* 21.0%), the expression of SREBP-1c, FAS and intrahepatic stearoyl CoA desaturase-1 (SCD-1) significantly decreased and the expression of PPAR-α was also significantly higher [119].

4.6.4. Sapindus Mukorossi Gaertn

Studies by Chinese have reported Sapindus mukorossi Gaertn skin is rich in saponins and has properties to regulate fat metabolism and to grant protection to the endothelial cells of blood vessels. However, researchs to provide detailed information about the efficacy of Sapindus mukorossi Gaertn in the prevention and treatment of NAFLD are scarce [120]. Peng *et al.* [120] evaluated in a rat model of NAFLD treatment with an alcohol extract of Sapindus mukorossi Gaertn (AESM) in high dosage (0.5 g/kg), moderate dosage (0.1 g/kg) and low dose (0.05 g/kg). The researchers found that high doses of AESM could relieve AST, ALT, TC, triglycerides, LDL-C, GGT, and also raise HDL-C. Also, the morphology of liver tissue and liver cells began to be normal with this treatment [120].

4.6.5. Sasa Borealis (SBS)

The medicinal benefits of Sasa Borealis Bamboo are mainly given by antidiabetic effects in improving insulin secretion as well as for their hypoglycemic and hypolipidemic, anti-obesogenic and antioxidants effects [121]. For Bamboo, the clinical use for the treatment of hypertension, atherosclerosis, cardiovascular disease and cancer has been reported [122]. However, there have been few studies that have investigated the effects of dietary supplementation with extracts of cane Sasa borealis (SBS) in NAFLD. A recent study examined the effect of supplementation with SBS (150 mg/kg/day) in the presence of a HFD for a cycle of action of 5-week in rats and found that the body weight, liver weight, TGs, TC and lipid accumulation in the liver was significantly lower in the HFD plus SBS group compared with only HFD group. Also in the group supplemented with SBS, the transcription factor PPAR-α is increased significantly and converocly SREBP-1c was suppressed in a meaningful way, in addition, supplementation with SBS lead to a significant reduction in hepatic levels of PPAR-γ mRNA, FAS, ACC1, and enzyme diacylglycerol and acyltransferase-2 (DGAT-2) [121].

Table 3. Studies on therapeutic agents used in non-alcoholic fatty liver disease (NAFLD).

Intervention	Model	Findings	Ref.
Tryptophan supplementation	Animal	Increased occludin concentrations and reduced ratios liver weight/body weight	[57]
Glutamine supplementation	Animal	Reduced oxidative stress in the liver; inhibition of the expression of p65 NF-κB (nuclear factor kappa-light-chain-enhancer of activated B cells), and hepatic steatosis improvement	[58]
L-carnitine supplementation	Animal	Prevention of NAFLD progression through upregulation of mitochondrial β-oxidation and the redox system	[59]
Docosahexaenoic acid (DHA) supplementation	Human	Improvement of hepatic steatosis in children with NAFLD. Doses of 250 and 500 mg/day appear to be equally effective in reducing liver fat content	[64]
Niacin supplementation	Animal	Decreased liver fat content, liver weight, liver oxidative products, and prevention of fatty liver. Inhibition of mRNA and protein expression and diacylglycerol acyltransferase (DGAT) activity. No effects on mRNA expression of sterol regulatory element binding protein 1c (SREBP-1c), acetylCoA carboxylase 1 (ACC-1), fatty acid synthase (FAS), and carnitinepalmitoil transferase 1 (CPT-1)	[67]
Vitamin E supplementation	Animal	Vitamin E combined with exercise exert hypolipidemic and hepatoprotective effects in the presence of an atherogenic diet	[70]
VSL mixture (Streptococcus, Bifidobacterium, Lactobacillus)	Animal	Reduction in total fatty acid content in the liver and in hepatic inflammation, with improvement of hepatic insulin sensitivity	[82]
Probiotic treatment	Animal	Down-regulation of the activity of the transcription factor NF-κB	[83]
Lactobacillus rhamnosus treatment	Animal	Attenuation of fat accumulation in the liver and in the concentration of portal alanine aminotransferase (ALT)	[86]
Lactobacillus casein cepa Shirota treatment	Animal	Suppression in NASH development, reduced serum concentrations of lipopolysaccharide (LPS), inhibition of liver inflammation or fibrosis, and diminished inflammation of the colon	[87]
Supplementation with synbiotic, probiotic and prebiotic cultures along with recommendations on healthy lifestyles	Human	The synbiotic supplementation combined with changes in lifestyle is greater than just changes in lifestyle alone for the treatment of NASH	[78]
Resveratrol supplementation	Human	Resveratrol supplementation together with changes in lifestyle is more effective than just changes in lifestyle alone. This is at least partially due to attenuation of inflammatory markers and hepatocellular apoptosis	[100]
Resveratrol supplementation	Animal	Improvement in lipid metabolism and decreased the pro-inflammatory profile of NAFLD in the liver of mice with diet-induced obesity	[101]
Green tea extract	Animal	Higher glutathione levels, lower protein and mRNA contents of inflammatory cytokines, and lower DNA binding activity of NF-κB in liver and adipose tissue of mice supplemented with a green tea extract 2%	[46]
Quercetin treatment	Animal	Total or partial prevention of hepatic steatosis, inflammatory cell accumulation, oxidative stress, and fibrosis caused by the a methionine-choline deficient (MCD)	[51]
Proanthocyanidins from grape seed (GSP) plus metformin	Animal	Improvement of lipid metabolism, but the effects were not additive to normalize lipid levels	[110]
Review of interventions with anthocyanidins (ACNs) in NAFLD patients	Human	Foods rich in ACNs may be promising for prevention of NAFLD and its complications. However, further studies are required	[111]
Seed tamarindus indica	Animal	Intervention has a therapeutic potential against NAFLD, acting in part through insulin sensitization, antioxidant, and anti-obesity mechanisms	[52]
Ostol treatment	Animal	Decreased intrahepatic fat content and in the expression of SREBP-1c, FAS and stearoyl-CoA desaturase-1 (SCD-1), with increased expression of peroxisome proliferator activated receptor α (PPAR-α)	[119]
Sapindus alcohol extract mukorossi Gaertn supplementation	Animal	Regulation of the level of blood fat and improvement in the pathological changes in liver tissue in a rat model of NAFLD	[120]
Sasa borealis (SB5) supplementation	Animal	Improvement in cholesterol metabolism, decreased lipogenesis, and increased oxidation of lipids in rats with high-fat diet (HFD)-induced hepatic steatosis	[121]

4.6.6. Silimarin

Milk thistle has been known for over 2000 years as a herbal medicinal that has been traditionally used for a variety of pathologies. It has been particularly used for handling to diseases related to the liver and gallbladder. Silibum marianum (Latin term for the plant) and its seeds are rich in a variety of natural compounds called flavonolignans. Silimarin is known as a mixture of these compounds, which is extracted after being processed with ethanol, methanol and acetone and contains mainly silibin A, silibin B, taxofolin, isosilibin A, isolsilibin B, silichristin A, silidianin, and other compounds in smaller concentrationes. Apart from its use in liver and gallbladder disorders, milk thistle has recently gained attention due to its hypoglycemic and hypolipidemic properties [123]. Loguercio et al. [124] carried out a multicenter, phase III, doubled-blind critical trial to asses RA (comprises the silybin phytosome complex (silybin plus phosphatidylcholine) coformulated with vitamin E) in individuals with NAFLD histologically documented. The participants were distributed (1:1) to receive active treatment (RA; active components: silybin 94 mg, phosphatidylcholine 194 mg, vitamin E acetate 50% (α-tocopherol 30 mg) 89.28 mg) or placebo (P; extrawhite saccharine replacing active components) with a daily dose of 2 times orally and for a period of 12 consecutive months, and the authors found that patients treated with RA showed relief in values of transaminases (AST, ALT) and GGT, insulin resistance and different histological features of the liver [124]. Similarly, a recent study compare the metabolic effects of the Mediterranean diet versus the diet associated with silybin, phosphatidylcholine and vitamin E complex (RE complex) in overweight patients with NAFLD and reported that the treatment for six months with the Mediterranean diet and the RE complex, exhibited improvement not only in anthropometric parameters (reduction in BMI and waits circumference) but also in insulin resistance and hepatic fat accumulation [125].

4.7. Miscellaneous Therapeutic Agents' Interventions in NAFLD: Astaxanthin, Cinnamon, and Coffee

Astaxanthin (ASTX) is a xanthophyll carotenoid this primarily in marine animals, among them in salmon and crustaceans [126], which is a potent antioxidant acting as a free radical scavenger including ROS [127] and peroxyl radicals, thus protecting PUFAs in biological membranes from lipid peroxidation [128]. Seeking to define an effective dose of dietary treatment with ASTX to address metabolic dysfunctions, male C57BL/6J mice were fed a HFD (35%) and were treated with 0, 0.003%, 0.01% or 0.03% of ASTX (w/w) for 12 weeks [129]. At the highest dosage used, ASTX significantly decreased plasma TGs, AST, and ALT concentrations, and increased expression of endogenous antioxidants genes in liver was observed, with lower sensitivity of isolated splenocytes to LPS stimulation, thereby suggesting that ASTX can have a role in preventing of obesity-associated metabolic disturbances and inflammation [129].

Askari et al. [130] designed a RCT to evaluate the effects of cinnamon supplementation in patients with NAFLD, involving 55 patients with NAFLD randomized supplemented either with 2 cinnamon capsules (each capsule containing 750 mg of cinnamon) or placebo capsule daily for 12 weeks, and all patients were instructed to implement a balanced diet and physical activity. Under these conditions, the treatment group exhibited significantly decreased HOMA, fasting blood glucose, TC, LDL-C, TGs, ALT, AST, GGT, hs-CRP, however, the serum levels of HDL-C and in both groups remained unaltered [130].

The coffee is regarded as the most consumed beverage worldwide. A recent large prospective study showed that consumption of pure and decaffeinated coffee is associated with decreased all-cause death [131]. Similarly, it has been reported that the intake of coffee reduces the risk of advanced liver disease and complications associated with this [132], and equally of hepatocellular carcinoma independent of the etiology [133]. However, despite the above benefits, the molecular mechanisms that contribute to the protective effect of coffee are not well clarified. In this regard, a study evaluated the effects of the administration of decaffeinated espresso coffee versus placebo in rats fed with HFD and changes in the proteomic profile of the liver. It was found that rats receiving HFD plus placebo developed periacinar steatosis, lobular inflammation, and average fibrosis; while those receiving HFD plus coffee exhibited only average steatosis. Coffee consumption increased the hepatic expression of chaperones of the endoplasmic reticulum and induced the expression of master regulators of redox state. In addition, coffee intake was associated with decreased expression of the α-subunit flavoprotein electron transfer, an element of the mitochondrial respiratory chain related with *de novo* lipogénesis [134].

5. Conclusions and Projections

Currently, an effective pharmacological therapy for the NAFLD treatment is not available. Lifestyle interventions involving diet and exercise remain the first line treatment (Figure 1), however, the weight loss long term has a low success rate as well as dietary restrictions adherence. This situation has prompted the exploration of new therapeutic agents for the prevention of hepatic steatosis and the progression of the disease. Scientific evidence of potential therapeutic agents remains lacking, partly because of the lack of clinical trials with based on evidence of liver histopathology data, but also due to the fact that NAFLD is a multifactorial disease involving deep and complex metabolic changes in the liver, which are in close relationship with other tissues such as adipose tissue and skeletal muscle, making the possibility of successfully respond to monotherapy unlikely. This situation points to the need for new therapeutic approaches considering the assessment of the effectiveness of combined bioactive compounds that have proven hepatoprotective actions, in order to find possible additive or potentiating effects in the prevention and treatment of NAFLD. In addition, it would be of importance to consider the effects of therapeutic agents in conjunction with other non-pharmacological therapies, such as those focused on behavioral therapies and surgical procedures, to evaluate the usefulness of complementary mechanisms of actions on NAFLD outcomes.

Acknowledgments: The authors are grateful to project (11140174) from Initiation FONDECYT (National Fund for Scientific and Technological Development) of Rodrigo Valenzuela, Department of Nutrition, Faculty of Medicine, Chile. And the Enlaza-Mundos Program of the Mayor of Medellin (Colombia)—Agency for Higher Education of Medellin-SAPIENCIA, for the support to co-finance postgraduate study abroad (Maria Catalina Hernandez-Rodas).

Author Contributions: Maria Catalina Hernandez-Rodas, Rodrigo Valenzuela and Luis A. Videla. Analysis of the information and writing the manuscript. All authors reviewed and approved the final version of the manuscript.

References

1.   Thoma, C.; Day, C.P.; Trenell, M.I. Lifestyle interventions for the treatment of non-alcoholic fatty liver disease in adults: A systematic review. *J. Hepatol.* **2012**, *56*, 255–266. [CrossRef] [PubMed]
2.   Browning, J.D.; Szczepaniak, L.S.; Dobbins, R.; Nuremberg, P.; Horton, J.D.; Cohen, J.C.; Grundy, S.M.; Hobbs, H.H. Prevalence of hepatic steatosis in an urban population in the United States: Impact of ethnicity. *Hepatology* **2004**, *40*, 1387–1395. [CrossRef] [PubMed]
3.   Bellentani, S.; Saccoccio, G.; Masutti, F.; Crocè, L.S.; Brandi, G.; Sasso, F.; Cristanini, G.; Tiribelli, C. Prevalence of and risk factors for hepatic steatosis in Northern Italy. *Ann. Intern. Med.* **2000**, *132*, 112–117. [CrossRef] [PubMed]
4.   Mitchel, E.B.; Lavine, J.E. Review article: The management of paediatric nonalcoholic fatty liver disease. *Aliment. Pharmacol. Ther.* **2014**, *40*, 1155–1170. [CrossRef] [PubMed]
5.   Lonardo, A.; Ballestri, S.; Marchesini, G.; Angulo, P.; Loria, P. Nonalcoholic fatty liver disease: A precursor of the metabolic syndrome. *Dig. Liver Dis.* **2015**, *47*, 181–190. [CrossRef] [PubMed]
6.   Centis, E.; Marzocchi, R.; di Domizio, S.; Ciaravella, M.F.; Marchesini, G. The effect of lifestyle changes in non-alcoholic fatty liver disease. *Dig. Dis.* **2010**, *28*, 267–273. [CrossRef] [PubMed]
7.   Giorgio, V.; Prono, F.; Graziano, F.; Nobili, V. Pediatric non alcoholic fatty liver disease: Old and new concepts on development, progression, metabolic insight and potential treatment targets. *BMC Pediatr.* **2013**, *13*, 40. [CrossRef] [PubMed]
8.   Vuppalanchi, R.; Chalasani, N. Nonalcoholic fatty liver disease and nonalcoholic steatohepatitis: Selected practical issues in their evaluation and management. *Hepatology* **2009**, *49*, 306–317. [CrossRef] [PubMed]

9.   Dixon, J.B.; Bhathal, P.S.; Hughes, N.R.; O'Brien, P.E. Nonalcoholic fatty liver disease: Improvement in liver histological analysis with weight loss. *Hepatology* **2004**, *39*, 1647–1654. [CrossRef] [PubMed]

10.   Catalano, D.; Trovato, G.M.; Martines, G.F.; Randazzo, M.; Tonzuso, A. Bright liver, body composition and insulin resistance changes with nutritional intervention: A follow-up study. *Liver Int.* **2008**, *28*, 1280–1287. [CrossRef] [PubMed]

11.   Trovato, G.M.; Catalano, D.; Martines, G.F.; Pirri, C.; Trovato, F.M. Western dietary pattern and sedentary life: Independent effects of diet and physical exercise intensity on NAFLD. *Am. J. Gastroenterol.* **2008**, *108*, 1932–1933. [CrossRef] [PubMed]

12.   Trovato, F.M.; Catalano, D.; Martines, G.F.; Pace, P.; Trovato, G.M. Mediterranean diet and non-alcoholic fatty liver disease: The need of extended and comprehensive interventions. *Clin. Nutr.* **2015**, *34*, 86–88. [CrossRef] [PubMed]

13.   Ghaemi, A.; Taleban, F.A.; Hekmatdoost, A.; Rafiei, A.; Hosseini, V.; Amiri, Z.; Homayounfar, R.; Fakheri, H. How Much Weight Loss is Effective on Nonalcoholic Fatty Liver Disease? *Hepat. Mon.* **2013**, *13*, 15227. [CrossRef] [PubMed]

14.   Musso, G.; Cassader, M.; Rosina, F.; Gambino, R. Impact of current treatments on liver disease, glucose metabolism and cardiovascular risk in non-alcoholic fatty liver disease (NAFLD): A systematic review and meta-analysis of randomised trials. *Diabetologia* **2012**, *55*, 885–904. [CrossRef] [PubMed]

15.   Bradford, V.; Dillon, J.; Miller, M. Lifestyle interventions for the treatment of non-alcoholic fatty liver disease. *Hepat. Med.* **2013**, *6*, 1–10. [PubMed]

16.   Franz, M.J.; VanWormer, J.J.; Crain, A.L.; Boucher, J.L.; Histon, T.; Caplan, W.; Bowman, J.D.; Pronk, N.P. Weight-loss outcomes: A systematic review and meta-analysis of weight-loss clinical trials with a minimum 1-year follow-up. *J. Am. Diet. Assoc.* **2007**, *107*, 1755–1767. [CrossRef] [PubMed]

17.   Zelber-Sagi, S.; Nitzan-Kaluski, D.; Goldsmith, R.; Webb, M.; Zvibel, I.; Goldiner, I.; Blendis, L.; Halpern, Z.; Oren, R. Role of leisure-time physical activity in nonalcoholic fatty liver disease: A population-based study. *Hepatology* **2008**, *48*, 1791–1798. [CrossRef] [PubMed]

18.   St George, A.; Bauman, A.; Johnston, A.; Farrell, G.; Chey, T.; George, J. Independent effects of physical activity in patients with nonalcoholic fatty liver disease. *Hepatology* **2009**, *50*, 68–76. [CrossRef] [PubMed]

19.   Sreenivasa Baba, C.; Alexander, G.; Kalyani, B.; Pandey, R.; Rastogi, S.; Pandey, A.; Choudhuri, G. Effect of exercise and dietary modification on serum aminotransferase levels in patients with nonalcoholic steatohepatitis. *J. Gastroenterol. Hepatol.* **2006**, *21*, 191–198. [CrossRef] [PubMed]

20.   Johnson, N.A.; Sachinwalla, T.; Walton, D.W.; Smith, K.; Armstrong, A.; Thompson, M.W.; George, J. Aerobic exercise training reduces hepatic and visceral lipids in obese individuals without weight loss. *Hepatology* **2009**, *50*, 1105–1112. [CrossRef] [PubMed]

21.   Wadden, T.A.; Butryn, M.L. Behavioral treatment of obesity. *Endocrinol. Metab. Clin. N. Am.* **2003**, *32*, 981–1003. [CrossRef]

22.   Bellentani, S.; Dalle Grave, R.; Suppini, A.; Marchesini, G.; Fatty Liver Italian Network. Behavior therapy for nonalcoholic fatty liver disease: The need for a multidisciplinary approach. *Hepatology* **2008**, *47*, 746–754. [CrossRef] [PubMed]

23.   Osland, E.J.; Powell, E.E.; Banks, M.; Jonsson, J.R.; Hickman, I.J. Obesity management in liver clinics: Translation of research into clinical practice. *J. Gastroenterol. Hepatol.* **2007**, *22*, 504–509. [CrossRef] [PubMed]

24.   Ovchinsky, N.; Lavine, J.E. A critical appraisal of advances in pediatric nonalcoholic Fatty liver disease. *Semin. Liver Dis.* **2012**, *32*, 317–324. [PubMed]

25.   Tappy, L.; Lê, K.A.; Tran, C.; Paquot, N. Fructose and metabolic diseases: New findings, new questions. *Nutrition* **2010**, *26*, 1044–1049. [CrossRef] [PubMed]

26.   Abid, A.; Taha, O.; Nseir, W.; Farah, R.; Grosovski, M.; Assy, N. Soft drink consumption is associated with fatty liver disease independent of metabolic syndrome. *J. Hepatol.* **2009**, *51*, 918–924. [CrossRef] [PubMed]

27.   Jin, R.; Welsh, J.A.; Le, N.A.; Holzberg, J.; Sharma, P.; Martin, D.R.; Vos, M.B. Dietary fructose reduction improves markers of cardiovascular disease risk in Hispanic-American adolescents with NAFLD. *Nutrients* **2014**, *6*, 3187–3201. [CrossRef] [PubMed]

28.   Carvalhana, S.; Machado, M.V.; Cortez-Pinto, H. Improving dietary patterns in patients with nonalcoholic fatty liver disease. *Curr. Opin. Clin. Nutr. Metab. Care* **2012**' *15*, 468–473. [CrossRef] [PubMed]

29.   Yang, H.Y.; Tzeng, Y.H.; Chai, C.Y.; Hsieh, A.T.; Chen, J.R.; Chang, L.S.; Yang, S.S. Soy protein retards the progression of non-alcoholic steatohepatitis via improvement of insulin resistance and steatosis. *Nutrition* **2011**, *27*, 943–948. [CrossRef] [PubMed]

30.   Leng, L.; Jiang, Z.Q.; Ji, G.Y. Effects of soybean isoflavone on liver lipid metabolism in nonalcoholic fatty liver rats. *Zhonghua Yu Fang Yi Xue Za Zhi* **2011**, *45*, 335–339. [PubMed]

31.   Kani, A.H.; Alavian, S.M.; Esmaillzadeh, A.; Adibi, P.; Azadbakht, L. Effects of a novel therapeutic diet on liver enzymes and coagulating factors in patients with non-alcoholic fatty liver disease: A parallel randomized trial. *Nutrition* **2014**, *30*, 814–812. [CrossRef] [PubMed]

32.   Bortolotti, M.; Maiolo, E.; Corazza, M.; van Dijke, E.; Schneiter, P.; Boss, A.; Carrel, G.; Giusti, V.; Lê, K.A.; Quo Chong, D.G.; *et al.* Effects of a whey protein supplementation on intrahepatocellular lipids in obese female patients. *Clin. Nutr.* **2011**, *30*, 494–498. [CrossRef] [PubMed]

33.   Cave, M.; Deaciuc, I.; Mendez, C.; Song, Z.; Joshi-Barve, S.; Barve, S.; McClain, C. Nonalcoholic fatty liver disease: Predisposing factors and the role of nutrition. *J. Nutr. Biochem.* **2007**, *18*, 184–195. [CrossRef] [PubMed]

34.   Bezerra Duarte, S.M.; Faintuch, J.; Stefano, J.T.; de Oliveira, M.B.; de Campos Mazo, D.F.; Rabelo, F.; Vanni, D.; Nogueira, M.A.; Carrilho, F.J.; de Oliveira, C.P. Hypocaloric high-protein diet improves clinical and biochemical markers in patients with nonalcoholic fatty liver disease (NAFLD). *Nutr. Hosp.* **2014**, *29*, 94–101. [PubMed]

35.   Garcia-Caraballo, S.C.; Comhair, T.M.; Verheyen, F.; Gaemers, I.; Schaap, F.G.; Houten, S.M.; Hakvoort, T.B.; Dejong, C.H.; Lamers, W.H.; Koehler, S.E. Prevention and reversal of hepatic steatosis with a high-protein diet in mice. *Biochim. Biophys. Acta* **2013**, *1832*, 685–695. [CrossRef] [PubMed]

36.   Vos, M.B.; Kimmons, J.E.; Gillespie, C.; Welsh, J.; Blanck, H.M. Dietary fructose consumption among US children and adults: The Third National Health and Nutrition Examination Survey. *Medscape J. Med.* **2008**, *10*, 160. [PubMed]

37.   Bergheim, I.; Weber, S.; Vos, M.; Krämer, S.; Volynets, V.; Kaserouni, S.; McClain, C.J.; Bischoff, S.C. Antibiotics protect against fructose-induced hepatic lipid accumulation in mice: Role of endotoxin. *J. Hepatol.* **2008**, *48*, 983–992. [CrossRef] [PubMed]

38.   Ouyang, X.; Cirillo, P.; Sautin, Y.; McCall, S.; Bruchette, J.L.; Diehl, A.M.; Johnson, R.J.; Abdelmalek, M.F. Fructose consumption as a risk factor for non-alcoholic fatty liver disease. *J. Hepatol.* **2008**, *48*, 993–999. [CrossRef] [PubMed]

39.   Girard, A.; Madani, S.; Boukortt, F.; Cherkaoui-Malki, M.; Belleville, J.; Prost, J. Fructose-enriched diet modifies antioxidant status and lipid metabolism in spontaneously hypertensive rats. *Nutrition* **2006**, *22*, 758–766. [CrossRef] [PubMed]

40.   Vos, M.B.; Lavine, J.E. Dietary fructose in nonalcoholic fatty liver disease. *Hepatology* **2013**, *57*, 2525–2531. [CrossRef] [PubMed]

41.   Targher, G. Non-alcoholic fatty liver disease, the metabolic syndrome and the risk of cardiovascular disease: The plot thickens. *Diabet. Med.* **2007**, *24*, 1–6. [CrossRef] [PubMed]

42.   Abenavoli, L.; Milic, N.; Peta, V.; Alfieri, F.; de Lorenzo, A.; Bellentani, S. Alimentary regimen in non-alcoholic fatty liver disease: Mediterranean diet. *World J. Gastroenterol.* **2014**, *20*, 16831–16840. [CrossRef] [PubMed]

43.   Parker, H.M.; Johnson, N.A.; Burdon, C.A.; Cohn, J.S.; O'Connor, H.T.; George, J. Omega-3 supplementation and non-alcoholic fatty liver disease: A systematic review and meta-analysis. *J. Hepatol.* **2012**, *56*, 944–951. [CrossRef] [PubMed]

44.   Ryan, M.C.; Itsiopoulos, C.; Thodis, T.; Ward, G.; Trost, N.; Hofferberth, S.; O'Dea, K.; Desmond, P.V.; Johnson, N.A.; Wilson, A.M. The Mediterranean diet improves hepatic steatosis and insulin sensitivity in individuals with non-alcoholic fatty liver disease. *J. Hepatol.* **2013**, *59*, 138–143. [CrossRef] [PubMed]

45.   Ayyad, C.; Andersen, T. Long-term efficacy of dietary treatment of obesity: A systematic review of studies published between 1931 and 1999. *Obes. Rev.* **2000**, *1*, 113–119. [CrossRef] [PubMed]

46.   Park, H.J.; Lee, J.Y.; Chung, M.Y.; Park, Y.K.; Bower, A.M.; Koo, S.I.; Giardina, C.; Bruno, R.S. Green tea extract suppresses NFκB activation and inflammatory responses in diet-induced obese rats with nonalcoholic steatohepatitis. *J. Nutr.* **2012**, *142*, 57–63. [CrossRef] [PubMed]

47.   Rector, R.S.; Thyfault, J.P.; Wei, Y.; Ibdah, J.A. Non-alcoholic fatty liver disease and the metabolic syndrome: An update. *World J. Gastroenterol.* **2008**, *14*, 185–192. [CrossRef] [PubMed]

48. Videla, L.A.; Rodrigo, R.; Araya, J.; Poniachik, J. Oxidative stress and depletion of hepatic long-chain polyunsaturated fatty acids may contribute to nonalcoholic fatty liver disease. *Free Radic. Biol. Med.* **2004**, *37*, 1499–1507. [CrossRef] [PubMed]

49. Pagano, G.; Pacini, G.; Musso, G.; Gambino, R.; Mecca, F.; Depetris, N.; Cassader, M.; David, E.; Cavallo-Perin, P.; Rizzetto, M. Nonalcoholic steatohepatitis, insulin resistance, and metabolic syndrome: Further evidence for an etiologic association. *Hepatology* **2002**, *35*, 367–372. [CrossRef] [PubMed]

50. Liu, Z.L.; Xie, L.Z.; Zhu, J.; Li, G.Q.; Grant, S.J.; Liu, J.P. Herbal medicines for fatty liver diseases. *Cochrane Database Syst. Rev.* **2013**, *8*. [CrossRef]

51. Marcolin, E.; San-Miguel, B.; Vallejo, D.; Tieppo, J.; Marroni, N.; González-Gallego, J.; Tuñón, M.J. Quercetin treatment ameliorates inflammation and fibrosis in mice with nonalcoholic steatohepatitis. *J. Nutr.* **2012**, *142*, 1821–1828. [CrossRef] [PubMed]

52. Sasidharan, S.R.; Joseph, J.A.; Anandakumar, S.; Venkatesan, V.; Madhavan, C.N.; Agarwal, A. Ameliorative potential of Tamarindus indica on high fat diet induced nonalcoholic fatty liver disease in rats. *Sci. World J.* **2014**, *2014*, 507197. [CrossRef] [PubMed]

53. Balunas, M.J.; Kinghor, A.D. Drug discovery from medicinal plants. *Life Sci.* **2005**, *78*, 431–441. [CrossRef] [PubMed]

54. Zhang, S.; Zheng, L.; Dong, D.; Xu, L.; Yin, L.; Qi, Y.; Han, X.; Lin, Y.; Liu, K.; Peng, J. Effects of flavonoids from Rosa laevigata Michx fruit against high-fat diet-induced non-alcoholic fatty liver disease in rats. *Food Chem.* **2013**, *141*, 2108–2116. [CrossRef] [PubMed]

55. Prior, R.L.; Cao, G. Antioxidant capacity and polyphenolic components of teas: Implications for altering *in vivo* antioxidant status. *Proc. Soc. Exp. Biol. Med.* **1999**, *220*, 255–261. [CrossRef] [PubMed]

56. Akiba, Y.; Takahashi, K.; Horiguchi, M.; Ohtani, H.; Saitoh, S.; Ohkawara, H. L-tryptophan alleviates fatty liver and modifies hepatic microsomal mixed function oxidase in laying hens. *Comp. Biochem. Physiol. Comp. Physiol.* **1992**, *102*, 769–774. [CrossRef]

57. Ritze, Y.; Bárdos, G.; Hubert, A.; Böhle, M.; Bischoff, S.C. Effect of tryptophan supplementation on diet-induced non-alcoholic fatty liver disease in mice. *Br. J. Nutr.* **2014**, *112*, 1–7. [CrossRef] [PubMed]

58. Lin, Z.; Cai, F.; Lin, N.; Ye, J.; Zheng, Q.; Ding, G. Effects of glutamine on oxidative stress and nuclear factor-κB expression in the livers of rats with nonalcoholic fatty liver disease. *Exp. Ther. Med.* **2014**, *7*, 365–370. [CrossRef] [PubMed]

59. Kerner, J.; Bieber, L. Isolation of a malonyl-CoA-sensitive CPT/β-oxidation enzyme complex from heart mitochondria. *Biochemistry* **1990**, *29*, 4326–4334. [CrossRef] [PubMed]

60. Lombardo, Y.B.; Chicco, A.G. Effects of dietary polyunsaturated n-3 fatty acids on dyslipidemia and insulin resistance in rodents and humans. A review. *J. Nutr. Biochem.* **2006**, *17*, 1–13. [CrossRef] [PubMed]

61. Araya, J.; Rodrigo, R.; Videla, L.A.; Thielemann, L.; Orellana, M.; Pettinelli, P.; Poniachik, J. Increase in long-chain polyunsaturated fatty acid n-6/n-3 ratio in relation to hepatic steatosis in patients with non-alcoholic fatty liver disease. *Clin. Sci.* **2004**, *106*, 635–643. [CrossRef] [PubMed]

62. Xin, Y.N.; Xuan, S.Y.; Zhang, J.H.; Zheng, M.H.; Guan, H.S. Omega-3 polyunsaturated fatty acids: A specific liver drug for non-alcoholic fatty liver disease (NAFLD). *Med. Hypothese.* **2008**, *71*, 820–821. [CrossRef] [PubMed]

63. Shapiro, H.; Tehilla, M.; Attal-Singer, J.; Bruck, R.; Luzzatti, R.; Singer, P. The therapeutic potential of long-chain omega-3 fatty acids in nonalcoholic fatty liver disease. *Clin. Nutr.* **2011**, *30*, 6–19. [CrossRef] [PubMed]

64. Nobili, V.; Alisi, A.; Della Corte, C.; Risé, P.; Galli, C.; Agostoni, C.; Bedogni, G. Docosahexaenoic acid for the treatment of fatty liver: Randomised controlled trial in children. *Nutr. Metab. Cardiovasc. Dis.* **2013**, *23*, 1066–1070. [CrossRef] [PubMed]

65. Ganji, S.H.; Qin, S.; Zhang, L.; Kamanna, V.S.; Kashyap, M.L. Niacin inhibits vascular oxidative stress, redox-sensitive genes, and monocyte adhesion to human aortic endothelial cells. *Atherosclerosis* **2009**, *202*, 68–75. [CrossRef] [PubMed]

66. Meyers, C.D.; Kamanna, V.S.; Kashyap, M.L. Niacin therapy in atherosclerosis. *Curr. Opin. Lipidol.* **2004**, *15*, 659–665. [CrossRef] [PubMed]

67. Ganji, S.H.; Kukes, G.D.; Lambrecht, N.; Kashyap, M.L.; Kamanna, V.S. Therapeutic role of niacin in the prevention and regression of hepatic steatosis in rat model of nonalcoholic fatty liver disease. *Am. J. Physiol. Gastrointest. Liver Physiol.* **2014**, *306*, G320–G327. [CrossRef] [PubMed]

68. Herrera, E.; Barbas, C. Vitamin E: Action, metabolism and perspectives. *J. Physiol. Biochem.* **2001**, *57*, 43–56. [CrossRef] [PubMed]

69. Wefers, H.; Sies, H. The protection by ascorbate and glutathione against microsomal lipid peroxidation is dependent on vitamin E. *Eur. J. Biochem.* **1988**, *174*, 353–357. [CrossRef] [PubMed]

70. Tzanetakou, I.P.; Doulamis, I.P.; Korou, L.M.; Agrogiannis, G.; Vlachos, I.S.; Pantopoulou, A.; Mikhailidis, D.P.; Patsouris, E.; Vlachos, I.; Perrea, D.N. Water Soluble Vitamin E Administration in Wistar Rats with Non-alcoholic Fatty Liver Disease. *Open Cardiovasc. Med. J.* **2012**, *6*, 88–97. [CrossRef] [PubMed]

71. Eslamparast, T.; Eghtesad, S.; Hekmatdoost, A.; Poustchi, H. Probiotics and Nonalcoholic Fatty liver Disease. *Middle East. J. Dig. Dis.* **2013**, *5*, 129–136. [PubMed]

72. Farrell, G.C. Is bacterial ash the flash that ignites NASH? *Gut* **2001**, *48*, 148–149. [CrossRef] [PubMed]

73. Maddur, H.; Neuschwander-Tetri, B.A. More evidence that probiotics may have a role in treating fatty liver disease. *Am. J. Clin. Nutr.* **2014**, *99*, 425–426. [CrossRef] [PubMed]

74. Tandon, P.; Garcia-Tsao, G. Bacterial infections, sepsis, and multiorgan failure in cirrhosis. *Semin. Liver Dis.* **2008**, *28*, 26–42. [CrossRef] [PubMed]

75. Yang, L.; Seki, E. Toll-like receptors in liver fibrosis: Cellular crosstalk and mechanisms. *Front. Physiol.* **2012**, *3*, 138. [CrossRef] [PubMed]

76. Miele, L.; Valenza, V.; La Torre, G.; Montalto, M.; Cammarota, G.; Ricci, R.; Mascianà, R.; Forgione, A.; Gabrieli, M.L.; Perotti, G.; *et al.* Increased intestinal permeability and tight junction alterations in nonalcoholic fatty liver disease. *Hepatology* **2009**, *49*, 1877–1887. [CrossRef] [PubMed]

77. Wigg, A.J.; Roberts-Thomson, I.C.; Dymock, R.B.; McCarthy, P.J.; Grose, R.H.; Cummins, A.G. The role of small intestinal bacterial overgrowth, intestinal permeability, endotoxaemia, and tumour necrosis factor alpha in the pathogenesis of non-alcoholic steatohepatitis. *Gut* **2001**, *48*, 206–211. [CrossRef] [PubMed]

78. Eslamparast, T.; Poustchi, H.; Zamani, F.; Sharafkhah, M.; Malekzadeh, R.; Hekmatdoost, A. Synbiotic supplementation in nonalcoholic fatty liver disease: A randomized, double-blind, placebo-controlled pilot study. *Am. J. Clin. Nutr.* **2014**, *99*, 535–542. [CrossRef] [PubMed]

79. Cani, P.D.; Bibiloni, R.; Knauf, C.; Waget, A.; Neyrinck, A.M.; Delzenne, N.M.; Burcelin, R. Changes in gut microbiota control metabolic endotoxemia-induced inflammation in high-fat diet-induced obesity and diabetes in mice. *Diabetes* **2008**, *57*, 1470–1481. [CrossRef] [PubMed]

80. Round, J.L.; Mazmanian, S.K. The gut microbiota shapes intestinal immune responses during health and disease. *Nat. Rev. Immunol.* **2009**, *9*, 313–323. [CrossRef] [PubMed]

81. Malaguarnera, M.; Greco, F.; Barone, G.; Gargante, M.P.; Malaguarnera, M.; Toscano, M.A. *Bifidobacterium longum* with fructo-oligosaccharide (FOS) treatment in minimal hepatic encephalopathy: A randomized, double-blind, placebo-controlled study. *Dig. Dis. Sci.* **2007**, *52*, 3259–3265. [CrossRef] [PubMed]

82. Li, Z.; Yang, S.; Lin, H.; Huang, J.; Watkins, P.A.; Moser, A.B.; Desimone, C.; Song, X.Y.; Diehl, A.M. Probiotics and antibodies to TNF inhibit inflammatory activity and improve nonalcoholic fatty liver disease. *Hepatology* **2003**, *37*, 343–350. [CrossRef] [PubMed]

83. Ma, X.; Hua, J.; Li, Z. Probiotics improve high fat diet-induced hepatic steatosis and insulin resistance by increasing hepatic NKT cells. *J. Hepatol.* **2008**, *49*, 821–830. [CrossRef] [PubMed]

84. Esposito, E.; Iacono, A.; Bianco, G.; Autore, G.; Cuzzocrea, S.; Vajro, P.; Canani, R.B.; Calignano, A.; Raso, G.M.; Meli, R. Probiotics reduce the inflammatory response induced by a high-fat diet in the liver of young rats. *J. Nutr.* **2009**, *139*, 905–911. [CrossRef] [PubMed]

85. Mencarelli, A.; Distrutti, E.; Renga, B.; D'Amore, C.; Cipriani, S.; Palladino, G.; Donini, A.; Ricci, P.; Fiorucci, S. Probiotics modulate intestinal expression of nuclear receptor and provide counter-regulatory signals to inflammation-driven adipose tissue activation. *PLoS ONE* **2011**, *6*, 22978. [CrossRef] [PubMed]

86. Ritze, Y.; Bárdos, G.; Claus, A.; Ehrmann, V.; Bergheim, I.; Schwiertz, A.; Bischoff, S.C. *Lactobacillus* rhamnosus GG protects against non-alcoholic fatty liver disease in mice. *PLoS ONE* **2014**, *9*, 80169. [CrossRef] [PubMed]

87. Okubo, H.; Sakoda, H.; Kushiyama, A.; Fujishiro, M.; Nakatsu, Y.; Fukushima, T.; Matsunaga, Y.; Kamata, H.; Asahara, T.; Yoshida, Y.; *et al.* Lactobacillus casei strain Shirota protects against nonalcoholic steatohepatitis development in a rodent model. *Am. J. Physiol. Gastrointest. Liver Physiol.* **2013**, *305*, G911–G918. [CrossRef] [PubMed]

88. Loguercio, C.; Federico, A.; Tuccillo, C.; Terracciano, F.; D'Auria, M.V.; de Simone, C.; del Vecchio Blanco, C. Beneficial effects of a probiotic VSL#3 on parameters of liver dysfunction in chronic liver diseases. *J. Clin. Gastroenterol.* **2005**, *39*, 540–543. [PubMed]

89. Vajro, P.; Mandato, C.; Licenziati, M.R.; Franzese, A.; Vitale, D.F.; Lenta, S.; Caropreso, M.; Vallone, G.; Meli, R. Effects of Lactobacillus rhamnosus strain GG in pediatric obesity-related liver disease. *J. Pediatr. Gastroenterol. Nutr.* **2011**, *52*, 740–743. [CrossRef] [PubMed]

90. Aller, R.; de Luis, D.A.; Izaola, O.; Conde, R.; Gonzalez Sagrado, M.; Primo, D.; de La Fuente, B.; Gonzalez, J. Effect of a probiotic on liver aminotransferases in nonalcoholic fatty liver disease patients: A double blind randomized clinical trial. *Eur. Rev. Med. Pharmacol. Sci.* **2011**, *15*, 1090–1095. [PubMed]

91. Ma, Y.Y.; Li, L.; Yu, C.H.; Shen, Z.; Chen, L.H.; Li, Y.M. Effects of probiotics on nonalcoholic fatty liver disease: A meta-analysis. *World J. Gastroenterol.* **2013**, *19*, 6911–6918. [CrossRef] [PubMed]

92. Malaguarnera, M.; Vacante, M.; Antic, T.; Giordano, M.; Chisari, G.; Acquaviva, R.; Mastrojeni, S.; Malaguarnera, G.; Mistretta, A.; Li Volti, G.; et al. *Bifidobacterium longum* with fructo-oligosaccharides in patients with non alcoholic steatohepatitis. *Dig. Dis. Sci.* **2012**, *57*, 545–553. [CrossRef] [PubMed]

93. Cardona, F.; Andrés-Lacueva, C.; Tulipani, S.; Tinahones, F.J.; Queipo-Ortuño, M.I. Benefits of polyphenols on gut microbiota and implications in human health. *J. Nutr. Biochem.* **2013**, *24*, 1415–1422. [CrossRef] [PubMed]

94. Fraga, C.G.; Galleano, M.; Verstraeten, S.V.; Oteiza, P.I. Basic biochemical mechanisms behind the health benefits of polyphenols. *Mol. Aspe. Med.* **2010**, *31*, 435–445. [CrossRef] [PubMed]

95. Baur, J.A.; Sinclair, D.A. Therapeutic potential of resveratrol: The *in vivo* evidence. *Nat. Rev. Drug Discov.* **2006**, *5*, 493–506. [CrossRef] [PubMed]

96. Schmatz, R.; Perreira, L.B.; Stefanello, N.; Mazzanti, C.; Spanevello, R.; Gutierres, J.; Bagatini, M.; Martins, C.C.; Abdalla, F.H.; Daci da Silva Serres, J.; et al. Effects of resveratrol on biomarkers of oxidative stress and on the activity of delta aminolevulinic acid dehydratase in liver and kidney of streptozotocin-induced diabetic rats. *Biochimie* **2012**, *94*, 374–383. [CrossRef] [PubMed]

97. Hou, X.; Xu, S.; Maitland-Toolan, K.A.; Sato, K.; Jiang, B.; Ido, Y.; Lan, F.; Walsh, K.; Wierzbicki, M.; Verbeuren, T.J.; et al. SIRT1 regulates hepatocyte lipid metabolism through activating AMP-activated protein kinase. *J. Biol. Chem.* **2008**, *283*, 20015–20026. [CrossRef] [PubMed]

98. Borra, M.T.; Smith, B.C.; Denu, J.M. Mechanism of human SIRT1 activation by resveratrol. *J. Biol. Chem.* **2005**, *280*, 17187–17195. [CrossRef] [PubMed]

99. Wang, G.L.; Fu, Y.C.; Xu, W.C.; Feng, Y.Q.; Fang, S.R.; Zhou, X.H. Resveratrol inhibits the expression of SREBP1 in cell model of steatosis via Sirt1-FOXO1 signaling pathway. *Biochem. Biophys. Res. Commun.* **2009**, *380*, 644–649. [CrossRef] [PubMed]

100. Faghihzadeh, F.; Adibi, P.; Rafiei, R.; Hekmatdoost, A. Resveratrol supplementation improves inflammatory biomarkers in patients with nonalcoholic fatty liver disease. *Nutr. Res.* **2014**, *34*, 837–843. [CrossRef] [PubMed]

101. Andrade, J.M.; Paraíso, A.F.; de Oliveira, M.V.; Martins, A.M.; Neto, J.F.; Guimarães, A.L.; de Paula, A.M.; Qureshi, M.; Santos, S.H. Resveratrol attenuates hepatic steatosis in high-fat fed mice by decreasing lipogenesis and inflammation. *Nutrition* **2014**, *30*, 915–919. [CrossRef] [PubMed]

102. Imai, K.; Nakachi, K. Cross sectional study of effects of drinking green tea on cardiovascular and liver diseases. *BMJ* **1995**, *310*, 693–696. [CrossRef] [PubMed]

103. Bose, M.; Lambert, J.D.; Ju, J.; Reuhl, K.R.; Shapses, S.A.; Yang, C.S. The major green tea polyphenol, (-)-epigallocatechin-3-gallate, inhibits obesity, metabolic syndrome, and fatty liver disease in high-fat-fed mice. *J. Nutr.* **2008**, *138*, 1677–1683. [PubMed]

104. Tuñón, M.J.; García-Mediavilla, M.V.; Sánchez-Campos, S.; González-Gallego, J. Potential of flavonoids as anti-inflammatory agents: Modulation of pro-inflammatory gene expression and signal transduction pathways. *Curr. Drug Metab.* **2009**, *10*, 256–271. [CrossRef] [PubMed]

105. Martínez-Flórez, S.; Gutiérrez-Fernández, B.; Sánchez-Campos, S.; González-Gallego, J.; Tuñón, M.J. Quercetin attenuates nuclear factor-kappaB activation and nitric oxide production in interleukin-1β-activated rat hepatocytes. *J. Nutr.* **2005**, *135*, 1359–1365. [PubMed]

106. Peres, W.; Tuñón, M.J.; Collado, P.S.; Herrmann, S.; Marroni, N.; González-Gallego, J. The flavonoid quercetin ameliorates liver damage in rats with biliary obstruction. *J. Hepatol.* **2000**, *33*, 742–750. [CrossRef]

107. Egert, S.; Bosy-Westphal, A.; Seiberl, J.; Kürbitz, C.; Settler, U.; Plachta-Danielzik, S.; Wagner, A.E.; Frank, J.; Schrezenmeir, J.; Rimbach, G.; et al. Quercetin reduces systolic blood pressure and plasma oxidised low-density lipoprotein concentrations in overweight subjects with a high-cardiovascular disease risk phenotype: A double-blinded, placebo-controlled cross-over study. *Br. J. Nutr.* **2009**, *102*, 1065–1074. [CrossRef] [PubMed]

108. Kobori, M.; Masumoto, S.; Akimoto, Y.; Oike, H. Chronic dietary intake of quercetin alleviates hepatic fat accumulation associated with consumption of a Western-style diet in C57/BL6J mice. *Mol. Nutr. Food Res.* **2011**, *55*, 530–540. [CrossRef] [PubMed]

109. Engelbrecht, A.M.; Mattheyse, M.; Ellis, B.; Loos, B.; Thomas, M.; Smith, R.; Peters, S.; Smith, C.; Myburgh, K. Proanthocyanidin from grape seeds inactivates the PI3-kinase/PKB pathway and induces apoptosis in a colon cancer cell line. *Cancer Lett.* **2007**, *258*, 144–153. [CrossRef] [PubMed]

110. Yogalakshmi, B.; Sreeja, S.; Geetha, R.; Radika, M.K.; Anuradha, C.V. Grape seed proanthocyanidin rescues rats from steatosis: A comparative and combination study with metformin. *J. Lipids* **2013**, *2013*, 153897. [CrossRef] [PubMed]

111. Valenti, L.; Riso, P.; Mazzocchi, A.; Porrini, M.; Fargion, S.; Agostoni, C. Dietary anthocyanins as nutritional therapy for nonalcoholic fatty liver disease. *Oxidative Med. Cell. Longev.* **2013**, *2013*, 145421. [CrossRef] [PubMed]

112. Prior, R.L.; Wu, X. Anthocyanins: Structural characteristics that result in unique metabolic patterns and biological activities. *Free Radic. Res.* **2006**, *40*, 1014–1028. [CrossRef] [PubMed]

113. Tsuda, T.; Horio, F.; Uchida, K.; Aoki, H.; Osawa, T. Dietary cyanidin 3-*o*-β-D-glucoside-rich purple corn color prevents obesity and ameliorates hyperglycemia in mice. *J. Nutr.* **2003**, *133*, 2125–2130. [PubMed]

114. Suda, I.; Ishikawa, F.; Hatakeyama, M.; Miyawaki, M.; Kudo, T.; Hirano, K.; Ito, A.; Yamakawa, O.; Horiuchi, S. Intake of purple sweet potato beverage affects on serum hepatic biomarker levels of healthy adult men with borderline hepatitis. *Eur. J. Clin. Nutr.* **2008**, *62*, 60–67. [CrossRef] [PubMed]

115. Zhang, L.; Xu, J.; Song, H.; Yao, Z.; Ji, G. Extracts from Salvia-Nelumbinis naturalis alleviate hepatosteatosis via improving hepatic insulin sensitivity. *J. Transl. Med.* **2014**, *12*, 236. [CrossRef] [PubMed]

116. Qi, Z.; Xue, J.; Zhang, Y.; Wang, H.; Xie, M. Osthole ameliorates insulin resistance by increment of adiponectin release in high-fat and high-sucrose-induced fatty liver rats. *Planta Med.* **2011**, *77*, 231–235. [CrossRef] [PubMed]

117. Zhang, Y.; Xie, M.L.; Xue, J.; Gu, Z.L. Osthole regulates enzyme protein expression of CYP7A1 and DGAT2 via activation of PPARalpha/gamma in fat milk-induced fatty liver rats. *J. Asian Nat. Prod. Res.* **2008**, *10*, 807–812. [CrossRef] [PubMed]

118. Zhang, J.; Xue, J.; Wang, H.; Zhang, Y.; Xie, M. Osthole improves alcohol-induced fatty liver in mice by reduction of hepatic oxidative stress. *Phytother. Res.* **2011**, *25*, 638–643. [CrossRef] [PubMed]

119. Nam, H.H.; Jun, D.W.; Jeon, H.J.; Lee, J.S.; Saeed, W.K.; Kim, E.K. Osthol attenuates hepatic steatosis via decreased triglyceride synthesis not by insulin resistance. *World J. Gastroenterol.* **2014**, *20*, 11753–11761. [CrossRef] [PubMed]

120. Peng, Q.; Zhang, Q.; Xiao, W.; Shao, M.; Fan, Q.; Zhang, H.; Zou, Y.; Li, X.; Xu, W.; Mo, Z.; Cai, H. Protective effects of Sapindus mukorossi Gaertn against fatty liver disease induced by high fat diet in rats. *Biochem. Biophys. Res. Commun.* **2014**, *450*, 685–691. [CrossRef] [PubMed]

121. Song, Y.; Lee, S.J.; Jang, S.H.; Ha, J.H.; Song, Y.M.; Ko, Y.G.; Kim, H.D.; Min, W.; Kang, S.N.; Cho, J.H. Sasa borealis stem extract attenuates hepatic steatosis in high-fat diet-induced obese rats. *Nutrients* **2014**, *6*, 2179–2195. [CrossRef] [PubMed]

122. Shibata, M.; Yamatake, Y.; Sakamoto, M.; Kanamori, M.; Takagi, K. Phamacological studies on bamboo grass (1). Acute toxicity and anti-inflammatory and antiulcerogenic activities of water-soluble fraction(Folin) extracted from Sasa albomarginata Makino et Shibata. *Nihon Yakurigaku Zasshi Folia Pharmacol. Jpn.* **1975**, *71*, 481–490. [CrossRef]

123. Kazazis, C.E.; Evangelopoulos, A.A.; Kollas, A.; Vallianou, N.G. The therapeutic potential of milk thistle in diabetes. *Rev. Diabet. Stud.* **2014**, *11*, 167–174. [CrossRef] [PubMed]

124. Loguercio, C.; Andreone, P.; Brisc, C.; Brisc, M.C.; Bugianesi, E.; Chiaramonte, M.; Cursaro, C.; Danila, M.; de Sio, I.; Floreani, A.; et al. Silybin combined with phosphatidylcholine and vitamin E in patients with nonalcoholic fatty liver disease: A randomized controlled trial. *Free Radic. Biol. Med.* **2012**, *52*, 1658–1665. [CrossRef] [PubMed]

125. Abenavoli, L.; Greco, M.; Nazionale, I.; Peta, V.; Milic, N.; Accattato, F.; Foti, D.; Gulletta, E.; Luzza, F. Effects of Mediterranean diet supplemented with silybin-vitamin E-phospholipid complex in overweight patients with non-alcoholic fatty liver disease. *Expert Rev. Gastroenterol. Hepatol.* **2015**, *9*, 519–527. [CrossRef] [PubMed]

126. Hussein, G.; Sankawa, U.; Goto, H.; Matsumoto, K.; Watanabe, H. Astaxanthin, a carotenoid with potential in human health and nutrition. *J. Nat. Prod.* **2006**, *69*, 443–449. [CrossRef] [PubMed]

127. Guerin, M.; Huntley, M.E.; Olaizola, M. Haematococcus astaxanthin: Applications for human health and nutrition. *Trends Biotechnol.* **2003**, *21*, 210–216. [CrossRef]

128. Goto, S.; Kogure, K.; Abe, K.; Kimata, Y.; Kitahama, K.; Yamashita, E.; Terada, H. Efficient radical trapping at the surface and inside the phospholipid membrane is responsible for highly potent antiperoxidative activity of the carotenoid astaxanthin. *Biochim. Biophys. Acta* **2001**, *1512*, 251–258. [CrossRef]

129. Yang, Y.; Pham, T.X.; Wegner, C.J.; Kim, B.; Ku, C.S.; Park, Y.K.; Lee, J.Y. Astaxanthin lowers plasma TAG concentrations and increases hepatic antioxidant gene expression in diet-induced obesity mice. *Br. J. Nutr.* **2014**, *112*, 1797–1804. [CrossRef] [PubMed]

130. Askari, F.; Rashidkhani, B.; Hekmatdoost, A. Cinnamon may have therapeutic benefits on lipid profile, liver enzymes, insulin resistance, and high-sensitivity C-reactive protein in nonalcoholic fatty liver disease patients. *Nutr. Res.* **2014**, *34*, 143–148. [CrossRef] [PubMed]

131. Freedman, N.D.; Park, Y.; Abnet, C.C.; Hollenbeck, A.R.; Sinha, R. Association of coffee drinking with total and cause-specific mortality. *N. Engl. J. Med.* **2012**, *366*, 1891–1904. [CrossRef] [PubMed]

132. Corrao, G.; Zambon, A.; Bagnardi, V.; D'Amicis, A.; Klatsky, A. Collaborative SIDECIR Group. Coffee, caffeine, and the risk of liver cirrhosis. *Ann. Epidemiol.* **2001**, *11*, 458–465. [CrossRef]

133. Montella, M.; Polesel, J.; La Vecchia, C.; Dal Maso, L.; Crispo, A.; Crovatto, M.; Casarin, P.; Izzo, F.; Tommasi, L.G.; Talamini, R.; *et al.* Coffee and tea consumption and risk of hepatocellular carcinoma in Italy. *Int. J. Cancer* **2007**, *120*, 1555–1559. [CrossRef] [PubMed]

134. Salomone, F.; Li Volti, G.; Vitaglione, P.; Morisco, F.; Fogliano, V.; Zappalà, A.; Palmigiano, A.; Garozzo, D.; Caporaso, N.; D'Argenio, G.; *et al.* Coffee enhances the expression of chaperones and antioxidant proteins in rats with nonalcoholic fatty liver disease. *Transl. Res.* **2014**, *163*, 593–602. [CrossRef] [PubMed]

Permissions

All chapters in this book were first published by MDPI; hereby published with permission under the Creative Commons Attribution License or equivalent. Every chapter published in this book has been scrutinized by our experts. Their significance has been extensively debated. The topics covered herein carry significant findings which will fuel the growth of the discipline. They may even be implemented as practical applications or may be referred to as a beginning point for another development.

The contributors of this book come from diverse backgrounds, making this book a truly international effort. This book will bring forth new frontiers with its revolutionizing research information and detailed analysis of the nascent developments around the world.

We would like to thank all the contributing authors for lending their expertise to make the book truly unique. They have played a crucial role in the development of this book. Without their invaluable contributions this book wouldn't have been possible. They have made vital efforts to compile up to date information on the varied aspects of this subject to make this book a valuable addition to the collection of many professionals and students.

This book was conceptualized with the vision of imparting up-to-date information and advanced data in this field. To ensure the same, a matchless editorial board was set up. Every individual on the board went through rigorous rounds of assessment to prove their worth. After which they invested a large part of their time researching and compiling the most relevant data for our readers.

The editorial board has been involved in producing this book since its inception. They have spent rigorous hours researching and exploring the diverse topics which have resulted in the successful publishing of this book. They have passed on their knowledge of decades through this book. To expedite this challenging task, the publisher supported the team at every step. A small team of assistant editors was also appointed to further simplify the editing procedure and attain best results for the readers.

Apart from the editorial board, the designing team has also invested a significant amount of their time in understanding the subject and creating the most relevant covers. They scrutinized every image to scout for the most suitable representation of the subject and create an appropriate cover for the book.

The publishing team has been an ardent support to the editorial, designing and production team. Their endless efforts to recruit the best for this project, has resulted in the accomplishment of this book. They are a veteran in the field of academics and their pool of knowledge is as vast as their experience in printing. Their expertise and guidance has proved useful at every step. Their uncompromising quality standards have made this book an exceptional effort. Their encouragement from time to time has been an inspiration for everyone.

The publisher and the editorial board hope that this book will prove to be a valuable piece of knowledge for researchers, students, practitioners and scholars across the globe.

List of Contributors

Carlo Smirne, Violante Mulas, Matteo Nazzareno Barbaglia, Venkata Ramana Mallela, Rosalba Minisini, Michela Emma Burlone, Mario Pirisi and Elena Grossini
Department of Translational Medicine, Università del Piemonte Orientale, via Solaroli, 17, 28100 Novara, Italy

Karolina Grąt and Olgierd Rowiński
Second Department of Clinical Radiology, Medical University of Warsaw, 02-097 Warsaw, Poland

Michał Grąt
Department of General, Transplant and Liver Surgery, Medical University of Warsaw, 02-097 Warsaw, Poland

Mei-Ju Hsu, Madlen Christ, Hagen Kühne, Sandra Nickel and Bruno Christ
Applied Molecular Hepatology Laboratory, Department of Visceral, Transplant, Thoracic and Vascular Surgery, University of Leipzig Medical Center, 04103 Leipzig, Germany

Isabel Karkossa, Kristin Schubert and Ulrike E. Rolle-Kampczyk
Department of Molecular Systems Biology, Helmholtz Centre for Environmental Research (UFZ), 04318 Leipzig, Germany

Ingo Schäfer and Peter Seibel
Molecular Cell Therapy, Center for Biotechnology and Biomedicine, Leipzig University, 04103 Leipzig, Germany

Stefan Kalkhof
Department of Molecular Systems Biology, Helmholtz Centre for Environmental Research (UFZ), 04318 Leipzig, Germany
Institute for Bioanalysis, University of Applied Sciences Coburg, 96450 Coburg, Germany
Department of Therapy Validation, Fraunhofer Institute for Cell Therapy and Immunology, 04103 Leipzig, Germany

Martin von Bergen
Department of Molecular Systems Biology, Helmholtz Centre for Environmental Research (UFZ), 04318 Leipzig, Germany
Institute of Biochemistry, Leipzig University, 04103 Leipzig, Germany

Nadia Barizzone
Department of Health Sciences, Università' del Piemonte Orientale, via Solaroli, 17, 28100 Novara, Italy

Benedetta Donati and Luca Valenti
Department of Pathophysiology and Transplantation, Università degli Studi di Milano, Fondazione IRCCS Ca' Granda Ospedale Policlinico Milano, 20122 Milano, Italy

Roberto Gambino, Chiara Rosso, Lavinia Mezzabotta, Silvia Pinach, Natalina Alemanno, Francesca Saba and Maurizio Cassader
Department of Medical Sciences, University of Turin, C.so Dogliotti 14, 10126 Torino, Italy

Gemma Aragonès, Sandra Armengol, Alba Berlanga, Esther Guiu-Jurado and Carmen Aguilar
Group de Recerca GEMMAIR (AGAUR)-Medicina Aplicada, Institut Investigació Sanitària Pere Virgili (IISPV), Departament de Medicina i Cirurgia, Universitat Rovira i Virgili (URV), 43007 Tarragona, Spain

Teresa Auguet and Cristóbal Richart
Group de Recerca GEMMAIR (AGAUR)-Medicina Aplicada, Institut Investigació Sanitària Pere Virgili (IISPV), Departament de Medicina i Cirurgia, Universitat Rovira i Virgili (URV), 43007 Tarragona, Spain
Servei Medicina Interna, Hospital Universitari Joan XXIII Tarragona, Mallafré Guasch, 4, 43007 Tarragona, Spain

Salomé Martínez and Joan Josep Sirvent
Servei Anatomia Patològica, Hospital Universitari Joan XXIII Tarragona, Mallafré Guasch, 4, 43007 Tarragona, Spain

Fátima Sabench, Mercé Hernández and Daniel Del Castillo
Servei de Cirurgia, Hospital Sant Joan de Reus, Departament de Medicina i Cirurgia, Universitat Rovira i Virgili (URV), IISPV, Avinguda Doctor Josep Laporte, 2, 43204 Tarragona, Spain

José Antonio Porras and Maikel Daniel Ruiz
Servei Medicina Interna, Hospital Universitari Joan XXIII Tarragona, Mallafré Guasch, 4, 43007 Tarragona, Spain

Mariana Verdelho Machado
Division of Gastroenterology, Department of Medicine, Duke University Medical Center, Durham, NC 27710, USA
Gastroenterology Department, Hospital de Santa Maria, Centro Hospitalar Lisboa Norte (CHLN), Lisboa 1649-035, Portugal

Anna Mae Diehl
Division of Gastroenterology, Department of Medicine, Duke University Medical Center, Durham, NC 27710, USA

Salvatore Petta
Gastroenterology, Di.Bi.M.I.S Policlinic Paolo Giaccone Hospital, University of Palermo, PC 90127 Palermo, Italy

Amalia Gastaldelli
Cardiometabolic Risk Unit—Institute of Clinical Physiology, CNR, PC 56124 Pisa, Italy

Eleni Rebelos
Department of Clinical and Experimental Medicine, University of Pisa, PC 56122 Pisa, Italy

Elisabetta Bugianesi
Gastroenterology and Hepatology, Department of Medical Sciences, Città della, Salute e della Scienza di Torino Hospital, University of Turin, PC 10122 Turin, Italy
Department of Medical Sciences, University of Turin, C.so Dogliotti 14, 10126 Torino, Italy

Piergiorgio Messa
Department of Nephrology, Urology and Renal Transplant—Fondazione IRCCS Ca', Granda, PC 20122 Milano, Italy

Luca Miele
Institute of Internal Medicine, Gastroenterology and Liver Diseases Unit, Fondazione Policlinico Gemelli, Catholic University of Rome, PC 00168 Rome, Italy

Gianluca Svegliati-Baroni
Department of Gastroenterology 1 and Obesity 2, Polytechnic University of Marche, PC 60121 Ancona, Italy

Luca Valenti
Metabolic Liver Diseases—Università degli Studi Milano-Fondazione IRCCS Ca', Granda via F Sforza 35, PC 20122 Milano, Italy

Maria Catalina Hernandez-Rodas and Rodrigo Valenzuela
Department of Nutrition, Faculty of Medicine, University of Chile, Santiago 8380453, Chile

Ferruccio Bonino
Department of Clinical and Experimental Medicine, University of Pisa, PC 56122 Pisa, Italy
Institute for Health, PC 53042 Chianciano Terme, Italy

Stefano Ballestri
Operating Unit Internal Medicine, Pavullo General Hospital, Azienda USL Modena, ViaSuore di San Giuseppe Benedetto Cottolengo, 5, Pavullo, 41026 Modena, Italy

Fabio Nascimbeni
Outpatient Liver Clinic and Operating Unit Internal Medicine, NOCSAE, Azienda USL Modena, Via P. Giardini, 1355, 41126 Modena, Italy
Department of Biomedical, Metabolic and Neural Sciences, University of Modena and Reggio Emilia, Via P. Giardini, 1355, 41126 Modena, Italy

Dante Romagnoli and Amedeo Lonardo
Outpatient Liver Clinic and Operating Unit Internal Medicine, NOCSAE, Azienda USL Modena, Via P. Giardini, 1355, 41126 Modena, Italy

Enrica Baldelli
Department of Biomedical, Metabolic and Neural Sciences, University of Modena and Reggio Emilia, Via P. Giardini, 1355, 41126 Modena, Italy

Giovanni Targher
Section of Endocrinology, Diabetes and Metabolism, Department of Medicine, University and Azienda Ospedaliera Universitaria Integrata of Verona, Piazzale Stefani, 1, 37126 Verona, Italy

Cristiane A. Villela-Nogueira, Nathalie C. Leite, Claudia R. L. Cardoso and Gil F. Salles
Department of Internal Medicine, Medical School and University Hospital Clementino Fraga Filho, Universidade Federal do Rio de Janeiro, Rua Croton 72, Rio de Janeiro 22750-240, Brasil

Stefano Gitto and Erica Villa
Department of Gastroenterology, Azienda Ospedaliero-Universitaria and University of Modena and Reggio Emilia, Via del Pozzo 1, 41124 Modena, Italy

Luigi Elio Adinolfi, Luca Rinaldi, Barbara Guerrera, Luciano Restivo, Aldo Marrone, Mauro Giordano and Rosa Zampino
Department of Medical, Surgical, Neurological, Metabolic, and Geriatric Sciences, Second University of Naples, Naples 80100, Italy

Luis A. Videla
Molecular and Clinical Pharmacology Program, Institute of Biomedical Sciences, Faculty of Medicine, University of Chile, Santiago 8380453, Chile

Index

Printed in the USA
CPSIA information can be obtained
at www.ICGtesting.com
JSHW051624061123
51533JS00005B/88